THE MEDITERRANEAN DIETS
IN HEALTH AND DISEASE

THE
MEDITERRANEAN DIETS
IN
HEALTH AND DISEASE

Edited by

Gene A. Spiller
Health Research and Studies Center
Los Altos, California
and
SPHERA Foundation

An **avi** Book
Published by Van Nostrand Reinhold
New York

An AVI Book
(AVI is an imprint of Van Nostrand Reinhold

Copyright © 1991 by Van Nostrand Reinhold
Library of Congress Catalog Card Number 90–41112
ISBN 0–442–00449–4

Printed in the United States of America.

Van Nostrand Reinhold
115 Fifth Avenue
New York, New York 10003

Chapman and Hall
2–6 Boundary Row
London, SE1 8HN, England

Thomas Nelson Australia
102 Dodds Street
South Melbourne 3205
Victoria, Australia

Nelson Canada
1120 Birchmount Road
Scarborough, Ontario MIK 5G4, Canada

16 15 14 13 12 11 10 9 8 7 6 5 4 3 2 1

QP
141
$.M35$
1991

Library of Congress Cataloging-in-Publication Data
The Mediterranean diets in health and disease/Gene A. Spiller,
  editor.
    p.   cm.
    ''An AVI book''—T.p. verso.
    Includes bibliographical references and index.
    ISBN 0–442–00449–4
    1. Nutrition. 2. Diet—Mediterranean Region. I. Spiller, Gene A.
QP141.M35   1991
613.2'09182'2—dc20   90–41112
                                                        CIP

To my father, who inspired me to understand the deep values of the Mediterranean cultures, and to the wise people of the Mediterranean region who chose a protective diet well before today's clinical research proved its value.

CONTENTS

Preface xi
Acknowledgments xiii
Contributors xv

PART I: OVERVIEW AND HISTORY

1. **Comparison of Current Eating Habits in Various
   Mediterranean Countries**   3
   Rosalba Giacco and Gabriele Riccardi

   Mediterranean Diet: Myth or Reality? 4
   Comparison Between the Present-Day Diet
     in Mediterranean Countries and Current Dietary
     Recommendations for CHD Prevention, 6

2. **Ancient Mediterranean Food**   10
   Thomas Braun

   The Evidence, 10
   Cereals, 16
   Fruit, 40

PART II: TYPICAL MEDITERRANEAN FOODS
AND THEIR PHYSIOLOGY

3. **Cereal Foods: Wheat, Corn, Rice, Barley, and Other
   Cereals and Their Products**   59
   Claudia Lintas and Aldo Mariani-Costantini

   General Characteristics of Cereals, 60
   Wheat, 61
   Rice, 84

Corn, 88
Barley, 93
Oats, 96

4. Legumes   **102**
Flaminio Fidanza

Production and Consumption, 102
Chemical Composition and Nutritive Value, 103
Toxic Substances, 106
Legumes in the Diet, 107

5. Vegetables and Fruits   **110**
Giulio Testolin, Ambrogina Alberio, and Ernestina Casiraghi

Fruit and Vegetable Consumption, 110
Classification and Technology of Fruits and Vegetables, 113
Diet and Nutrition, 115

6. Edible Fats and Oils   **125**
Enzo Fedeli and Giulio Testolin

Fats and Oils Consumed in Italy and in Other
    Mediterranean Countries, 128
Technologies, 129

7. Dairy Products   **135**
Giorgio Ottogalli and Giulio Testolin

Statistical Data, 136
Technology, 136
Dairy Microbiology and Hygiene, 145
Nutrition and Diet, 148

**8. Grains, Legumes, Fruits, and Vegetables: Lente
Carbohydrate Sources in the Mediterranean Diet**   **160**
*Thomas M. S. Wolever, Alexandra L. Jenkins, Peter J. Spadafora,
and David J. A. Jenkins*

Physiological Effects of Slow Release Carbohydrate
    Foods, 161
Effects of Individual Foods, 167

9. **Physiological Effects of Monounsaturated Oils**   182
   Gene A. Spiller

   Olive Oil Studies, 184
   Olive and Peanut Oil Studies, 187
   Almond Studies, 188
   Canola Oil Study, 188

PART III: CLINICAL ASPECTS AND EPIDEMIOLOGY

10. **Lipids**   195
    *Luciano Cominacini, Ulisse Garbin, Anna Davoli, Beatrice Cenci,
    and Ottavio Bosello*

    Epidemiology, 195
    Mediterranean Diet Characteristics and EURATOM Study
       Results, 198
    Effects of Dietary Carbohydrates on Plasma Lipids, 200
    Effects of Dietary Fats on Plasma Lipids, 203
    Effects of Dietary Proteins on Plasma Lipids, 206
    Effects of Dietary Fibers on Plasma Lipids, 207

11. **Hypertension**   219
    Pasquale Strazzullo and Alfonso Siani

    Epidemiological Aspects, 220
    Intervention Studies, 222
    Experimental Studies, 227

12. **Cardiovascular Diseases**   232
    Alessandro Menotti

    Early Hospital Observations, 233
    Mortality Data, 234
    The Seven Countries Study, 235
    Recent Trends, 244
    Intervention, 245

13. **Obesity**   252
    Ottavio Bosello, Fabio Armellini, and Mauro Zamboni

    Epidemiology: Prevalence of Obesity, 253
    Influence of Various Nutrients in Energy Balance, 256

Comparison of Dietary Habits in Different Countries, 266
Intervention, 270

14. Diabetes   277
Gabriele Riccardi and Angela Rivellese

Epidemiology, 278
Intervention, 281

15. Diet and Cancer   287
Adriano Decarli and Carlo La Vecchia

Summary of Knowledge, 287
Characteristics of Mediterranean Diet, 290
Gastric Cancer and Diet in Italy, 291
A Case-Control Surveillance Study in Northern Italy, 294

Index   305

PREFACE

It is difficult to find the moment when the idea for a book is first born. For this book, the basic concept was probably born during conversations I had in Parma, Italy, with Dr. Riccardi of the University of Naples and Dr. Jenkins of the University of Toronto (Canada). Later, in a conference room at the University of Verona (Italy) School of Medicine, I had a day-long meeting with Drs. Bosello and Cominacini of the University of Verona, and Drs. Jenkins and Riccardi and their co-workers. After an intense working day, the general plan of this book was completed.

The title Mediterranean *diets* rather than *diet* was appropriately chosen as there is more than one Mediterranean diet, a point discussed in chapter 1. This chapter focuses on the definition of a Mediterranean diet and no matter what the reader's interest may be, it is imperative that this first chapter be carefully read.

We should always remember that there are—from a preventive medicine point of view—good and poor Mediterranean diets. The best example is probably the difference between the high olive oil, high carbohydrate, low meat diet of southern Italy and the high saturated fat, higher meat diets of the northern Italians. Prevalence of disease parallels these differences.

Chapter 2 covers some ancient history in an easy-to-read manner that is instructional as well as fascinating even for the nonmedical scientist or the nonhistorian.

In part II, chapters 3 to 7 cover some basic foods of the Mediterranean region: cereals, legumes, vegetables and fruits, oils, and dairy products. In the second half of part II cereals, legumes, fruits and vegetables (chapter 8) and monounsaturated oils (chapter 9) are discussed for their physiological effects. These two groups of foods were singled out because they are so typical of good Mediterranean diets.

Part III covers the medical and epidemiological aspects of the Mediterranean diets as they relate to the major degenerative diseases: lipids (chapter 10), hypertension (chapter 11), cardiovascular diseases (chapter 12), diabetes (chapter 13), obesity (chapter 14), and cancer (chapter 15). Some points previously covered in chapters 8 and 9 (physiological aspects) are sometimes presented again in part III with a different perspective that helps the reader to grasp the magnitude of the questions that need to be answered.

With the growing interest in North America—both by medical researchers and by the population in general—in diets of Mediterranean type, with the disturbing knowledge that the better Mediterranean diets may be losing ground to other less desirable diets in the very countries where they were born, it is hoped that this book will help to foster an understanding of how valuable to better health these ancient diets can be.

Could it be that all the knowledge we need for better health and disease prevention is there, already tested not by a few months or years of clinical research but by centuries of use? You may be able to answer this question after you have read this book.

ACKNOWLEDGMENTS

I wish to thank Drs. Ottavio Bosello, Luciano Cominacini, David Jenkins, and Gabriele Riccardi for their assistance and advice as this book evolved from an idea to a finished manuscript.

A special acknowledgment goes to Dr. Ancel Keys, whose work and publications have been the foundation of a better understanding of diet and health and, in particular, of the Mediterranean diet. His name and his work will be quoted frequently in this book, a book that might never have been possible without his research.

Finally, I wish to thank Rebecca Carr and Alethe Echols for their assistance in various phases of manuscript editing and production.

CONTRIBUTORS

Ambrogina Alberio, Università di Milano, Dipartimento di Scienze e Tecnologie Alimentari e Microbiologiche, Milano, Italy

Fabio Armellini, Policlinico di Borgo Roma, Istituto di Clinica Medica, Università di Verona, Verona, Italy

Ottavio Bosello, Policlinico di Borgo Roma, Istituto di Clinica Medica, Università di Verona, Verona, Italy

Thomas Braun, Merton College, Oxford, United Kingdom

Ernestina Casiraghi, Università di Milano, Dipartimento di Scienze e Tecnologie Alimentari e Microbiologiche, Milano, Italy

Beatrice Cenci, Istituto di Clinica Medica, Università di Verona, Verona, Italy

Luciano Cominacini, Istituto di Clinica Medica, Università di Verona, Verona, Italy

Aldo Mariani-Costantini, Istituto Nazionale della Nutrizione, Roma, Italy

Anna Davoli, Istituto di Clinica Medica, Università di Verona, Verona, Italy

Adriano Decarli, Università di Milano, Istituto Biometria Statistica Medica, Milano, Italy

Enzo Fedeli, Università di Milano, Dipartimento di Scienze e Tecnologie Alimentari e Microbiologiche, Milano, Italy

Flaminio Fidanza, Università degli Studi di Perugia, Dipartimento di

Scienze e Tecnologie, Istituto di Scienza dell' Alimentazione, Perugia, Italy

Ulisse Garbin, Istituto di Clinica Medica, Università di Verona, Verona, Italy

Rosalba Giacco, Università di Napoli, Facoltà di Medicina e Chirurgia, Istituto di Medicina Interna e Malattie Dismetabliche, Napoli, Italy

Alexandra L. Jenkins, University of Toronto, Department of Nutritional Science, Faculty of Medicine, Toronto, Canada

David J. A. Jenkins, University of Toronto, Department of Nutritional Science, Faculty of Medicine, Toronto, Canada

Carlo La Vecchia, Institute of Social and Preventive Medicine, University of Lausanne, Switzerland; Ist. Ricerche Farmacologiche M. Negri, Milano, Italy

Claudia Lintas, Istituto Nazionale della Nutrizione, Roma, Italy

Alessandro Menotti, Istituto Superiore di Sanità, Laboratorio di Epidemiologia e Biostatistica, Roma, Italy

Giorgio Ottogalli, Università degli Studi di Milano, Dipartimento di Scienze e Tecnologie Alimentari e Microbiologiche, Milano, Italy

Gabriele Riccardi, Università di Napoli, Falcoltà di Medicina e Chirurgia, Istituto di Medicina Interna e Malattie Dismetabliche, Napoli, Italy,

Angela Rivellese, Università di Napoli, Facoltà di Medicina e Chirurgia, Istituto di Medicina Interna e Malattie Dismetabliche, Napoli, Italy

Alfonso Siani, Università di Napoli, Napoli, Italy

Peter J. Spadafora, University of Toronto, Department of Nutritional Science, Faculty of Medicine, Toronto, Canada

Gene A. Spiller, Health Research and Studies Center, Los Altos, California

Pasquale Strazzullo, Università di Napoli, Facoltà di Medicina e Chirugia, Istituto di Medicina Interna e Malattie Dismetaboliche, Napoli, Italy

Giulio Testolin, Università di Milano, Dipartimento di Scienze e Tecnologie Alimentari e Microbiologiche, Milano, Italy

Thomas M. A. Wolever, University of Toronto, Department of Nutritional Science, Faculty of Medicine, Toronto, Canada

Mauro Zamboni, Policlinico di Borgo Roma, Istituto di Clinica Medica, Università di Verona, Verona, Italy

THE MEDITERRANEAN DIETS
IN HEALTH AND DISEASE

Part I

OVERVIEW AND HISTORY

Comparison of Current Eating Habits in Various Mediterranean Countries

Rosalba Giacco
Gabriele Riccardi

The Mediterranean diet, as a model of a healthful diet, has been the subject of several studies since World War II. The term *Mediterranean diet* was first used by Ancel Keys, an American physiologist, in his book *How to Eat Well and Stay Well: the Mediterranean Way* (Keys and Keys 1975). At the end of World War II, the Keyses' theory regarding the importance of a well-balanced diet in maintaining health began to solidify: They proposed a relationship between the eating habits of populations of different geographical areas and the distribution of morbidity and mortality from cardiovascular diseases. Prof. Keys's insight was confirmed by the results of the Seven Countries Study, which showed that the Mediterranean countries, where cardiovascular disease morbidity and mortality are low, have particularly low serum cholesterol levels compared to countries such as Finland and the United States, where the incidence of cardiovascular diseases is higher. These diversities can be partly explained by the difference in the intake of saturated fatty acids in the various populations (Keys 1970; Keys et al. 1986).

Intervention studies on eating habits have greatly strengthened acceptance of the role played by diet in the etiology of cardiovascular diseases. In a study conducted in northern Karelia, Finland, a group of middle-aged volunteers was invited to replace their usual diets, rich in saturated fatty acids, with a typical Mediterranean diet (with a low content of saturated fatty acids) for six weeks. The results showed a significant decrease in plasma cholesterol concentrations, but these returned to their previous high levels when the subjects returned to their customary diets (Ehnholm et al. 1982). At about the same time, a complementary study with a similar methodology was being conducted in the area of Cilento in southern Italy. Its aim was to evaluate the effects of tempo-rarily replacing the habitual Mediterranean diet with a typical northern European diet. In this case, plasma cholesterol levels declined to their initial values when the participants returned to their usual diets. This study further confirms the relationship between dietary habits and plasma lipid levels (Ferro-Luzzi et al. 1984).

MEDITERRANEAN DIET: MYTH OR REALITY?

Although the Mediterranean diet has often been proposed as a model of healthful eating habits, many uncertainties still exist concerning the nutritional characteristics of this type of diet. A research study carried out by the European Atomic Energy Community (EURATOM) in the 1960s represents one of the major sources of information on the quality and quantity of food intake in Europe. This study showed remarkable dissimilarities among the different countries studied, in particular, con-sumption of more cereals, fruit, and vegetables and less meat, sugar, milk, and dairy products in Italy than in other European countries. It was particularly interesting to note that in Italy, the quantity of fat con-sumed was the same as that of other countries, but it was very different in terms of quality: almost exclusively olive oil, with irrelevant quantities of margarine, butter, and lard (Cresta et al. 1969).

Unfortunately, when speaking of the Mediterranean diet, we are in-clined to conceive of it as a homogeneous nutritional model, although there are several Mediterranean nations with varied cultures, traditions and, probably, dietary habits as well. On first consideration, it would not seem correct to extrapolate the eating habits in Greece or southern Italy to all the other Mediterranean countries; but further reflection sug-gests that beyond the apparent diversities, some nutritional characteris-tics could be common to all or most of the Mediterranean area.

Ferro-Luzzi and Sette (1989) provided further information on this is-sue by means of a study that compared the nutritional intakes of 16 Mediterranean and 12 northern European countries from 1961 to 1963. This research confirms the results of the EURATOM study on the differ-ent intakes of fat in the two groups of countries compared. However, the study does not give much additional information as to other charac-teristics of the Mediterranean diet, although it seems to indicate that consumption of vegetables in both northern Europe and the Mediterra-nean area is similar. Moreover, it investigated the eating habits of the Mediterranean countries only from 1961 to 1963, and it is possible that modifications in eating styles did occur as a consequence of socioeco-nomic evolution, making the present diet in Mediterranean countries more similar to that of highly industrialized countries with higher cardiovascular risk.

Therefore, we have undertaken a nutritional study aiming at (1) defining the nutritional characteristics of all the countries in the Mediterranean area through evaluation of their food intakes, and (2) examining the possibility that there is a common nutritional pattern for all Mediterranean countries that could be defined as "Mediterranean diet" and determining whether this type of diet corresponds to the current recommended allowances for the prevention of coronary heart disease (CHD).

We have adopted the 1979 to 1981 Food Balance Sheets published by FAO (FAO 1984) to gain information on the dietary intake of 14 Mediterranean countries (Portugal, Spain, France, Italy, Yugoslavia, Greece, Malta, Israel, Libya, Algeria, Tunisia, Turkey, Egypt, and Morocco) and, for comparison, of the United States, chosen as an example of a typical industrialized country at high risk for cardiovascular diseases. The Food Balance Sheets show for each country the foods available (produced and/or imported) but do not take into account the losses that may occur before consumption. Despite this limitation, the FAO report represents the only standard source currently available for a comparison of food consumption among countries.

Our research shows that the consumption of eggs, milk, and dairy products is lower in all Mediterranean countries (62–430 g/d) than in the United States (505 g/d). The result is in good agreement with previous studies and confirms that a lower intake of these food items is still a constant feature of the present-day Mediterranean diet. A high consumption of olive oil (Fig. 1-1) represents another important characteristic of this type of diet, although the intake varies greatly from country to country. The importance of olive oil as a substitute for animal fat in the diet has been demonstrated by clinical and biological research; the results support its role in preventing cardiovascular diseases (Trevisan et al. 1990).

Our study has led to another interesting result concerning the high intake of cereals in the Mediterranean countries. These countries derive 30–60% of their daily caloric intake from cereals, whereas in the United States, the average is only 19%. The high consumption of food rich in starch in the Mediterranean countries is similar to that reported for the Far East, where cardiovascular mortality risk is also low. Another typical aspect of the dietary habits of the Mediterranean area is the low consumption of meat, although people from European countries tend to eat more meat than do North African people: 89 ± 44 g/d versus 78 ± 64 g/d (means ± standard deviation).

As expected, the intake of legumes, which are rich in soluble fiber and complex carbohydrates, is also higher in the Mediterranean area as

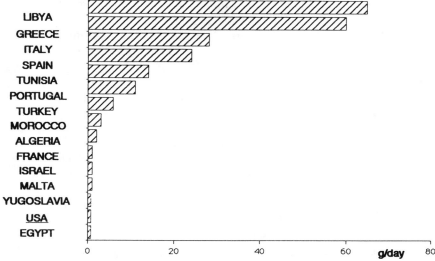

Figure 1-1.   Per capita consumption of olive oil in Mediterranean countries and United States.

compared to the United States, 6 g/d, with the exception of France, 5 g/d; the levels range from a maximum of 21 g/d for Yugoslavia to a minimum of 7 g/d for Malta. However, the intake of legumes is lower than expected, averaging a portion less than twice a week. This result raises the possibility that changes in eating habits have occurred in recent decades because of the improvement in socioeconomic conditions. This phenomenon can help to explain the absence of very striking differences between the United States and the Mediterranean countries regarding consumption of other foods usually believed to be typical of the Mediterranean diet, namely fruit and vegetables.

In summary, the Mediterranean diet is characterized by a high intake of cereals and olive oil and a low intake of animal fat and meat.

COMPARISON BETWEEN THE PRESENT-DAY DIET IN MEDITERRANEAN COUNTRIES AND CURRENT DIETARY RECOMMENDATIONS FOR CHD PREVENTION

In analyzing the composition of the diet in Mediterranean countries (Fidanza and Versiglioni 1987), we have expressed the nutrients as percentage of total daily calories (Fig. 1–2) and compared their distribution with the current allowances recommended by the European Atherosclerosis

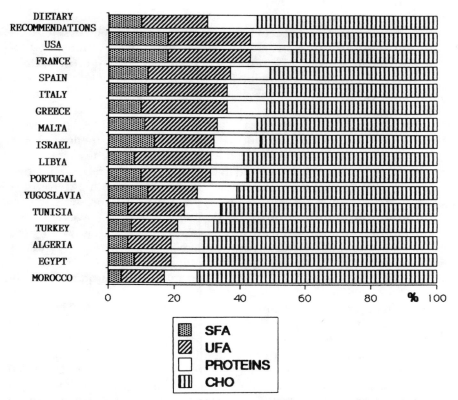

Figure 1-2.   Diet composition in Mediterranean countries and United States.

Society (EAS) for the prevention of cardiovascular diseases (Study Group of the EAS 1987). These recommendations can be summarized as follows:

- Limit the total fat intake to less than 30% of caloric intake.
- Reduce saturated fatty acids to less than 10% and cholesterol to less than 300 mg/d.
- Keep the intake of complex carbohydrates above 50% of total caloric intake, especially of foods rich in fiber and of vegetable origin.

In addition, avoidance of overweight and moderation in salt intake are also recommended.

For eight of the Mediterranean countries, saturated fatty acids represent less than 10% of the total caloric intake; for five of them, the intake ranges between 11% and 14%, whereas for France it is 18%, the same as that reported for the United States. Total fat represents less than 30% of total energy intake in six countries: Yugoslavia, Tunisia, Turkey, Algeria, Egypt, and Morocco. It is just slightly above the recommended intake, between 31% and 37%, for seven countries: Spain, Portugal, Italy, Libya, Greece, Israel, and Malta. The only country to have a very high fat intake (43%) is France, this figure again being the same as that for the United States. With the exception of France, populations in the Mediterranean countries use chiefly unsaturated fat, which does not contribute to the risk of cardiovascular diseases (Grundy and Bonanome 1987). The consumption of cholesterol is lower in the Mediterranean countries, with the exception of France, than in the United States (656 mg/d). However, it falls within the recommended allowance (< 300 mg/d) for only five countries: Egypt, Algeria, Morocco, Tunisia, and Turkey.

The carbohydrate fraction in the Mediterranean diet, however, corresponds to the recommended allowance, > 50%. The exception once again is France, where carbohydrate intake is 43% of total energy and is similar to that reported for the United States, 44%.

In all the Mediterranean countries and in the United States, protein allowance is in line with the EAS recommendations. It is mainly of vegetable origin for North African countries.

Contrary to our expectations, the daily intake of fiber, which is known to have beneficial effects on glucose and lipid metabolism and also to contribute to cancer prevention (Jenkins et al. 1979; Rivellese et al. 1980), seems to be lower than the recommended intake, 20 g/1000 kcal/d, in the whole Mediterranean area. It varies from 7 g/1000 kcal/d in Malta to 11 g/1000 kcal/d in Turkey, quantities that do not differ greatly from those reported for the United States, 7 g/1000 kcal/d.

In short, there is a common nutritional profile for the Mediterranean countries characterized by low intake of saturated fat, moderate intake of total fat with prevalence of monounsaturated fat, and high intake of complex carbohydrates. These characteristics confirm the adequacy of the Mediterranean diet for preventing cardiovascular diseases and other chronic degenerative diseases typical of industrialized countries (Stamler 1985; Riccardi et al. 1988).

The socioeconomic development that has occurred in this area in the last few decades has unfortunately begun, probably, to bring with it some poor dietary habits, particularly the high intake of cholesterol and the low intake of vegetable fiber by people of the whole Mediterranean area. It is hoped that awareness of the nutritional value of the Mediterranean diet will help maintain and spread these beneficial dietary practices and possibly reverse the dangerous trend, caused by urbanization and socioeconomic progress, toward discarding this model of a healthful diet.

REFERENCES

Cresta, M., S. Ledermann, A. Garnier, E. Lombardo, and G. Lacourly. 1969. *Etude des consommations alimentaires des populations de onze régions de la communauté européenne en vue de la détermination des niveaux de contamination radioactive.* Rapport établi au Centre d'Etude Nucléaire de Fotenay-aux-Roses, France: EURATOM, Commissariat à l'énergie atomique (CEA).

Ehnholm, C., J. K. Huttunen, P. Pietinen, et al. 1982. Effect of diet on serum lipoprotein in a population with a high risk of coronary heart disease. *New Engl. J. Med.* **307**:850–855.

FAO (Food and Agriculture Organization of the United Nations). 1984. *Food Balance Sheets, 1979–1981 Average.* Rome.

Ferro-Luzzi, A., and S. Sette. 1989. The Mediterranean diet: an attempt to define its present and past composition. *Eur. J. Clin. Nutr.* **43**(suppl. 2):13–29.

Ferro-Luzzi, A., P. Strazzullo, C. Scaccini, et al. 1984. Changing the Mediterranean diet: effects on blood lipids. *Am. J. Clin. Nutr.* **40**:1027–1037.

Fidanza, F., and N. Versiglioni. 1987. *Tabelle di Composizione Degli Alimenti.* Naples: Idelson.

Grundy, S. M., and A. Bonanome. 1987. Workshop on Monounsaturated Fatty Acids. *Arteriosclerosis* **6**:644–648.

Jenkins, D. J. A., A. R. Leeds, B. Slavin, et al. 1979. Dietary fiber and blood lipids: reduction of serum cholesterol in type II hyperlipidemia by guar gum. *Am. J. Clin. Nutr.* **32**:16–18.

Keys, A. 1970. Coronary heart disease in seven countries. *Circulation* **41**(1):1–211.

Keys, A., and M. Keys. 1975. *How To Eat Well and Stay Well the Mediterranean Way.* New York: Doubleday.

Keys, A., A. Menotti, M. J. Karvonen, et al. 1986. The diet and 15 year death rate in Seven Countries Study. *Am. J. Epidemiol.* **124**:903–915.

Riccardi, G., A. A. Rivellese, and M. Mancini. 1988. Current dietary recommendations for coronary heart disease prevention. *Diab. Nutr. Metab.* **1**:7–9.

Rivellese, A., G. Riccardi, and A. Giacco, et al. 1980. Effect of dietary fibre on glucose control and serum lipoproteins in diabetic patients. *Lancet* **2**:447–450.

Stamler, J. 1985. The marked decline in coronary heart disease mortality rates in USA 1968–1981; summary of findings and possible explanations. *Cardiology* **72**:11–22.

Study Group, European Atherosclerosis Society. 1987. Strategy for prevention of coronary heart disease: a policy statement of European Atherosclerosis Society. *Eur. Heart J.* **8**:77–88.

Trevisan, M., V. Krogh, J. Freudenheim, et al. 1990. Consumption of olive oil, butter, and vegetable oils and heart disease risk factors. *JAMA* **263**(5):688–692.

2

Ancient Mediterranean Food

Thomas Braun

THE EVIDENCE

Our survey of ancient Mediterranean food deals with the world of the Bible, the Greeks, and the Roman Empire, covering a period of fifteen hundred years from the beginning of the first millennium B.C. to the barbarian invasions of the fifth century A.D. The ecologically distinct river civilizations of Egypt and Mesopotamia cannot be fully taken into account, although the Nile flows into the Mediterranean and the lands of the eastern Mediterranean were, from time to time during this period, under the same rulers as Mesopotamia. Nor is there scope to consider at length the adaptation of Mediterranean civilization by central and northwestern Europe and Britain while under Roman rule. But the evidence from these neighboring regions is sometimes relevant.

The greatest innovations of human history had been successfully completed thousands of years earlier. Since the beginning of Neolithic times hunting, fishing, and fowling had been supplemented by agriculture and husbandry; how this had come about, and how the transport of goods by sea had further transformed the diet of the Mediterranean peoples, was already beyond human memory. Sophocles in *Antigone* (332–352) ponders these achievements:

> Wonders are many, and none more wonderful than man,
> who crosses the sea, driven by the stormy south wind,
> making his path under engulfing waves.
> The oldest of the gods, Earth,
> imperishable, unwearied, he wears away,
> as his ploughs go up and down, year by year,
> turning the soil with the offspring of horses.
>
> And the blithe race of birds he snares,
> the tribes of beasts, and the brood of the salt sea,

in the twisted mesh of his nets, this cunning man;
and by his craft he controls the beasts of the open country
who roam the hills; the shaggy-maned horse
he tames, putting the yoke around his neck,
and the tireless bull of the mountain. . . .

New archaeological techniques in our own generation have given us the knowledge of these remote beginnings that the biblical and classical world lacked. Mediterranean agriculture—the cultivation of wheat and barley and domestication of sheep, goats, pigs, and, where possible, cattle—can today be traced back some six thousand years before the beginning of Hebrew and Greek literature. What people ate, and when, can now be deduced from the leftovers of animal food, from material that has been carbonized or waterlogged, and from the impressions and silica skeletons of grains in mudbrick or pottery. Jane Renfrew's *Palaeoethnobotany* (1973) and N. W. Simmonds's *Evolution of Crop Plants* (1976) provide excellent comprehensive surveys of the development of cultivated vegetable foods. By the time these were completed, this kind of evidence had transformed our knowledge of the diet of prehistory but had not been fully utilized for historical times: Excavators of Greek and Roman sites had not been much concerned with food remains. Paleoethnobotany is a fast-changing subject. The detailed work of the past fifteen years needs to be brought together in an updated survey: The account here presented is the worse for its absence but has benefited from the evidence presented by M. S. Spurr (1986), "Arable Cultivation in Roman Italy 200 B.C.—c. A.D. 100." Archaeology can provide help: Food preparation is often represented in ancient art, and deductions can be made from finds of tableware, cooking vessels, and the equipment of food processing. An outstanding example is L. A. Moritz's (1958) *Grain Mills and Flour in Classical Antiquity*. But the literary evidence is fullest of all, even more than for the two thousand years of literate Egyptian and Near Eastern civilization that precede our chosen period. Much that archaeology today confirms was already known from ancient texts when Victor Hehn put together his great work on the migration of domestic plants and animals from Asia to Europe, *Kulturpflanzen und Haustiere*, which went through many editions in the last century.

Except for mathematical and technical treatises, it would be hard to

---

Editor's Note: In this chapter the references to ancient works (e.g., *Odyssey*, XIX 113) are placed within the text rather than at the end of the chapter. References to recent works are listed at the end of the chapter. This format was chosen as more appropriate for the historical perspective given here.

find a book in the enormous corpus of Greek literature that does not at some point touch on food. The same is true of the smaller body of Roman literature and of the books of the Bible. Some caution is admittedly needed. In literature of a high moral or poetical tone there may be a certain lack of realism. Fitzgerald's translation of the *Rubaiyat* of Omar Khayyam contains a famous quatrain describing a desert picnic in medieval Iran:

> A jug of wine, a loaf of bread, and thou
> Beside me, singing in the wilderness.

Fitzgerald was more faithful to his original than is generally realized; but in this case he could not bear to include the third item in Omar's original menu, a leg of mutton. His readers would have thought this unpoetic. But in real life bread and wine alone make an unsatisfying picnic, even in the company of the most tuneful beloved. The same considerations affect Homer. An ancient critic noticed that the Homeric heroes never ate fish, except once when Odysseus's men were stranded on the Island of the Sun God where they had been forbidden to touch the god's cattle. The poet thought roast meat more appropriate for heroes: it cost him nothing to provide it. But Odysseus (*Odyssey* xix 113) speaks of the fish of the sea as a gift comparable to wheat and barley, tree-fruit, and sheep. Similarly, boiled meat must have been thought to fall below the dignity of Epic, as it is never served to Homeric heroes; but boiling occurs in Homeric similes. By contrast, the Gospels are strikingly matter-of-fact in this as in other respects: one of their most vivid scenes is in the 21st chapter of John, where the risen Christ is seen cooking fish and bread for His breakfast over a charcoal fire.

But there was plenty of far-from-elevated literature in which food was described with relish and in detail. It was a favorite topic for Greek comedy, where the comic action frequently ends in feasting and fun, and the audience—which, especially in times of war, might be hungry—enjoyed down-to-earth but mouth-watering descriptions of the feasting. Comedy had occasion to mention the diet of the poor as well. Among the stock characters of New Comedy, from the fourth century B.C. onward, was the comic cook: He would be expected to talk about the items of his trade. And comedy provided much wistful looking back to the Golden Age, imagined to have preceded the days of hard work and slavery, when every kind of delicacy had been there for the taking. There were many hundreds of Greek comedies. Only a few survive complete, but thousands of fragments (quoted in this chapter from Kock's *Comicorum Atticorum Fragmenta*) are preserved in other texts. The fragments about food mostly derive from Athenaeus's *Deipnosophistai*

(Wise Men at Dinner), ca. A.D. 200, a work of fifteen books (each ancient book or papyrus roll comprising about a quarter of an octavo volume), of which 60% survives. The work is cast in the form of a conversation of thirty wiseacres about every aspect of eating. Athenaeus, who had the run of the Library of Alexandria, scoured not only ancient comedy but a number of other books, many of them now lost, for his purpose. There were cookery books among them, but his standpoint is that of a consumer of good writing rather than of the food itself and certainly not that of a food producer or cook. His interest is by no means confined to the excesses of the rich. The array of citations he presents gives an impression of the Greeks as a highly literate but on the whole frugal people, accepting with gusto many far from luxurious items. It also leaves numerous problems of exact translation. When all the references to an obscure gastronomic term have been set out, its meaning may still puzzle us.

Greek scientists assessed food more objectively. Valuable information comes from medical writers, whose drugs were almost entirely derived from plants and fruits, and who were seriously concerned with diet, on the basis of careful observation. The Hippocratic corpus of the classical Greek era (fifth and fourth century B.C.) recommended restraint for the healthy and barley gruel and barley water for the sick. Athenaeus quotes the sensible verdicts on different foods given in his *Diet for the Sick and Well* by Diphilus of Siphnos, the physician of King Lysimachus (who died in 281 B.C.). The pharmaceutical work of the army doctor Dioscorides in the first century A.D. and several treatises by the great medical writer Galen in the second show what Greek doctors considered to be healthy eating in the days of the Roman Empire. Their approach lacks what we consider a sound scientific basis: The theory of the humours led to assessments of what foods are cooling or heating, moistening or drying, but there was no knowledge of calories, proteins, or vitamins (as indeed there was not until the first decades of this century). But observation had led to sound views on the nourishing, laxative, and emollient properties of certain foods and on the merits of moderate food consumption and balanced living. How much the layman absorbed can be seen in Plutarch's essay "On keeping one's health" (*Moralia* 122B ff). It contains excellent advice that would have been ahead of its time in England or America a generation ago. Greek botanical science dealt systematically with food plants: The surviving *Enquiry into Plants* by Aristotle's successor Theophrastus (371–287 B.C.) remained authoritative until Linnaeus.

In science, the Romans could only follow the Greeks. The extensive *Natural History* of the Elder Pliny, in 37 books, completed in A.D. 77, at times misunderstands Theophrastus. Pliny, a busy man of insatiable curiosity who hated to waste time and had books read to him even when dining, sunbathing, and traveling, got many things wrong, though he remains indispensable. In practical matters, however, the Romans rightly prided themselves on their superiority. One of the consequences of their destruction of Carthage in 146 B.C. was the authorized translation into Latin of the standard Carthaginian work on agriculture by Mago in 28 books. This work is lost, but a series of Roman agricultural manuals survives. They date from the second century B.C. to imperial times: The most accessible are the short treatise of Cato the Censor, ca. 160 B.C., the more polished treatise of Varro, begun in his eightieth year, 36 B.C., the methodical work of Columella, compiled A.D. 60–65, and the manual of Palladius (fourth century A.D.), which has an introduction, one book for each month of the year, and a verse appendix on grafting. The exquisite verses of Virgil's *Georgics* (36–29 B.C.) profess to give instruction on agriculture and beekeeping. We have, also, the complete text of a cookery book for epicures ascribed to the gourmet Apicius. It does not indicate quantities, but enthusiastic experiment has latterly supplied them: Compare *The Roman Cookery Book,* translated by Barbara Flower and Elisabeth Rosenbaum (1958) with *The Roman Cookery of Apicius,* translated and adapted for the modern kitchen by John Edwards (1984).

Verse satirists mocked greed and bad manners at banquets; and in a surviving fragment of a sprawling picaresque novel by Petronius (first century A.D.) there is the description of a preposterous feast given by the parvenu Trimalchio, planned to amuse as well as gorge the guests. The menu is a parody, though sometimes quoted in all seriousness. It is again a joke when the *Augustan History* asserts that the emperor Elagabalus (A.D. 212–218) served up the brains of six hundred ostriches at one of his banquets (30,2), and fed his dogs with *foie gras* (21,1). But there was some truth in such lampoons, as can be seen, for instance, from the genuine extant menu of a grand priestly dinner on 24 August, some time between 73 and 63 B.C., when Julius Caesar and a number of vestal virgins were among the diners (Macrobius, *Saturnalia* xiii 10–12). Roman literature in its totality, however, is not as biased toward upper class practices as might be expected. The satirists knew the bitterness of poverty. They and the love poets also had a romantic penchant for rustic life, and there are charming accounts of simple meals in the country: the poet may himself extend an invitation to one.

Such information is necessarily anecdotal. In the absence of thoroughgoing statistics our survey of the different kinds of food available may not satisfy all modern readers. How frequent and serious, they will ask, were food shortages? What was the calorie and protein content of the diet of a pauper in Rome, eligible for the dole, or of an Italian peasant or agricultural slave, or of a Roman legionary soldier? When Jacques André wrote his useful survey, *l'alimentation et la cuisine à Rome* (1961), these difficult questions were not normally tackled. A start has now been made. Peter Garnsey's *Famine and Food Supply in the Graeco-Roman World* (1988) has broken new ground with excellent results. An authoritative study of ancient diet is expected from K. D. White, author of *Roman Farming* (1970) and *Greek and Roman Technology* (1984), which throw valuable light on food production and processing. Meanwhile, he has whetted our appetite with his ''Food requirements and food supplies in classical times in relation to the diet of the various classes,'' White (1976). Unfortunately, it was brought to my attention too late to be fully used for these chapters. An up-to-date study of the diet of the Roman army is provided by a chapter in Roy Davies's *Service in the Roman Army* (1989). Like all efficient armies, the Roman army proves to have been fed, mostly at the taxpayer's expense, very well indeed.

There were movements within the Mediterranean area throughout this period. In the Bronze Age, the Myceneans of mainland Greece had already been trading with southern Italy and the Levant. From the eighth century B.C. onward Greek and Phoenician settlers brought the cultivation of vines and olives westward to Sicily, Italy, North Africa, and the coastlands of Gaul and Spain. From the late seventh century B.C. wheat was imported from the Ukraine and Egypt to Greece. This trade came to be Athens's lifeline. Later, Sicily, Sardinia, North Africa, and then Egypt sent wheat to Rome. There was much shipping of other sought-after products that would keep: salt fish, wine, olive oil, raisins, and dried figs. How much, and along what routes, will become increasingly clear now that thermoluminescent tests can help to detect the provenance of the coarse, broken pottery of wine and storage vessels which, unlike painted ware, largely used to be discarded by archaeologists.

The Mediterranean was also in continuous contact with other zones. As Hehn (1870) demonstrated, many staple Mediterranean food products were of Asian origin. Some that could not be acclimatized were imported from afar. The Greeks were using cassia by ca. 600 B.C. (Sappho fr 44, 30 Lobel-Page) and buying cinnamon from the Arabs in Herodotus's time (iii 110–111). It has been thought that these spices came all the way from Indonesia to the African coast by outrigger canoe to be sold to Arab middlemen (Miller 1969, 153–172). The price of disbelieving this is to conjecture that by cassia and cinnamon the Greeks meant something other than what we do (Crone 1987, 253–263). In Roman times, pepper and other spices were shipped from South India at a large profit by traders who had learned to take advantage of the monsoon winds. They also brought samples of rice and Indian millet. To the south and east, the Mediterranean borders on the African and Asian deserts. Readers of the Bible are constantly reminded of how close the grapes, figs, olives, and pomegranates of Palestine were to the Jericho date palms, with Mesopotamia, where the staple oil is sesame instead of olive, not far away. To the north of the Mediterranean stretch the temperate lands of Europe, linked by trade to the Mediterranean basin long before the Roman conquest and eager to import its products, but also consuming foods alien to it, such as butter, beer, rye bread, and Atlantic fish. Our subject cannot be treated in isolation; and the two brief sections that follow, covering only a part of ancient Mediterranean diet, can hardly do justice to its many complexities.

CEREALS

Barley-meal and wheaten flour are "the marrow of men," says Homer (*Odyssey* xx 108). Long before the beginning of our period, varieties of barley and wheat, originally introduced from the Near East, were being sown along the shores of the Mediterranean and throughout barbarian Europe, with the exception of certain tracts, such as western Ireland, where soil and climate were too hostile. In northern Europe meat has nevertheless always figured large in the diet: readers of the Authorized Version of the Bible will remember that in it "meat" is used, in a wider sense, for food. But in the Mediterranean, food meant cereals first and foremost. In Hebrew and Greek the words for food in general are לֶחֶם (*leḥem*) and σῖτος (*sitos*), which specifically mean grain or bread.

Although wheat was always preferred for human food, *barley* must be considered first. The Egyptians, when speaking of both, always gave barley precedence (Währen 1965, 16). Pliny (*NH* xviii 72) held barley to be the oldest cereal. This belief explains why it was used in the most ancient Greek sacrifices: The gods dislike innovation (Plutarch, *Greek Questions 6 = Moralia* 292). Modern research tends to show that the cultivation of wheat and barley had begun at much the same time, in the eighth millennium B.C. But barley was providing the staple diet for most people at the beginning of our period, especially in Greece. It long remained the food of poor folk without access to subsidized wheat imports, because barley grows well not only on the well-drained, fertile deep soil that it likes best but also on the thin limestone soil characteristic of Greece and the Judaean hills, as well as many other parts of the Mediterranean world. It is not nearly as fastidious as wheat with respect to rain supply while germinating, and takes a shorter time to mature, so that it is less likely than wheat to suffer from disease and can endure in regions both hotter and colder. It will consequently flourish from sea level up to nearly 5,000 feet.

Of cultivated barley, the husked two-rowed *Hordeum distichum* L. was being grown in Palestine, Syria, and Turkey by the seventh millennium B.C. It could be sown as a spring crop if autumn-sown cereals had failed. Evidence of naked two-rowed barley in antiquity has been hard to come by. Naked six-rowed barley, *Hordeum vulgare* L. var. *nudum*, which can be threshed and therefore is the most convenient as human food, was domesticated in Anatolia before 7000 B.C. and had spread to Greece by 6000 B.C. Surprisingly, hooded six-row barley, *Hordeum vulgare* L. var. *trifurcatum*, seems to occur somewhat later, although early samples are found all the way from southwest Iran to Thessaly. Moritz (1955, 129–134) argued that most barley in ancient times was husked, as opposed to naked barley—i.e., barley whose grain needs only to be separated from the chaff. I find this hard to believe. Theophrastus's claim that "barley has the most naked seed of all" (*H.P. viii.* 4.1) is on the face of it clear-cut. Since Moritz wrote, naked barley has been found at Aquileia, at the head of the Adriatic (Spurr 1986, 14). In ancient Egypt and biblical Palestine, as later in Greece, Italy, and other Mediterranean lands, there is ample evidence for threshing with oxen. The procedure is so familiar as to be taken for granted in literature, but Xenophon (*Oeconomicus* xviii 3–5) and Varro (*RR* i 52) describe it. The ears were strewn on the threshing floor and yoked oxen driven round it in a circle. They trampled the ears with their hooves or pulled a drag over them. The next stage was winnowing with fan or shovel to separate the grain from the chaff. It is not always specified what kind of grain is meant; but Boaz winnowed his barley (Ruth 3:2), and the *Iliad* (xx 495–6) refers to "yoked oxen, threshing white barley on the well-made threshing floor." Threshing and winnowing imply naked barley; husked barley would have had to be pounded in a mortar instead.

The Book of Ruth, probably written in the fifth century B.C. but telling a story whose dramatic date is in the eleventh, describes how Naomi and her husband and two sons left Bethlehem for the land of Moab, east of Jordan, because of a food shortage. After ten years, having lost her husband and sons, Naomi returned, destitute, with Ruth, one of her new Moabite daughters-in-law, because she had heard that God had given his people *lehem:* The word, as we have noted, means "bread" specifically but also food in general. In accordance with the humane provisions of Jewish law, Ruth was allowed to glean after the harvesters employed by her rich kinsman, Boaz. Boaz invited her to join the reapers, to eat some *lehem* and dip a morsel into the wine (here *lehem* must literally mean bread). He gave her enough roasted grain to satisfy her hunger, and she took home an *ephah* (bushel) of barley. She went on gleaning until the end of the barley harvest and the wheat harvest. Then, in her best clothes, she crept to the threshing floor, where Boaz, after he had eaten and drunk and his heart was merry, had gone to lie down at the end of the heap of grain. Here she asked him to marry her as next of kin. To show his approval, Boaz filled her mantle with six measures of barley to take to her mother-in-law. The narrative embodies several features of ancient cereal production to which we shall now turn.

First, food shortage. In many places the main barley crop might fail once or twice in a lifetime. Food shortage in the days of the Patriarchs had driven Jacob and his sons to buy grain from the government stores in Egypt (Gen. 42) and had later driven Naomi's family to Moab. Other families had no doubt migrated for a while, used stored grain, or bought it from others, for Bethlehem was not left derelict: Naomi's contemporaries were there to recognize her on her return. It was not a famine like the recent one in Ethiopia or that caused by the locust plague in Edessa, a long way east of the Mediterranean, in 811 A.D. The problem of food shortages, which is the subject of Peter Garnsey's *Famine and Food Supply in the Graeco-Roman World*, will be discussed at the end of this section.

Secondly, we should note how well the Book of Ruth documents the predominance of barley at the outset of our period. True, the impoverished Ruth could not afford to wait with the gleaning, and the barley harvest precedes the wheat harvest. (In temperate Italy barley was reaped in June, wheat in July [Palladius vii 2, viii 1]; in Palestine the harvests would be in May and June respectively.) But the wheat harvest is mentioned briefly and in passing not only because it came later but also because wheat was a minor crop. Leavened wheaten bread had long been familiar: The point of the custom of eating unleavened bread at the Passover was that the Children of Israel, when they left Egypt in haste (Exod. 12:14–20) in the second millennium B.C., had had no time to bake their normal leavened loaves. But, outside certain favored areas, wheat was a scantier and riskier crop than barley. The Judaean hills will have been an even less favorable environment for wheat than Attica, the Athenian hinterland; and for Attica we have figures. An inscription recording firstfruits offered at Eleusis in 329/8 B.C. indicates that Attica's harvest in that year produced 11,371,420 kg of barley but only 1,082,500 kg of wheat (*IG* ii^2 1672, analyzed by Garnsey 1988, 98). The statistics for 1931–1960, the last period before modern methods transformed agriculture, show that wheat in Attica could be expected to fail more than one year in four, but barley only one year in twenty (Garnsey 1988, 10). Admittedly, there are grounds to think that 329/8 B.C. may have been an atypical year for Attica. Even so, Boaz could not have risked devoting much of his land to wheat.

Barley does not contain the necessary gluten-forming proteins to make a well-risen loaf. But there were ways of making barley acceptable as human food. It is a simple matter to roast grain, before it has hardened, on a pan to make it palatable. The roasted grain that the reapers shared with Ruth during the barley harvest must have been barley, though wheat can be treated in the same way. Roasted grain was a common article of diet in Old Testament times (cf. Lev. 23:14; 1 Sam. 17:17, 25:18, 2 Sam. 17:28) as it still is in the Near East today.

The Greeks, too, roasted barley. Every Athenian bride was required by a law of Solon (594 B.C.) to take to her wedding a *phrygetron*, barley-roaster (Pollux i 246). This was evidently a shallow pan with a handle in the shape of a loop into which the thumb was inserted, the fingers spreading out on the underside (Sparkes 1962, 128, Plate IV 6). It would be hung up with the pots (Polyzelus fr. 6, Kock i 791). On a large scale, the general Nicias recommended transport ships carrying wheat and roasted barley to feed the Athenian expedition against Syracuse in 415 B.C. (Thucydides vi 22). But it does not seem that the Greeks ate the roasted grains without further preparation. Roasting could be preliminary to making *alphita*, barley-meal. The best barley-meal, according to Galen (VI 507 Kühn) was from roasted fresh barley. Roasting was part of the porridge-making process described by Pliny:

> The Greeks soak the barley-grain in water, leave it overnight to dry, and the next day roast and then grind it. But some shake the barley from its ears while they are still green, clean it, pound it wet in a mortar, wash it in baskets, dry it in the sun, pound it again, clean it and grind it. Whichever way it has been prepared, they add to twenty pounds of barley three of linseed and half of coriander and a small cupful of salt; and having first roasted everything they mix it in the mill. Those who want to keep it for some time keep it in new earthenware jars with fine wheat-flour and its own bran (*NH* xviii 72–74).

Pliny's Greek porridge was being enjoyed for its own sake by people who could afford wheaten bread, as the use of fine wheat flour for preserving it makes clear. Pliny continues ". . . experience has condemned barley-bread, though it was anciently much used; it is now mostly fed to animals." By the time of the Roman Empire, imported wheat was being doled out to the proletariat of Rome. Barley-bread betokened rural poverty. It was with this that Jesus miraculously fed the Five Thousand, who were humble Galileans (John 6:9). Barley-cakes had been common in Old Testament times (Judg. 7:13; 2 Kings 4:42; Ezek. 4:12). They were easy to make. The grains were crushed into groats, and these were kneaded, often just with water, and baked (Ezek. 4:12), or perhaps on occasion only dried. No leaven was used: it would have made little difference. The result was barley-cakes like those that have survived at Wangen, Untersee in Switzerland. They are only about one and a half inches high, and four to five inches in diameter, of a dough consisting of grains of barley more or less crushed (Renfrew 1973, 81). Two bowls, one containing a flat barley-cake, and the other with a number of small, lozenge-shaped ones, of coarsely crushed grain, have been found in Egypt in a pharaonic tomb of the 21st century B.C. (Wittmack in Steindorff 1896, 41–42). In the Metropolitan Museum of Art, New York, and the British Museum, London, are rough Egyptian barley-cakes of the 21st century and ca. 1500 B.C. respectively. They are triangular, each side measuring about seven inches (illustrated by Währen 1965, 27, fig. 15).

The usual Greek word for barley-cake is μᾶζα (maza), from μάσσω, "knead," always distinguished from the wheaten loaf, ἄρτοσ (artos). At Scolus in Boeotia there were statues of Megalomazos and Megalartos, Great Barley-cake and Great Wheat-loaf (Polemon from Athenaeus iii 109B). An old harvest song, preserved among the Homeric *Epigrams* (xv), shows that *maza*, as well as barley-porridge (flavored with sesame this time, not coriander and linseed), was thought a sign of wealth:

> Let us turn to the house of a man of great power and
>   outstanding,
> lasting fortune! Plenty of Wealth will come in, and with
>   Wealth,
> flourishing Joy and noble Peace. Let all bins be full,
>   and the . . .
> *maza* always overflow the kneading-trough! And now the
>   cheerful
> barley-porridge, full of sesame. . . .

It is surprising how appreciative the early Greeks were of barley-cakes, though they never claimed that they were better than wheaten bread. Ἀγαθὴ καὶ μᾶζα μετ᾽ ἄρτον, "next to bread, barley-cake is good too," ran the proverb (Zenobius i 12). With few wheat-growing areas of their own, they put up cheerfully with the second best. Hesiod, in up-country Boeotia, was a hardy farmer subsisting on his own produce, even though lowland Boeotia, one of the rare Greek wheatlands, was not far away. He describes a picnic at the height of summer. It is an idyllic one, with wine imported from Thracian Biblis to go with good home farm produce: goat's milk, veal and kid, and with it a *maza amolgaiē* (*Works and Days* 590). The adjective *amolgaiē* has puzzled commentators. Martin West's *Commentary* (1978) is surely right in deriving it from *amolgē*, milking (though a Greek farmer would smile at his supposing that "it might be most convenient to milk a goat directly onto the flour"). It makes sense to knead groats with milk, or for that matter with oil or honey, for an improved product. The *kammata* that were served after dinner to Spartan boys were cakes of barley-meal soaked in oil and baked and served on laurel leaves (Nicocles the Spartan, *FGH* 587 F1, quoted by Athenaeus iv 140D). Archilochus in the mid-seventh century B.C., like Hesiod, washed down his *maza* with Thracian wine, the very best (see below, page 50): "in my spear is my kneaded *maza*, in my spear my wine of Ismaros" (Fr. 2 West). *Maza*-eating did not shame a warrior any more than a farmer. Its merit must have lain in its convenience: it was easier to prepare on campaign than leavened wheaten bread, which requires time and skill. That must be why Telemachus, a King's son who has wheaten loaves served in the palace (*Odyssey* xvii 343, xviii 120) and a staff of a dozen women to prepare them (*Odyssey* xx 105f), takes on board his ship not wheaten flour but twenty measures of mill-crushed barley-groats in leather bags (ii 349–355) while not stinting the wine, which is to be the best sweet wine the housekeeper can supply.

In a law of 594 B.C., Solon ruled that those who dined at state expense at the town hall—the most signal honor Athens could provide—should receive a *maza* on ordinary days and wheaten bread only during festivals. Barley was the staple food, with oil and wine, in early Sparta (Plutarch, *Lycurgus* 8). In the mid-sixth century B.C. Hipponax of Ephesus describes a man who has wasted his inheritance and, unlike the Prodigal Son, cannot avoid digging: he "eats mediocre figs and a barley *kollix*, slaves' fodder" (fr. 26 West, from Athenaeus vii 304B). But this does not imply, as is often supposed, that the Greeks had already anticipated Pliny's wholesale condemnation of barley-cake. The Ephesians, with the rare advantage of the wheatlands of the Cayster valley, could afford to be more fastidious than other Greeks; the *kollix*, moreover, was coarse (Archestratos, *Gastronomy*, Kock ii 548, quoted by Athenaeus iii 112AB). Barley-cakes came in different qualities. The worst were black, with chaff mixed in the kneading, "prepared with a view to cheapness." (The chaff is another indication of naked barley.) A vegetarian ascetic of the school of Pythagoras might make a meal of these low-grade barley-cakes for only an obol (Antiphanes, Kock ii 76, quoted by Athenaeus iv 161B). Destitute folk would eat them with a few figs and wild plants such as sow-thistle and mushrooms (Poliochus, Kock iii 390, and Antiphanes, Kock ii 111, from Athenaeus ii 60B–D). But other kinds of barley-cake were highly esteemed. The barley-cakes provided at the Athens town hall were "Achillean," from a superlative barley (so the ancient commentator on Aristophanes' *Knights* 819), by contrast to the coarse-ground Athenian *phystē* and other kinds (Athenaeus iii 111EF). "We take care," says the comedy-writer Alexis in a context of banqueting with snow-cooled drink, "that the *maza* we eat regularly should be as white as possible" (Kock ii 348, from Athenaeus iii 124A). The *maza* of Teos, like that of Eretria, "city of white barley-meal," was famous (Athenaeus iv 160A). Lesbos's barley-meal was supreme. Antiphanes (loc. cit.) praises it in an encomium of wheaten loaves. He must have barley-cakes in mind when he says:

> The best one can get, the best of all
> of rich barley, all cleanly sifted,
> comes from Lesbos, the wave-washed breast [i.e., hill]
>   of Eresos,
> whiter than snow from the sky. If the gods eat barley-meal,
> then Hermes must go there and buy it for them!
> There is satisfactory barley-meal in seven-gated Thebes,
> and in Thasos and some other cities, but theirs are
>   grape-stones
> compared to those of Lesbos. Understand this clearly!

The comparison with grape-stones is worth noting. When barley is prepared for human consumption today, it is often reduced to the grape-stone sized pieces called pearl barley. Repeated grindings or crushings will produce meal. Barley-meal is still a dietary staple in some parts of the world: it is the present-day Tibetan *tsampa*. Barley-meal can occasionally be fine: the medical writer Erotianus speaks of *palē* as the "whitest and finest of barley-meal" (111,9), using a word which with its variants *palēmation, paipalē*, is sometimes applied to fine barley-meal by other writers (Hippocrates *Womens' Diseases* i 64 = VIII 132 Littré; Archigenes, quoted by Galen, XII 791 Kühn; Polyaenus, *Strategemata* iv 3,22). But it is normally used for the finest wheat-flour (Scholiast on Aristophanes' *Clouds* 262, Pollux vi 62) and equated with wheat-flour "dust" (Hesychius, sv. πάλη), equivalent to the Latin *pollen* (see below, page 29); and even the finest barley-meal cannot compete with *pollen*. L. A. Moritz (1949) argued that *alphita* was the Greek word for coarse meal, and *aleura* for fine flour, regardless of what grain these were made from. True enough, the Hippocratic Corpus writes of coarse wheat-meal as "wheaten *alphita*" (*Regimen in Acute Diseases* [Sp.] 53 = I 173 Kühlewein) and of "*alphita* of beans and vetch" (On *Internal Affections* 23 = VII 226 Littré), as Galen notes (VI 76 Kühn). But these are exceptional usages. It normally makes sense to translate *alphita* as barley-meal and *aleura* as wheaten flour. Moritz, reluctant to believe that the staple food of the

Homeric Greeks was barley-meal, hoped by freeing the word *alphita* from its association with barley to resolve the paradox that in Greek Epic it is mentioned only as human food, whereas horses are fed with emmer as well as barley (*Iliad* v 196, *Odyssey* iv 41) and even wheat (*Iliad* viii 188), which is also given to geese (*Odyssey* xix 536, 556). But the contrast here is between the food of ordinary folk and the fodder ascribed to the horses of mythical heroes; and the wheat-fed geese were being fattened for the royal table.

The Greeks were content with their barley-cakes. Most of the allusions to *maza* in Athenian Comedy are friendly. A Megarian, starving because of Athenian depredations in the Peloponnesian War, is seen coming to Athens during the fantasy truce of Aristophanes' *Acharnians* (425 B.C.): he tries to sell his daughters as piglets, being tempted among other things by an Athenian *maza*, though figs, garlic, and salt are also attractions. This is frugal bait, but it should be remembered that figs had become a luxury for the Athenians themselves because of the War (see the section on Indigenous Mediterranean Fruits, below, page 52). A *maza* steeped in sweetened wine was palatable and gave the impression of being more nourishing than it really was (Galen, *On the strength of foods* i 11   = VI 510 Kühn). Athenion the Aristotelian, the leader of Athens's revolt from Rome in 88 B.C., was criticized during the siege for his distributions of a *choinix* of barley every four days because it was "chicken-feed, not human food" (Posidonius *FGH* 87 F 36, from Athenaeus iv 214F). That has been taken to show that the Athenians had by this time come to reject barley altogether (Moritz 1967), but the Athenians' resentment was surely because the ration was too scanty. A *choinix* was normally one day's allowance (Herodotus vii 187, Diogenes Laertius viii 18). It does not look as if the Greeks ever turned against barley on principle. But none of them will have doubted the verdict of Aristotle that wheat was more nourishing than barley (*Problems* xxi 2. 927[a]18), endorsed by the dietician Diphilus of Siphnos, who pronounced in the early third century B.C. that wheaten loaves were "superior to those of barley for nourishment and digestibility and altogether better" (Athenaeus iii 115c). An unidentified quotation in Athenaeus runs "we do not care for *alphita*, for the town is full of (wheaten) loaves" (iii 113A). That must come from an imaginary scene of feasting and merriment in a comedy. In real life in an ordinary Greek city people could not be so choosy.

Barley-gruel, by contrast to barley-cakes, was highly esteemed as food for the sick. Hippocrates, *Regimen in acute diseases* (10–20, 23–27) recommends a decoction from the finest barley: either thick (*oulai ptisanai*) or a strained juice (*chylos*). This was valued as lubricant, thirst-quenching, easy of evacuation, not harmful to the bowels. Careful instructions were given about how and when to administer it. Barley-gruel continued to be recommended for the sick even though it was not rated highly for nourishment: it is preferable to wheat-gruel for the sick because cooler, according to Aristotle, *Problems* i 37, 863^{b}6, even though he notes that those engaged in processing barley are paler and more subject to catarrh than those who process wheat (*Problems* xxi 24. 929^{b}27–28, xxxviii 10, 967^{b}2). The emollient qualities of barley-water continued to recommend themselves to Dioscorides (ii 108) in the first century A.D. and to Galen (VI 507 Kühn) in the second, who notes that barley-meal in water, or mixed with must or sweet wine, is also a good drink for healthy people in summer in advance of bathing.

Barley beer, unflavored by hops, was extensively used in ancient Egypt, which was not an ideal land for grapes and bought good wine from Greece (see below, page 50). Beer was known in parts of Gaul and Spain, and was extensively brewed for the Roman army along the Rhine frontier and in Britain; but it played no part in the diet of the Mediterranean proper.

The sacramental drink of the Eleusinian Mysteries, supposedly first offered to the goddess Demeter, was of barley-meal mixed with water and mint. But additional nourishment might well be added to a barley-meal posset, *kykeōn*. In the Homeric epics, Nestor proffered Pramnian wine mixed with barley-meal, grated cheese, and honey (*Iliad* xi 639–640), and Circe bewitched Odysseus's men with the same draught (*Odyssey* x 234–235). Hippocrates writes of possets of barley-meal mixed with water, wine, honey, or milk, which last can be goat's, cow's, mare's, or donkey's milk (*Regimen* ii 41, VI 538 Littré). Barley-meal could be mixed with the meal of other grains and of pulses to make solid food. Ezekiel (4:9) speaks of wheat and barley, beans and lentils, millet and emmer, put into a single vessel to make bread: This is allegorical, but would make no sense if no mixture had been used for bread in ordinary life. Pliny says that the Roman barley-bread, *panis hordaceus,* used to be made with a modest proportion of leaven from the flour of chick-pea or vetch (*NH* xviii 104). Could the basic flour of *panis hordaceus* have been a mixture too? The meal of vetch or chick-peas, already mentioned in the Hippocratic Corpus, would add body to barley-meal: chick-pea meal makes *hummus,* that excellent food, today in the Levant. If *panis hordaceus* was a mixture, that would explain why the Romans should have fed it to gladiators, who were consequently known as *hordacei,* barley-men (Pliny *NH* xviii 72). Gladiators were an investment and it would have been folly to underfeed them.

The question is worth raising, because it does not seem that barley bread on its own was valued as human food by the Romans at any time. Barley rations in place of wheat were a serious collective punishment in the normally well-fed Roman army as early as 214 B.C. (Frontinus, *Strategemata* iv 1.25, cf. Livy xxiv 18) and 209 B.C. (Livy xxvii 13.9, Plutarch *Marcellus* 25), and again in the second century B.C. (Polybius vi 38,3). Antony inflicted it on his troops in 36 B.C. (Frontinus, *Strategemata* iv 1.37), and Octavian two years later (Dio xlix 38,4); recruits were fed on barley instead of wheat if they failed in their tasks (Vegetius i 13). *Polenta*, barley groats, are mentioned occasionally in Latin literature: the word has survived unchanged into modern times, although today's *polenta* is made from maize. But Ovid's legend of the poor old Sicilian woman who offered a drink sprinkled with roasted *polenta* (*Metamorphoses* v 448–461) implies the direst poverty; and we otherwise find it not as a food but as an additive to cabbage-water medicine (Cato 156,5) or medicinal wine (Celsus iv 18.3). The Romans of Pliny's day thought of barley bread as fodder for animals (*NH* xviii 74). Unlike the Greeks, the Romans and most Italians had evidently been fed on products of emmer wheat from the beginnings of our period. Even slaves were fed on wheaten bread by the exploitative Cato (*RR* 56). Columella recommended a mixture of high-grade white meal from two-rowed Galatian barley with wheat to feed the slaves (ii 9.16). Ulpian (*Digest* xxxiii 9.3.8) mentions barley stored to feed pack-animals or slaves: when fed to slaves this, too, may have been mixed. Only in times of scarcity can we be sure that the Romans resorted to barley alone. Columella (ii 9.14) concedes that when food is scarce, the six-rowed variety called *cantherinum* (horse-barley) is better for humans than bad wheat.

Emmer, the traditional Roman staple, is a hulled wheat. There was one other kind of hulled wheat in antiquity: the diploid einkorn wheat (*Triticum monococcum*, Greek *tiphē*), which was being farmed in upland Anatolia and Kurdistan around 7000 B.C. and had spread into Europe in the fifth millennium, although never into the irrigated plains of Mesopotamia and Egypt. It is still grown today in some mountainous areas of Anatolia. Einkorn is described by Theophrastus (*HP* viii 4.1), who notes that as a plant with slight yield it will grow in light soil (viii 9.2). But the slightness of the yield meant that its importance had been much reduced by classical times. The Romans did not even have a word of their own for it. By contrast, the tetraploid emmer (*Triticum turgidum* var. *dicoccum*) was highly valued. It was spreading over the Near East in the seventh millennium and became the main wheat crop of Mesopotamia in the sixth, and of the Nile valley and the Mediterranean basin during the fifth and fourth. The Greeks knew it as ζειά (*zeia*), with a variety ὀλύρα (*olyra*, Theophrastus *HP* viii 4.1; 9.2). For Homer, fertile land is the "emmer-bearing glebe," *zeidōros aroura*; but by Herodotus's time emmer ("*olyrai* which some call *zeiai*," ii 35,2), as opposed to wheat and barley, was thought of as typically Egyptian. For the Romans it was typical too. In Pliny's time it was being grown from Egypt to Gaul (*NH* xviii 81–82, 109), presumably because it had not been completely ousted by bread-wheat in Egypt and had been introduced to Gaul by the Romans. They called it *far:* It had been their only crop for three hundred years (Verrius, from Pliny *NH* xviii 63). Just as barley had been a traditional Greek sacrifice, the most ancient sacrifices of the Romans were of emmer pottage, *puls fitilla* (Pliny *NH* xviii 84) or emmer grain and salt (Vergil, *Æneid* v 745, Horace *Odes* iii 23, 20, Ovid *Fasti* ii 520, iii 284). Emmer was widely grown throughout Roman Italy until at least the fourth century A.D. (Spurr 1986, 12–13), because it was more robust than naked wheat, tolerating a variety of soils, and germinating even if autumn rains were late (cf. Columella ii 8,5; 9,3; Pliny *NH* xviii 83). Its husks gave protection from disease and insects, both when growing and in store. Modern cultivation under ancient conditions has produced a surprisingly high yield (Reynolds 1979, 60–64).

From emmer, the Romans made porridge, *puls,* their national dish. "Porridge-eating barbarians" they called themselves in fun (Plautus, *Mostellaria* 828, cf. *Poenulus* 54). Moritz (1955, 129–134) argued that emmer-porridge was eaten because toasting was essential to make the hulls brittle before they could be removed by pounding. Toasting, he thought, must have destroyed the gluten-forming proteins that would otherwise have enabled the pounded emmer-flour meal to rise when leavened. So porridge was all that emmer-flour was good for. This view has been frequently repeated, most recently by Spurr (1986, pp. 11–12). But it cannot be right. Egyptian leavened bread, of which examples have been found in Tutankhamen's tomb (Währen, op. cit. [see p. 1] 26, fig. 14), had been emmer-bread. If the Egyptians could hull emmer without destroying its gluten-forming proteins, so, surely, could the Romans. Fred Martin of Newport, Gwent, has baked bread from parched emmer: A sample is in the Abergavenny Castle Museum. Nor is it clear that toasting/parching was essential for hulling. Pliny indeed says "emmer . . . cannot be cleaned [i.e., hulled] unless toasted, which is why emmer grains are sown with their husks still on"(*NH* xviii 61). But too much, perhaps, has been built on this sentence. Peter Reynolds, who has grown emmer at the Butser Iron Age Farm in Hampshire, tells me that one can pound the hulls off untoasted emmer with an iron-capped pestle and a hollowed tree-trunk mortar, a practice known to Pliny (*NH* xviii 105) and still common in North Africa. Jane Renfrew (1985, 26–27) illustrates the big grain-drying kilns attached to Roman-British villas, "thought to have been used for drying and parching the hulled wheats to facilitate the threshing of the grain from the spikelets." But these are more likely to be malting floors (Reynolds and Langley 1979), which explains why there are no comparable kilns in Italy, where above all we should expect them. Toasting was certainly part of porridge-making; but Varro (*RR* i 63) suggests that the emmer could be pounded first and toasted afterwards.

Porridge from emmer-groats was, more probably, eaten by the early Romans because they liked it better, and because it was simpler to prepare than bread. Moritz thought that as the taste for bread grew, bread-wheat replaced emmer; but the finds, as we have seen, may rather indicate that emmer was being grown in Italy throughout the Imperial period. The Latin word for flour, *farina*, derives from *far*, emmer (Pliny *NH* xviii 88). This surely confirms that flour could be made from pounded emmer as well as from naked wheats. There are classical as well as Egyptian references to emmer-bread. Tryphon of Alexander wrote of bread from *olyra* and meal-bread from *zeiai* (Athenaeus iii 109C). Dioscorides, who was an army doctor under Claudius and Nero, knows of emmer-bread, which he says is more nourishing and digestible than barley-bread although not as good as wheaten bread (ii 108). Pliny says the most delicate or sweetest (*dulcissimus*) bread is made of *arinca*, which he identifies with *olyra* (*NH* xviii 92), although the identification is not quite certain because Pliny seems confused at this point (he thinks *arinca* is naked in Italy and Egypt but not in Greece, *NH* xvii 61, 92). That Roman bakers were called *pistores*, "pounders," confirms that they originally made bread from emmer rather than from naked wheat. The first *pistores* set up shop in Rome in 171–168 B.C. Women before then had done the work at home (Pliny *NH* xviii 107).

In Pliny's time plenty of bread was being consumed, but the traditional liking for porridge had continued. Pliny says little of bread-making but a good deal about *alica*, the excellent emmer-groats produced in a number of places in Italy and best of all in Campania, whose volcanic fertile ground was sown twice a year with emmer and once with millet. Pliny notes with astonishment that chalk from White Earth Hill near Pozzuoli was added to it (*NH* xviii 109–114). This is not as shocking as it sounds. Present-day British law requires all except whole meal flour to contain between 235 and 390 mg of calcium carbonate per 100 grams, in the form of *creta praeparata*. But Pliny also describes spurious *alica*, made from an inferior emmer grown in Tunisia, which had the immoderate proportion of 25% gypsum (hydrous calcium sulphate)—a reminder that, despite ancient towns having market overseers, there was little protection against adulteration of food (see also below, page 51, on adulterated wine). It is not a modern failing to adulterate food with chemicals. What is modern is adequate consumer protection.

Alica was needed not only for porridge but for *placenta*, a ponderous Roman cheese-cake for which Cato gives a recipe (*RR* 76). It required 6 lb of wheaten flour, 2 lb of Alica, 14 lb of sheep's cheese, sweet and fresh, 4½ lb of fine honey, and no eggs. To make a *libum*, a kind of flat cake, 1 lb of flour only was used, 2 lb of cheese, no honey, and a single egg (*RR* 75). These cakes were used in sacrifices; so the priests and their staff ate them in the end. It was a pleasing paradox that the runaway slave of a priest would prefer ordinary bread to either (Horace *Epistles* x 10–11). "Punic porridge" was compounded of 1 lb *alica*, 3 lb cheese, ½ lb honey, and one egg (*RR* 75). Cato's recipes, unlike Mrs. Beeton's, are so sparing of eggs that the products must have been heavy. Another use for *alica* was "Picene bread," prepared in the neighborhood of Ancona: It was steeped for nine days, then kneaded with raisin wine on the tenth into the shape of a long roll, baked in earthenware pots that were broken in the process, and only used for food when soaked with milk or sweet wine (Pliny *NH* xviii 106).

Bread-wheat, believed to derive from emmer by a series of mutations, was certainly being cultivated in the Near East at an early stage. Threshing and winnowing is attested throughout antiquity, of wheat as well as barley. Long before King David's time, Gideon is described winnowing his wheat (Judges 6:11). Free-threshing wheat, *pyros*, was distinguished from emmer and barley (*Odyssey* iv 604); the Latin name for it, *triticum*, means "threshable." But, as we have noted, it was a risky crop. Unlike barley, wheat required rain in the period of germination: A Mediterranean farmer could lose his wheat crop if there were no autumn showers shortly after planting. It was especially vulnerable to grubs (Theophrastus *HP* viii 10,4) and rust. The Romans appeased the god Robigus in the hope that he would ward off rust, *robigo;* rust was a greater danger to wheat than to barley (Pliny *NH* xviii 79, *pace* Theophrastus *HP* viii 10, 2). The god had a festival of his own on 25 April and was propitiated by the sacrifice of a puppy and a sheep (Ovid, *Fasti* iv 901–942).

Wheat did not take well to the thin soil of the limestone ridges that predominate in the Mediterranean. But we have noticed Boaz' wheat harvest in the stony fields of Bethlehem. Wheat-growing was widespread, though in most places on a modest scale, with thin planting promising at best a meager harvest. For good yields, rich moisture-retaining soil was required. This soil was available on lacustrine plains such as Thessaly, Boeotia, and upland Lycia; in the volcanic region of Campania; and in alluvial valleys such as those of the Po, the Maeander (adjoining Miletus), the Caicus (adjoining Ephesus), the Hermus (near Sardis) and the Scamander, river of Troy. Carbonized wheat was found in quantities at Troy, although barley was absent (Schliemann 1880, 320; Wittmack 1890, 614f). Only specially favored regions produced a wheat surplus: the Hauran northwest of Palestine, lowland Cilicia, the Thracian coast, Sicily, parts of southern Italy, Sardinia and Spain, tracts of

North Africa, and above all, outside the Mediterranean climatic region, the Ukraine and Egypt. The wheat trade was the reason for Greek colonization of Olbia and other Black Sea ports from ca. 615 B.C. on. Xerxes saw merchant ships carrying corn from the Ukraine to the Peloponnese in 480 B.C. (Herodotus vii 147). The Ukraine was the chief source of wheat imports to classical Athens: the sea route from the Crimea through the Bosporus and Dardanelles to the Aegean was Athens' lifeline. Egypt also supplied wheat to Greece. Naucratis, the Greek treaty port, also dates from ca. 615 B.C. Bacchylides in the first half of the fifth century B.C. describes how

> wheat-carrying ships over the gleaming sea
> bear from Egypt the greatest wealth (Fr.20B 14–16 Snell).

Cleomenes of Naucratis, given control over Egypt after its conquest by Alexander, made gigantic profits out of his wheat monopoly, to the detriment of Athens and other Greek states ([Aristotle], *Oeconomica* ii 2 1352ª16–23, 1352ᵇ14–20,[Demosthenes] lvi 7). After Egypt was annexed to the Roman Empire in 30 B.C., massive supplies of wheat—almost certainly free-threshing wheat by now, not emmer—were shipped to Rome.

There were many varieties of free-threshing wheat (see Theophrastus *HP* viii 4, 3–6, Pliny *NH* xviii 63–70). The chief distinction seems to be between common or bread wheat, *Triticum aestivum* L. = *Triticum vulgare* Host., and hard wheat, *Triticum durum* Desfontaines. Bread wheat, *siligo,* is found to have been grown in various parts of the Near East and Anatolia in the seventh millennium B.C.; it penetrated into Mesopotamia in the sixth and spread into the Nile Valley and Mediterranean lands in the fifth. It is from its ever-increased varieties that modern bread is made. The flour of bread-wheat was called *siligo* by the Romans; its finest, most powdery form was "the flower of *siligo,*" *flos siliginis,* or *pollen.* The "tender loaf, snowy white" was "made from soft *siligo*" (Juvenal, *Satire* v 70). Hard wheat (*triticum* par excellence) is attested in the Egyptian Fayyum in Ptolemaic times and was better suited than bread-wheat to some Mediterranean climates, such as that of southern Italy. Today it is often known as macaroni wheat and is grown for *pasta* and semolina. *Pasta* was unknown in ancient times, though semolina (*similago*) had many uses for cooking and baking. It is, however, possible to get yellow bread-flour out of the flint-hard grains of durum wheat by repeated grindings: hence a heavier but nourishing loaf.

There are difficulties in equating Greek words for flour with Roman. *Sētaneios* (*sitanios*) is one word for fine wheaten flour, derived either from *sētes,* "this year's," that is, spring-sown wheat, or from *sēthō,* "sift." The equivalent of *pollen* would seem to be *palē, palēmation,* or *paipalē* (see above, page 22) or *gyris* (Athenaeus iii 115D). Another word for fine flour is *semidalis*, which derives from the Assyrian *samîdu*, Aramaic *sem-idâ*; bread made from it was *artos semidalitēs*. *Sētaneios* is usually equated by modern scholars with *siligo*, and *semidalis* with *similago*. However, Moritz's argument in connection with *aleura* and *alphita* (see above, pages 22–23) would seem to apply with even greater force to these words for flour. They were used to describe the flour's quality. The consumer will not necessarily have known which grain produced a type of flour, still less loaves and cakes. According to Galen (VI 483–484 Kühn) there is no equivalent at all—except for the barbarism *silignis*—in Greek for *siligo*, by which name he says the Romans denote the finest flour.

The quality of flour will also have depended on cleaning—for the threshing oxen must have left droppings—and on how well the grains had been separated from weed-seed and milled. The Enemy, according to a parable of Jesus, sows tares (*zizania*) among the wheat (Matt. 13:25); Vergil describes how crops are vulnerable not only to rust, thistles, burrs, and caltrops but also to being interspersed with "luckless darnel (*lolium*) and barren oats" (*Georgics* i 154). Darnel and tares are thought to be identical. The Master in the parable got the reapers to sort out the wheat sheaves from the tares. But grain samples of the first century A.D. from two Roman sites on the German frontier show a high proportion of weed seeds (Hopf, 1963). Columella in passing mentions a *cribrum loliarium*, a darnel-sieve, and a *cribrum viciarium*, a vetch-sieve (viii 5, 16).

Next came milling. The definitive study by Moritz (1958), *Grain Mills and Flour in Classical Antiquity*, shows how the art developed. The original mill, attested from about 3000 B.C. in Egypt and used in Greece until the end of the classical era, was the saddle-quern. The "maidservant who is behind the mill" (Exod. 10:5) knelt behind a sloping slab of stone and ground the grain with an upper stone somewhat like a rolling pin. It will have been at such saddle-querns that the girls were employed to grind barley-meal and wheaten flour in Odysseus' palace (*Odyssey* xx 106–111). A bad woman was one who "will not touch the mill or lift the sieve" (Semonides of Amorgos, fr. 7, 59–60 West). Mortars were used side by side with saddle-querns—both were found at Troy—presumably because emmer and husked barley had to be pounded in a mortar before grinding. In Greece, between the sixth and third centuries B.C., the saddle-quern was improved. We find a "hopper-rubber" with a slit in the upper stone and herring-bone grooving on the lower. The slit controlled the feed and the grooves the size of the milled granules. By the second century B.C. the rotary mill had come in: Pliny says it was invented in Volsinii in Etruria (*NH* xxxvi 155). Cato mentions a "turning-mill" and a "pushing-mill" for use on the estate, though for olives and grapes, not grain (*RR* 10,11): These could be turned by slaves or donkeys (Plautus, *Asinaria* 708–709). Donkey-mills survive in the baking establishments at Pompeii and are depicted on certain Roman tombstones. The massive, hour-glass-shaped millstones were made of hard, porous stone. At Pompeii the local volcanic rock from Vesuvius was well-suited; elsewhere people might be prepared to import millstones by sea, for we learn that the Aegean island of Nisyros was famous as a source (Strabo x 488, *Anth. Pal.* ix 21.5). It is a donkey-millstone which, in a saying of Christ, hangs around the neck of the child-corruptor (Matt. 18:6). Meanwhile, small rotary mills replaced the saddle-quern where portability was needed—in the home or for the use of mobile army units. The *Moretum*, a poem ascribed to Vergil, gives a description of bread-making by a poor cottage-dweller: he uses a small rotary mill. Animals continued to be used for many big mills despite the invention of the geared water mill in the first century B.C. (Vitruvius x 5,2). The Diocletianic Price Edict of 301 A.D. shows water mills, donkey mills, and small hand-turned rotary mills all in use, not because the saving of labor was undervalued: A famous poem in the *Palatine Anthology* commends the water mill for this (ix 418). More probably it was because of the capital outlay and maintenance required and the lack of suitable year-round running water in many regions. Windmills were not invented until the Middle Ages.

The fineness of milling could not be varied as in a modern roller mill; but Pliny refers to techniques such as grinding grain when dry—which he says gives more flour—or when sprinkled with salt water, which results in a whiter but lower yield, with more being kept back in the bran (*NH* xviii 87). To get fine flour, if the nature of the grain allowed it, it would seem to have been necessary to repeat the grinding process and to sift with the flour-sieve, *cribrum farinarium*. In Pliny's time there were sieves of horsehair, invented in Gaul; of flax, invented in Spain; and of papyrus and rush from Egypt. We also hear of a *cribrum pollinarium*, evidently needed for the finest flour of all, *pollen* (*NH* xviii 108). But standards of processing will have varied. A rough stone lurking in cereal food can hurt the teeth, says Lucretius (iii 694). Horace (*Satires* i 5, 89–91) says that the bread in an unnamed little town on the main route from Rome to Brindisi is so good that the shrewd traveller will carry a supply with him, to avoid the notoriously gritty bread of Canusium (Canosa) next on the road. Grit in bread, well known as the cause of the worn teeth of mummified Egyptians, may have resulted from unsuitable millstones and have been hard to eliminate by sieving. It is worth remembering, in this context, the high cost of inland transport by pack animals. Millstones were the heaviest load of all.

Like milling, kneading and baking were originally done at home. But the trade of professional bakers grew up in cities. When Jeremiah was under arrest in Jerusalem early in the sixth century B.C., he was given a loaf of bread daily from the bakers' street (Jer. 37:21). Bread shops were thought a normal feature of a Greek town in the fifth century B.C. (Aristophanes, *Frogs* 112). Before the first bakers' shops at Rome in 171–168 B.C., the work had been done at home by the women, "as is the case even now among most peoples" (Pliny, *NH* xviii 107). In Imperial times we find aspects of the trade illustrated on the tombs of prosperous Roman bakers, usually men of slave origin with Greek surnames: such are the contractor M. Vergilius Eurysaces, whose cenotaph stands outside the Porta Maggiore at Rome, and P. Nonius Zethus, whose sarcophagus is now in the Chiaramonti collection in the Vatican. The corn-dole, as we shall see, was handed out in the form of grain: The urban proletariat, living in cramped quarters in multistory tenement buildings, will often have had to take their grain, despite their own poverty, to the bakers' establishments, where the entire work of bread-making was carried on, from milling to baking. In Rome's port of Ostia only two such establishments have been found, but these are large: one covers the space of six normal shops, the other is bigger still. One of the bakeries probably had a contract to supply the local police and fire brigade, the *vigiles* (Meiggs 1960, 274). At Pompeii the trade was in the hands of a series of smaller establishments, each catering for a district of the town.

Leaven has symbolic force in many of the sayings of Jesus; one can imagine him as a boy watching His mother make bread by using a piece of fully fermented dough left over from the previous day's baking—the normal method, according to Pliny (*NH* xviii 104). In the Mediterranean climate, spontaneous fermentation will take place within 24 hours. The technique had been evolved long before our period begins, though the use of unleavened bread for Jewish cereal offerings (Lev. 2:4–5,11, 7:12, 8:2; Num. 4:15) may hark back to a yet more remote time when leaven had not yet been introduced: sacrifices, as we have seen are deeply conservative. Pliny (*NH* xviii 102–104) mentions more sophisticated methods, such as kneading millet or fine wheat bran with must at vintage time: the resulting leaven would last a year. Another method, also recommended by Palladius (xi 21) was to knead wheat bran with must and dry it in the sun. In Spain and Gaul there was a leaven that was a by-product of beer manufacture (Pliny, *NH* xviii 68). There is one reference to the short cut of using bicarbonate of soda (*nitron*) instead of leaven to make soda bread (*Geoponica* ii 33,1).

Kneading dough is tedious. A terra-cotta group from Thebes, now in the Louvre, shows four women kneading to the sound of a reed-pipe (H. Blümner, *Technologie und Terminologie der Gewerbe und Künste bei den Griechen und Römern* i² (Leipzig 1912, fig. 25). Anaxarchus, a sophist of the fourth century B.C., had his bread maker wear a mask and gloves when kneading the dough to prevent it from being contaminated by breath and sweat. These sensible precautions were thought overindulgent, as was Anaxarchus's employment of a beautiful naked female wine pourer (Clearchus of Soli, *Lives, FHG* ii 308, quoted by Athenaeus xii 548C). Several bakeries at Pompeii had kneading machines (Mau 1899, 384 and plate 214, reproduced by Blümner, 1912, fig. 26). But most housewives in the Greek countryside were kneading by hand when I traveled there in the 1950s. After kneading came the task of shaping the dough. Occasionally, for ritual reasons or for fun, special shapes were produced: for instance, male or female genitalia (Martial xiv 69, Petronius 60,4, Martial ix 2,3). There were many different shapes, from rolls to twist-bread, and a great number of names to describe them. But there is much to be said for the standard shape of the loaves sold at Pompeii—round, stackable, and with incisions in the crust radiating from the center, so that the bread could be conveniently broken. It was His manner of breaking bread that caused the disciples to recognize the risen Jesus at Emmaus (Luke 24:30). Ancient bread was not normally sliced.

The Greek thesaurus compiled by Pollux lists varieties of bread (vi 72), as does Athenaeus in a lengthy excursus (iii 108F–116F). Athenaeus's citations are taken from a variety of sources including works on dietetics, gastronomy, and baking, but mostly, as is his habit, from plays. As usual, his is a purely literary viewpoint. Our difficulties of translation are exacerbated by Athenaeus's not always himself knowing the meaning of the names he quotes. *Obelias* loaves, for instance, he thinks could either be bread sold for the low price of an obol or else bread baked on an *obeliskos*, spit. But some of Athenaeus's varieties can be identified for certain, either because the names tell their own story unambiguously or because we have good supplementary information from elsewhere.

The main distinction was in the method of baking. Greek practices are to some extent identifiable with those of the Bible. The most primitive method produced *enkryphias*, ash-bread (Athenaeus iii 111A). It was baked on hot stones while covered with ashes. This word was used by the Septuagint translators for the bread vouchsafed to Elijah in the Wilderness (עֻגַת רְצָפִים I Kings 19:6). The Vulgate correctly renders it *panis subcinericus*. It was not good for the digestion because the baking was uneven (Diphilus of Siphnos, quoted by Athenaeus iii 115E). Somewhat less primitive is *escharitēs*, bread fired in a brazier or on a grill, probably equivalent to the griddle-bread of Leviticus 4:5, although the Septuagint did not think so. It was made of flour mixed with oil and when ready was dipped hot into sweet wine. *Obelias* bread was indeed baked on a spit: the second of Athenaeus's conjectures, spit-baked bread, is right, as is shown by Hippocrates *Regimen* ii 42 = VI 540 Littré.

Such loaves could be very long if meant to be carried on spits in religious processions (Pollux vi 75). *Tēganitēs* bread was made of dough fried in oil in a frying pan, *tēganon*, and shaken and folded like a pancake; it could be prepared with sea salt or honey (Galen VI 490–492 Kühn), flavored with sesame (Hipponax 26a,2 West, quoted by Athenaeus xiv 645C), or cooked with cheese (Hesychius s.v.). What the Romans called *panis testuacius* was baked under a dome-shaped pottery cover, *pnigeus*, Latin *testu* (Varro, *Lingua Latina* v 106, cf. Cato *RR* 74, [Vergil] *Moretum* 51, Seneca, *Letters* xc 23). To judge by modern Balkan practice, the cover was placed over lighted coals until hot then the coals were swept to one side, the dough set on the warm floor and recovered, and the coals heaped over the cover's side (Sparkes 1962, 128, plate IV 2). But none of these methods resulted in even baking (Galen VI 489 Kühn).

The best bread was that baked in ovens. There were portable open-fronted ones. Egyptian models of the third millennium B.C. show a woman in front of a portable oven, turning the contents with a stick (see Währen 1965, 19, illustrations 3–5). An oven of this kind must be what is meant by the *tannûr* (תַּנּוּר) in the Old Testament. The Greeks called such an oven *klibanos* or *kribanos*. Sparkes provides a photograph of one (1962, plate V 1). Numerous Greek terra-cottas, showing a woman minding a *klibanos*, closely resemble the Egyptian representation (see Blümner 1912, fig. 30, Louvre; Sparkes 1962, 127, plate VIII 4 Berlin). The oven-minder's care was necessary, for Galen complains that even *klibanos*-baked bread could be imperfectly baked: the heat might not reach the deepest part (VI 489 Kühn). The best baked bread was *ipnitēs*, from large ovens, *ipnoi*. The Romans improved these so greatly that the Latin term for a "furnace" oven, *furnus*, became a Greek loan-word, φοῦρνος. Such ovens can be seen in the baking establishments of Pompeii. They are admirable: brick built, with a firing chamber for charcoal under a vaulted oven space, enclosed by a smoke chamber, with two openings above for the draught and an ashpit (Mau 1899, 283, plate 213; Blümner, 1912, 71–72, fig. 32).

Athenaeus distinguishes bread from fine flour, *semidalitēs*, from meal-bread, *chondritēs*, which is coarser and has some bran, and whole meal bread, *synkomistos* or *autopyros*. The laxative properties of whole meal bread were acknowledged; but it was thought—reasonably enough, since bran has no food value in itself—less nourishing, and there was a universal prejudice, reminiscent of the prevalent view in England until recent times, in favor of bread as white as possible. White is always a word of praise in our sources (e.g., Aristophanes, Kock i 422, quoted by Athenaeus iii 109E). To refine by removing the bran was to "cleanse;" hence gray (φαιος) bread was called ρυπαρός, dirty (Athenaeus iii 114D). But the gray bread may have been literally dirty too. The difficulties of cleaning and refining flour were connected. When Plato the comic writer contrasts "big Cilician loaves" with "the nice clean kind" (Kock i 624, quoted by Athenaeus iii 110D), we may think of how the present-day tourist in Egypt gets nice clean white boring bread on board his Nile cruise boat and may be tempted by the big brown loaves sold cheaply on land, until he realizes how very dirty they are. "Dirty bread," *panis sordidus,* is mentioned as the food of the poor (Plautus *Asinaria* 142, Seneca *Letters* xviii 7) and is not to be distinguished from black bread (Terence, *Eunuch* 938–939, Martial xi 56,7–8), plebeian bread (Seneca, *Letters* cxix 3), *panis secundus* (Horace, *Epistles* ii 1, 122–123) or *panis cibarius,* plain bread given to slaves (Isidore xx 2). Galen says a test of clean, good bread is that it will not sink in water (VI 494 Kühn); "dirty" bread presumably did. The poor might have to make do with stale and dry bread. Juvenal contrasts the snowy loaf of soft *siligo* reserved for the mean patron Virro with the bread that is served to his clients: "a loaf broken with difficulty, lumps of solid dough already mouldy, which exercise your jaws but will not permit a bite." If the low-class guest tries to help himself to the patron's bread, he is told: "be so good as to help yourself from your usual basket, and know the colour of your bread" (Juvenal *Satire* v 67–75).

Artoi dipyroi were "twice fired." There must have been different kinds; compare biscuits and *biscottes.* A quotation given by Athenaeus (iii 110a) refers to them as luxurious and eaten hot; on the other hand, Justin, a peasant's son who was to become emperor, walked with two friends from their Balkan village all the way to Constantinople with only homemade *artoi dipyroi* in their cloaks (Procopius, *Secret History,* vi 2). *Lagana* (Athenaeus iii 110B) were thin and broad: the Septuagint translators used this word for Jewish unleavened bread (Lev. 2:4). If from an oven, they would have been made by the technique of spreading the dough thinly on the oven wall.

Different kinds of bread had different additives. Halfway between unleavened and leavened bread came lightly leavened bread, *akrozymos* (Galen XIII 173 Kühn) or *leviter fermentatus* (Isidore xx 2,15). Bread could be made without salt (Aristotle, *Problemata* xxi 5 927ᵃ35) or with more salt than usual (Hesychius, s.v. ἀγλευκίτας· ἄρτος ἄλιμος). Oil was added to *tēganitēs* bread; that was also true of "fatty bread," *aleipohatitēs* (Epicharmus, quoted by Athenaeus iii 110B). Chrysippus of Tyana in Cappadocia, in his book *Bread-making,* quoted by Athenaeus iii 113A–C and deriving from the period of the Roman Empire, writes of "delicate bread made with a little milk and oil and sufficient salt. The dough must be slack. This bread is called *Cappadocian* because that is where delicate bread is mostly made. The Syrians call such bread *lakhma* [compare Hebrew *lehem*]. It is found most serviceable in Syria because eaten very hot." The same writer describes *boletus* bread. "It is shaped like a boletus mushroom, which is kneaded in a trough greased and sprinkled with poppy-seed, so that it does not stick to the trough when rising. When it is put into the *furnus,* coarse meal is spread over the earthenware pan. The loaf is then laid on it and gets an excellent colour, like smoked cheese.'' The device of sprinkling with seeds was an old one. Alcman, a poet in Sparta ca. 600 B.C. or a little later, describes a banquet with

> seven couches set out and as many tables
> crowned with poppy-seed loaves
> and of linseed and sesame. . . .
> (fr. 19 Page, quoted by Athenaeus iii 111A)

Correlations with kinds of bread known in modern Europe and the Near East could be taken further. There may even be a modern equivalent to the Syrian bread made from sycamore fruit, which according to Andreas the physician (Athenaeus iii 115EF) caused those who ate it to lose their hair. Bread with dried fruit in it is at any rate baked in modern Switzerland, where *Birnenbrot,* pear bread, is a favorite.

People did not eat bread by itself if they could help it. To this day the Greek notion of a meal is of bread with something to go with it, archetypally cheese and olives. Their practice is analogous to that of smørrebrod-eating Scandinavians, or Germans whose morning and evening meals consist of bread with various delicacies such as sausage and cheese. But the Greeks' passion was for *opsa* with their bread. An *opson,* relish, meant something cooked (Athenaeus vii 276A). It could be something simple, such as the onion—surely a cooked onion—which was offered in Nestor's tent as an *opson* to go with wine (*Iliad* xi 630). But it was natural for Homer to attribute to the heroes *opsa* of roast meat (*Iliad* ix 489, *Odyssey* iii 480, v 267, vii 77). In classical Greece, however, fish, available in wonderful variety, was the relish *par excellence.* That was the verdict of the company in Plutarch's *Questions of the Symposium* (iv 2, *Moralia* 661 F), endorsed by Athenaeus. A gourmet was a relish eater, an ὀψοφάγος: the word was applied to fish enthusiasts but not to lovers of beef, figs, or grapes (Athenaeus vii 276F). From the diminutive *opsarion* comes the modern Greek word for fish, *psari,* which has ousted the classical *ichthys.*

Ever since Egyptian times it had been the practice to add milk, eggs, honey, and spices to flour to produce *cake.* The Greeks had always been fond of honey-cakes. Aethiops, one of the pioneers who sailed from Corinth to found Syracuse in 733 B.C., was remembered for having sold his future plot of land for a honey-cake on board (Archilochus, fr. 293 West, from Athenaeus iv 167D). In Greek and Italian towns there were cake makers, *pemmatourgoi, plakountopoioi, libarii, placentarii, fictores.* The term *fictor* indicates skill in producing different shapes of cake: these were often in the shape of animals, as a substitute for animal sacrifice in ritual. A famous example is among the reliefs of the god Horus harpooning the evil god Seth, who is represented as a hippopotamus, on an inner wall of the Ptolemaic temple of Edfu in Upper Egypt: the final scene shows the Seth-hippopotamus being sliced to pieces, but what is being sliced is a hippopotamus-shaped cake, to be distributed to the worshippers. We have mentioned the ponderous *placenta* for which Cato gives a recipe. Another of his recipes, once again without eggs, is for *mustaceus*, must-cake (*RR* cxxi): "moisten 1 peck of *siligo* flour with must, add aniseed, cummin, 2 lbs lard, 1 lb cheese, and the scraping from a laurel twig. Mould and put laurel leaves under while baking" (the same method as used for Spartan *kammata*). Athenaeus provides a lengthy excursus on different names for cakes, comparable with that on bread and once again making use of the work on baking by Chrysippus of Tyana (xiv 643E–648A). It is good to find that the Argives had wedding cake, baked over charcoal and brought from the bride to the groom, to be served with honey (Athenaeus xiv 645D). "They do not," according to a melancholy line from a comedy, "bake wedding-cake in the land of the dead" (Philetaerus, *Oenopion*, Kock ii 234, quoted by Athenaeus vii 280D).

Spelt (*Triticum spelta*) often appears instead of emmer in translations of classical works, which is a mistake. Spelt had indeed been cultivated in the Near East from about 2000 B.C., but in classical times it was not being grown in the Mediterranean basin, although it was a useful crop in colder regions to the north such as the Upper Rhine and Britain.

Rye (*Secale cereale* L.), called βρίζα (*briza*), *secale* or *centenum*, is more amply attested. It, too, is a northern crop, but it was grown south of the Alps around Turin in Pliny's time. It had an excellent yield, but for him it is "terrible food, only useful for averting famine . . . and even if mixed with emmer to mitigate its sourness, it is most unacceptable to the stomach" (*NH* xviii 140). It was being grown in Macedonia and Thrace in Galen's time, and dark bread was being made from it (VI 514 Kühn). Its appearance in the Diocletianic price edict of 301 A.D. shows that by then it had gained in importance. Although Americans call rye bread "Jewish bread," the Jews of Palestine and the Mediterranean in ancient times may not even have heard of it. The modern name is due to nineteenth-century immigrants bringing it from their native Poland.

Oats (*avena sativa* L.), βρόμος (*bromos*), *avena*, are better suited to the climate of the Mediterranean, but were long held to be weeds (Theophrastus, *HP* viii 9,2, Vergil, *Georgics* i 154). For shepherds they served as reed-pipes, referred to by Vergil in the introductory lines telling of his transition from the *Georgics* to the *Æneid*. But Columella mentions oats as a hay and fodder crop (ii 10, 32). They could be used for medicinal gruel (Hippocrates, *Regimen* ii 43). Boiled in vinegar, they removed warts (Pliny *NH* xxii 137). Galen says they were grown extensively in Asia Minor and especially in Mysia, above Pergamum, and were fed to draft animals but not to human beings except in times of extreme famine (VI 522–523 Kühn). But Pliny (*NH* 149) knew of Germanic peoples who sowed oats as a food crop and lived on oatmeal porridge!

There were two kinds of *millet* in the ancient Mediterranean, not identical with the finger and bulrush millets grown as main crops today in India and Africa. The varieties known to the Greeks and Romans were common millet, *panicum miliaceum* L., which they called κέγχρος (*kenchros*), *milium*, and foxtail millet, *setaria Italica* L., which they called μελίνη (*meline*), *panicum*. But these were not always clearly distinguished: the names can be interchanged. There was a Thracian people known as "millet-eaters" in the region of the present Turkish-Bulgarian frontier (Xenophon, *Anabasis* vii 5.12); millet and emmer were kept in Thracian granaries (Demosthenes x 16). Millet with its tiny grains was the food of backward peoples on the fringes of the Graeco-Roman world; for the Greeks and Romans it was a secondary crop. It needed both heat and moisture, rarely combined in the Mediterranean region except in the Nile and Po valleys and lowland Cilicia. Its main merit was that it could be sown in the spring if other crops had failed, for it took forty days or less to ripen (Theophrastus viii 2.6, Pliny *NH* xviii 60). "It is the greatest cure for famine: it stands up to all weathers and can never fail even if there is a shortage of every other grain" says Strabo in his description of the Po valley (v 218). It could be made into porridge. Pliny describes an exotic black millet, with a large grain and a reedlike stalk growing to seven feet, introduced in the last decade (i.e., 67–77 A.D.) from India. This was during a period when there was a flourishing trade across the Indian Ocean with South India and Ceylon, attested by many coin finds and costing the Roman Empire, according to Pliny, some 550,000 gold pieces a year (*NH* xii 84). Pepper was the main import in exchange for bullion. But, for a price, some exotic grains might also now be imported, for consumption or experimental planting.

The Mediterranean world had already heard of *rice* (*oryza*). Megasthenes, the Seleucid ambassador at the court of Chandragupta in Patna in 302–291 B.C., had reported on Indian meals based on boiled rice, recognizably similar to what they are today (*FGH* 715 F2, quoted by Athenaeus iv 153D). In Roman imperial times imported rice is occasionally attested. It was thought good for invalids (Celsus ii 18; 20; 24), and a decoction of it was recommended for strengthening the stomach but was very dear (Horace, *Satires* ii 3.155–157). Apicius's cookery book, which spares no expense, three times recommends rice for thickening sauces (ii 3.9; excerpts 7; 9). The account of Elagabalus (A.D. 218–222) in the *Augustan History* (21.3) cheerfully attributes to that debauched emperor a banquet of rice with pearls, which is supposed to have made a change from peas with gold beads and beans with amber. But this must be fantasy.

Maize, an American cereal, was unknown.

Intermittent *food shortages* occurred throughout ancient times. Food shortages in those days meant grain shortage. A number of overseas Greek colonies of the eighth and seventh centuries B.C. are said to have been settled because of scarcity of food at home. Later, food shortages are a recurrent phenomenon in city-states. In democratic Athens food shortages were mitigated, but never wholly prevented, by stringent state regulations to corner grain imports and regulate the sale of grain on arrival. Athens could occasionally offer a free handout to citizens, as when in 445/4 B.C. Psammetichus of Egypt sent a large supply of wheat, presumably in the hope of help against Persia (Schol. Aristophanes, *Wasps* 718, following Philochorus *FGH* 328 F 130). A common occurrence in many states was for grain merchants to hold on to their stores until prices peaked. Riots would ensue, and government would try to make the merchants disgorge at fair prices. In 189 B.C. Livy (xviii 35) says that the curule aediles of Rome fined the curmudgeonly merchants ("cornmudgins," Holland's translation of A.D. 1600 calls them) for holding back their grain. In a letter to the town council of Pisidian Antioch in A.D. 93 the Roman governor of Galatia imposed penalties on any merchants who did not sell their grain at a reasonable price after a fixed date (McCrum and Woodhead 1961 No. 458). In Tiberius's reign, the holy Apollonius of Tyana used moral force to make the grain hoarders of Aspendos disgorge (Philostratus's *Life* i 15). Dio Chrysostom, a notable of Prusa, devotes his 46th discourse, after having been the target of a riot, to explaining that he is *not* a grain hoarder.

State granaries, Joseph's solution as accepted by Pharaoh in the second millennium B.C. (Gen. 41:48–49) could counterbalance private hoarding: Rome instituted such granaries in 122 B.C. (Roman granary buildings, public and private, are discussed by Rickman 1971). From then on, too, intermittent arrangements were made to distribute subsidized and imported grain, which in 58 B.C. became a free dole to those on the list. That did not prevent—perhaps it exacerbated—the grain-supply crisis of 57 B.C., to deal with which Pompey was given special powers (see Rickman 1980, p. 52–53). The dole continued through many political vicissitudes. No ruler could afford to abolish it, although Julius Caesar reduced the number of recipients. Augustus, who in 30 B.C. had secured the wheat of Egypt, established a Prefect of the Grain Supply in about 4 B.C.: the prefect, C. Turranius, resisted dismissal (Seneca,

Dialogue x 20, 3) and was still holding office as a nonagenarian in A.D. 48 (Tacitus *Annals* xi 31). The emperor Claudius gave special privileges to grain merchants and built Ostia harbor to receive grain ships from Egypt (Suetonius, *Claudius* 19–20); it was on one of these that St. Paul was transported to Rome (Acts 25). But there was a grain shortage in A.D. 51 when an angry mob pelted Claudius with stale crusts by way of protest (Tacitus, *Annals* xii, 43.2). Aurelian in 270/275 A.D. was the first to distribute bread instead of grain (Zosimus i 61,3), although the *Historia Augusta* is perhaps only joking when it claims that he arranged for the dole to be of bread baked from *siligo,* with free pork, oil, and wine in the bargain (*Aurelian* 35, 48). In Constantine's New Rome state bakeries provided free bread, the *panis civilis* (see B. Kübler *Real-Encyclopädie* s.v.). Doles were sometimes provided in other towns: recent papyrus finds attest to registrations for the corn dole in Egyptian Oxyrhynchus in the third century A.D. (Rickman, 1980, 177–178). But even the dole recipients, a privileged minority in ancient Mediterranean lands, lived uncomfortably close to the bread-line.

FRUIT

Nonindigenous Fruits

We shall begin with an account of the fruits that did *not* originally grow in Mediterranean lands but were by degrees transplanted to them from further East.

Many of the names for Mediterranean fruits are loan-words that illustrate the story of their transplantation. The word *orange* is a good example. The bitter Seville orange, *Citrus Aurantium amarum,* from which the marmalade is made that today appears on every British breakfast table, originated in India and came in early times to Persia. *Narang* is the ancient Persian name for the fruit. The Arabs took over orange-growing from the Persians in the Middle Ages, and the Seville orange traveled through the Arab world, which extended from the borders of Persia westward to Morocco, until it came to Spain where it flourishes today. From Arabic *naranj* came the Spanish *naranja;* the loss of the initial letter has resulted in the French and English *orange.* But not all European nations call the fruit by a word derived from *naranj.* Dutch *Sinaasappel,* German *Apfelsine,* and Russian *Appelsin* tell a different story: In these languages the orange is the "apple of China." For the sweet orange, *Citrus Aurantium dulce,* indeed comes from the Far East. It came to Europe later than the Seville orange. There may have been some early arrivals in fifteenth century Italy, but the best ones were brought by the

Portuguese after Vasco da Gama had opened up the sea route around the Cape of Good Hope in 1498. Hence the modern Greek name, *porto-kali* or "Portugal fruit." The first sweet-orange tree from China was planted in a Lisbon garden in 1548 and was a tourist curiosity there for many years.

The various words for orange all illustrate a negative point: In ancient times there were no oranges in the Mediterranean. Indeed, there were few citrus fruits of any kind: no mandarins, tangerines, or grapefruit; and lemons were a rarity until the late Roman Empire. It is difficult for us to imagine ancient Italy without them. Lemons, like oranges, seem to us to be quintessentially a part of Italy.

> Know'st thou the country where the lemons bloom,
> and oranges gleam gold in leafy gloom?

So runs one of the most famous of Goethe's poems. But even today the lemon tree can be grown only in certain favored parts of Italy. It was a slow and arduous process to bring it from its homeland in India and Persia and acclimatize it in Europe.

Only after Alexander the Great conquered the Persian Empire did Europeans first hear of the *lemon*. Then Theophrastus (*HP* iv 4 2–3) first gave a description of this astonishing tree, whose "Median or Persian fruit"—so it was at first called—could not be eaten outright but was thought to be an effective antidote against poison, to protect clothes against moths, and, when cooked, to sweeten the breath. From his careful description of its cultivation—first in pots and then planted out—it is certain that Theophrastus is speaking of the lemon tree but only from hearsay. Subsequently a few precious lemons found their way into Mediterranean markets; but in Pliny's time the tree itself was still said to resent transplantation from its homeland (*NH* xii 16). So stories of the lemon's miraculous power against poison persisted. The "fortunate Median fruit," with its sour juice of lingering taste, is said by Vergil (*Georgics* ii 126–128) to be the best possible antidote for a child against its stepmother's poison. A story was later told of condemned criminals in Egypt, to whom a street seller gave some lemons out of pity when they were being dragged off to the amphitheater to be stung to death in public by snakes. The lemons miraculously saved their lives. Their efficacy was subsequently confirmed by controlled experiments on other condemned criminals (Athenaeus iii 84D–85A). It was only in the last years of the Roman Empire that lemon trees were acclimatized in Italy, and greater familiarity led to a more sober appraisal of the lemon's powers. Lemon trees were now planted against south-facing walls, well watered, and protected by matting in winter. In some especially warm places, on fertile soil and favored by mild sea air, they could grow in the open, as they do today (Florentinus, 3rd century A.D., quoted by Cassianus Bassus, *Geoponica* 10,7).

By Roman times, an especially large variety of lemon, the אֶתְרֹג (*etrog*), had come to play a part in Jewish ritual. In their October Feast of Tabernacles, the Jews had been instructed to make use of "the fruit of goodly trees," *nadarim* (Lev. 23:40). Rabbinical interpretation came round to taking this to mean "citrus trees," perhaps just because they were exotic and hard to get. They must have been brought by caravan across the Syrian desert. An unusually expensive demonstration took place in Jerusalem shortly before 90 B.C., when the brutal priest-king of the Jews, Alexander Jannaeus, was pelted at the Feast with ritual lemons (Josephus, *Antiquities of the Jews* xiii 372). Once the lemon had been naturalized in Italy and Corfu, special *etrog* groves were started to cater for Jewish needs. From the Middle Ages until recent times, the Jews of central and eastern Europe got their ritual lemons every year from the Mediterranean, thanks to those Jewish peddlers who trudged from village to village with their sacks of lemons. The surname *Citron* is borne by some of these peddlers' descendants.

The *peach* is another fruit at first unknown in Mediterranean lands and then imported from Asia. Its name derives through French from the Latin *Persica,* "the Persian fruit." Peaches and apricots travel less easily than citrus fruits and remained unknown longer in the Mediterranean. There is no mention of peaches in the Bible; had they existed, can we doubt that the writer of the *Song of Songs* would have compared his beloved to a peach? It must have been when Pompey's conquests extended Roman power to the neighborhood of Armenia and the Caspian in 66–65 B.C. that the peach tree was first brought from Persia and the apricot from its home in what is now Soviet Central Asia. There was not much difficulty in transplanting them. There were Gallic and Adriatic peaches in the first century of our era (Pliny *NH* xv 39). The modern Greek name for apricots, βερύκοκα (*verikoka*), is derived from the Latin *praecoquia,* "maturing early." Latin, being later and poorer, often borrows from Greek: Greek has less occasion to borrow from Latin. That it has done so in this instance confirms that the apricot was a comparatively late Roman import.

The *dessert cherry, Prunus cerasus,* is another importation. The barely palatable bird cherry, *Prunus avium,* had long been known in Europe: Stones have been found in the rubbish deposits of neolithic Swiss Lake dwellings. The bird cherry, *kerasos,* is described by Theophrastus (*HP* iii 13.1–3). The dessert cherry was brought to Italy by Lucullus, whom Pompey supplanted as general, from Asia Minor (Pliny *NH* xv 102). It was also called *kerasos;* hence the Latin *cerasum,* French *cérise,* English *cherry.*

The *melon* is yet another fruit that was unknown in Biblical times and is first mentioned in the first century. By the second, the melon, μηλοπέπων, latinized as *melopepo*, was common. Pliny (*NH* xix 67) says that *melopepones* derive from the seeds of a freak cucumber recently produced in the region of Naples, looking more like a quince than a cucumber and with a delightful fragrance. If Pliny is right, this would be a striking example of mutation. But melons were certainly at home in Persia and Central Asia during the Middle Ages: Marco Polo (I xxiii) praises the melons of Afghanistan, the best in the world, he says, and sweeter than honey. It may well be, therefore, that the melon, like so many other fruits, is also an ancient import from Asia, even though no classical writer says so. But if the melon really did originate in Italy, and the melons of medieval Central Asia derive from Europe, this would be a unique example of a fruit traveling from west to east instead of the other way around.

Modern enterprise has enabled the *banana* to grow in Crete, and the South American *avocado pear* in Israel, but these fruits were totally unknown to the ancient Mediterranean peoples, as was the *pineapple*, a native of tropical South America. An Italian scholar has claimed to have seen a pineapple in a Pompeii wall-painting, but the published photograph carries no conviction. Pineapplelike objects in ancient Mediterranean art are pinecones. The *watermelon*, now commonly grown in the Balkans, Greece, and Turkey, is a latecomer, originating from southern Africa.

Native European Fruit: Apples, Pears, and Plums

So far we have been discussing the fruits that came to the Mediterranean from the East. Now we turn to those that, in the classical period, were already at home in Mediterranean lands. The discussion falls into two parts. First, the trio of fruits that had been known in the region since prehistoric times but flourish even better in Northern Europe: apples, pears, and plums. Then comes the quartet of indigenous fruits that cannot grow beyond certain northern limits: olives, grapes, figs, and pomegranates. Here there is also a story of transplantation from East to West, although within the Mediterranean area. By the first century B.C. Varro (*RR* i 6) could speak of Italy as "a vast orchard"; but in earlier times it was a land of grain, timber, and cattle. Greek and Phoenician influence, from the eighth century B.C. onward, helped to bring these fruits to Sicily, Italy, and the western Mediterranean; Roman cultivators enthusiastically followed their lead.

The *apple* is archetypal. The Greek word *mēlon*, like the Latin *malus*, applies specifically to the apple but by extension to any tree fruit. It may be because of the Greek and Latin translations of the Bible that it is commonly assumed that it was an apple

> . . . whose mortal taste
> brought Death into the world, and all our woe.

But the Hebrew word in *Genesis* means "fruit" and has no specific application. There are only two allusions to apples in the Old Testament. One is in the *Song of Songs* (2:3–4):

> As the apple tree among the trees of the wood
> so is my beloved among the sons.
> I sat down under his shadow with great delight
> and his fruit was sweet to my taste.

The New English Bible translates the Hebrew word here, תַּפּוּחַ (*tappûah*), as "apricot," but this is hard to accept. There is no proof that the apricot, unmentioned in classical literature before Roman times, came to Palestine so early. The corresponding word in Arabic, *tuffâh*, means "apple." Perversely, the New English Bible retains the translation "apple" for תַּפּוּחַ in the other passage where it occurs, in a list of standard fruit trees (Joel 3:12). Apples, it would seem, did grow in ancient Palestine, but not well; and the Bible has nothing at all to say about the other two members of the trio, the pear and the plum.

Apples, pears, and plums are believed to derive ultimately from Asia; but apple pips and plum stones have been found in the middens of neolithic lake dwellings in Switzerland, and at the outset of our period we find these trees already cultivated in Europe. Apples play a greater part in Greek than in Hebrew literature—especially the magic apples of fable. Who has not heard of Paris's apple for which the three goddesses contended? The Greeks loved to tell of Hercules's labor of bringing from the far west the golden apples of the Hesperides and of the maiden Atalanta, whose suitors had to outrun her in a foot race or lose their lives. She was at last won by a young man who delayed her three times by dropping in her path a golden apple for which she could not help stooping. There are pleasing descriptions of real apples in Greek poetry. Sappho invites the Goddess of Love to come to her sacred apple grove

> where cold water trickles through the boughs
> of apple trees, and all the place is shaded
> with roses, and from quivering leaves
> slumber drops down." (fr. 2 Lobel-Page)

In a wedding song she compares the bride to an apple:

> As the sweet apple reddens upon the topmost bough
> higher than all the rest, which the pickers forgot somehow
> or rather, did not forget, but could not reach till now. (fr. 105
> Lobel-Page)

Sappho's word for sweet apple, *glykymēlon*, appears more than two thousand years later in Greek folk poetry, with much the same metaphor: one wishes a bride seven stalwart sons "and one sweet-apple daughter."

But apples in classical Greece were not always sweet or even healthy. Athenaeus's literary quotations contain warnings about green apples, sharp apples "with a disagreeable and mischievous juice," and harsh and sour apples and the risks they bring of bile, tremors, indigestion, and internal corrosion. It is noteworthy that among the few he praises are the "Matian" apples cultivated on the foothills of the Alps near modern Trieste (iii 80E–82E). It was in these more temperate latitudes that better apple trees could be found and imported into central Italy, where, in orchards with a carefully chosen aspect, Roman growers could develop improved varieties. The need was for the establishment of the tree's root system. This could not easily be done for seedlings or cuttings without much watering, which reduced the quality of the fruit. But cleft grafting and bark grafting on wild apple stock was producing good results in the second century B.C. (Cato *RR* 40–41). Columella (v 11.8) in the first century A.D. adds a Roman invention, the "very subtle" process of patch budding. By this time the wild apples "of horrible sourness, so powerful that it will blunt the edge of a sword," had given place to many new and delectable cultivars. "Nothing is so small that it cannot win glory," says Pliny the Elder (*NH* xv 49). The people who gave their names to new varieties ranged from the freed slave who discovered the round Sceptian apple to Caesar's friend Caius Matius, inventor of the exquisitely scented Matian apple also praised by Athenaeus, and the patrician Appius Claudius who, by grafting a quince, produced the popular *Appianum*.

Athenaeus (xix 650DE) offers fewer quotations about *pears* than you would expect in view of the fact that the pear tree appears in the earliest Greek poetry. There was a tall pear tree in the vineyard of Odysseus' father, and it was beside it that Homer has Odysseus find him, dressed in old clothes and devoting his declining years to the cultivation of fruit (*Odyssey* xxiv 226–234). The development of pears by the Romans parallels that of apples. Pliny in the first century A.D. gives 39 varieties of pear and 23 of apple (*NH* xv 47–56).

Apples and pears are part of a Greek summer scene in one of the idylls of Theocritus (vii 141–146):

> The larks and linnets sang, there moaned the turtle-dove; the brown bees hovered around the water springs. Everything smelt of rich summer, smelt of ripeness. Pears were at our feet, and at our sides apples rolled bountifully, and the spreading boughs were weighed down to the ground with βράβυλα.

The βράβυλον (*brabylon*) is normally a sloe; but ancient commentators (the Scholiast on this passage and Clearchus the Peripatetic according to Athenaeus ii 49F) say that in Theocritus's dialect it means *plum*, for which the usual Greek word is *kokkymēlon*, cuckoo-apple. Elsewhere, Greek allusions to plums are infrequent and unenthusiastic. Diphilus of Siphnos is quoted by Athenaeus (ii 50B) as saying that they are ''juicy, go bad easily, are easily excreted and give little nourishment.'' Here again, the Romans made progress by importing foreign kinds and by grafting. Cato mentions the plum only once, in a list of fruit trees to be grown from seedlings. But in the time of Vergil (*Georgics* iv 145) and Horace (*Epistles* i.16.8–9) they were evidently being grafted on thorn bushes (i.e., sloes) and wild cherry. Two generations later, Pliny (*NH* xv 41–42) speaks of plums grafted on nut trees and, in southern Spain, on apple stock. He names nine varieties, including the Armenian plum, the only one that is recommended by its fragrance. Purple and waxen plums he describes as comparatively small but well spoken of. Among those who speak well of waxen plums is Vergil's shepherd Corydon, who gives plums to his beloved (*Eclogue* ii 53): ''I will add waxen plums; this fruit, too, shall be honoured.'' The epithet derives from their sheen (Ovid, *Metamorphoses* xiii 817–818): ''Plums, not only livid with black juice, but also noble and looking like new wax.''

One variety of plum, the damson, comes, as its name suggests, from Damascus. It is accurately described by Athenaeus:

> There is a great quantity of plum trees in the territory of the Damascenes, and as they are cultivated there with exceeding care, the tree itself has got to be called a Damascene, as being a plum different from those found in other countries (ii 49DE). . . . This [Damascene]

plum is smaller in circumference than other plums, though in flavour it is very like them, except that it is a little sharper (ii 50A).

Pliny (*NH* xv 42) observes that the damson does not dry into wrinkles like other plums; from this we infer the production of prunes.

Indigenous Mediterranean Fruits: Olives, Grapes, Figs, Pomegranates

Far more important for all the peoples of the ancient Mediterranean was the quartet of indigenous fruits, foreign to the North, that is named in God's great promise to Moses. His people, we learn in the Book of Deuteronomy (7:8), was to be brought to "a land of vines, and fig trees, and pomegranates; a land of olive oil, and honey." Something must now be said about each of these four fruits. The *olive* and its oil figure largely throughout the Bible. When the Flood first subsided, Noah's dove brought him back an olive branch (Gen. 9:11), which has become a symbol of peace for mankind. "Thou anointest my head with oil," says the best-loved of the Psalms (23:5). The Mount of Olives outside Jerusalem, where Jesus was accustomed to go and where He spent His last hours of prayer before His arrest (Luke 23:39), is dear to millions who have never seen it. For the Greeks, too, the olive had special symbolism. The Athenians set store by the myth of their country's origin. The sea god Poseidon and the goddess Pallas Athena, they claimed, had once contended for the rule of their land. The other gods decreed victory for whoever of them produced the best gift for mortals. Poseidon struck the ground with his trident, producing the horse, but Athena won by planting the olive. Athens was named after her; an olive sprig figured with the head of Athena on Athenian coins. A jar of olive oil was the prize for the victor at Athens' chief athletic competitions. The archaic seated statue of Athena on the Acropolis was of olive-wood, still revered on the Acropolis after Pheidias in the 430s B.C. had made the famous standing Athena in gold and ivory.

Why all this reverence for the olive? In the ancient Mediterranean world quantities of olive oil were used daily. It provided the fat that is essential in diet. It was necessary for almost all cooking. At the same time, it was used for washing. The ancients knew about soap—Greek medical writers mention it as a cure for acne—but although they bathed a good deal, they used not soap but olive oil, which they carried in little flasks, smeared on themselves, and then scraped off again. Olive oil was a necessary part of perfumes and unguents. Since it keeps well, although not for ever, it was an important article of trade. Olive groves, for instance, grew in large areas of Syria to supply less favored parts of the Mediterranean. When trade links broke down with the fall of the Roman Empire, Syrian olive production no longer paid. With the neglect and loss of the olive trees, the desert encroached. The "dead towns of Syria," well-preserved ruins of late Roman towns, testify to the region's former prosperity, and the remains of olive presses with their stone rollers to how it was maintained.

The Greeks preferred olive oil to butter, though the absence of butter was principally due to lack of good pasture for dairy cattle. They disapproved of butter-eating by northern barbarians. The comic writer Anaxandrides (Kock ii 151, quoted by Athenaeus iv 131B) describes a Thracian wedding feast in the 380s B.C. as attended by

> butter-eaters
> with dirty hair, tens of thousands of them!

The Mediterranean remained butterless, just as India has always been cheeseless. This rejection of butter in favor of olive oil no longer seems a mere prejudice to ourselves as it would have done a generation ago.

Jeremiah, in a parable that has many variants, speaks of God having called his erring people "a green olive tree, fair, and of goodly fruit; with the noise of a great tumult He hath kindled fire upon it, and the branches of it are broken." That was a strong metaphor for those who knew the nature of the olive's cultivation. Its merit was that it would grow on poor stony soil like that of Attica. Vergil (*Georgics* ii 179–181) writes:

> Difficult ground and hostile hills,
> where there is lean clay and gravel in thorny fields,
> rejoice in Pallas' woods of long-lived olive.

The olive tree's slow growth made it a long-term investment, although not one out of the reach of poor farmers, because they could intercrop with grain. Once established, it was worth great efforts at rehabilitation if it bore badly (Columella v 9, 16–17). To destroy an olive tree was a last measure to be taken only when all else had failed.

The promise to Moses included the *vine* among the good things of Palestine. Two spies (Num. 13:23) crossed into the Promised Land and returned to the Children of Israel, encamped in the desert, with a bunch of grapes slung on a pole, as well as pomegranates and figs. The vineyards, grapes, and wine of Palestine constantly recur in biblical imagery, as in the New Testament parable of the laborers in the vineyard, and the story told by Jesus in the Temple of the Lord of the Vineyard and the ungrateful husbandmen (Luke 20:9–19). "I am the Vine, ye are the branches," Jesus said to His disciples at the Last Supper (John 15:5). Not for nothing do Christians have in their communion service

> the divine
> strong brother in God and last companion, wine.

Wine, said Jotham in a story that embraces all the chief fruit trees of the Holy Land, "cheereth God and man" (Judg. 9:13). That there was something divine about wine was a deep-rooted notion among other Mediterranean peoples. Dionysus or Bacchus, the god of wine, could, if crossed, be terrible. Euripides' *Bacchae* tells how Dionysus took revenge on a Greek ruler who defied him; at the same time the play treats the Bacchic cult with reverence. Dionysus was the god of the Athenian tragic theatre. At other times, the cult could be the occasion for good-natured fun, even at the god's expense, as we find in Aristophanes' comedy *The Frogs*. Later, kings and warlords ventured to impersonate Dionysus: Demetrius, besieger of cities, had himself hailed as the "new Dionysus" when he freed Athens at the end of the fourth century B.C., and so did Antony nearly three centuries later when he feasted at Athens with Cleopatra. The crazy emperor Caligula dressed up as Bacchus. In this connection we even find a Jewish writer speaking respectfully of Bacchus, as if he were a real god. Bacchus, said Philo of Alexandria (*Embassy to Gaius* 88–89) had brought men the blessing of wine and the good fellowship that goes with it; but Caligula was no Bacchus and had done nothing but harm!

Wine, like bread, was a daily staple as well as a god-given blessing. "Bread and wine give strength and courage," says Homer (*Iliad* ix 706, xix 161). Wine was not drunk, as ale was in seventeenth century England, because water was mistrusted. Greece has excellent springs: The Greeks normally mixed their wine with water. The modern Greek word for wine, κρασί (*krasi*) derives from the root "to mix." Drinking wine neat, as did those dirty-haired, butter-eating barbarians of the North, was thought dangerous. A Spartan king who had learned the habit from a delegation from South Russia—whose people, then as now, had a bad name for heavy drinking—was said to have gone mad in consequence and cut himself into little pieces (Herodotus vi 84.1). Some modern scholars have concluded that Greek wine must have been strong, like whisky, and also syrupy, like orange squash cordial. This has never been proved. The Greeks, though their upper-class social life revolved around wine parties, *symposia*, were mostly temperate; their dilution of

wine with water was like present-day Italian practice. The proportion of
water depended on the quality of the wine. The *Odyssey*, doubtless with
poetic license, describes wine from Thracian Ismaros so wonderful that
it was mixed with twenty parts of water (ix 196–211). Brandy and other
spirits, it may be added, were unknown in the ancient world. Distilling
was as yet an undiscovered art. But liqueur-type wine was produced by
letting the grapes first dry in the sun (Pliny *NH* xiv 81), a practice already
known to Hesiod (*Works and Days* 609–624): the raisin wine (*passum*) of
Crete was especially good (Martial xiii 106, Juvenal xiv 270–271). It was
Roman practice to boil wine to make a sweetening agent that was called
caroenum, defrutum or *sapa*, depending on how much of its volume it had
lost (Palladius xi 18 c.f. Pliny *NH* xiv 80). *Mulsum*, Greek *melikraton*, was
wine mixed with honey (Columella xii 41)—preferably dry wine (Pliny *NH*
xxii 113–114)—drunk as an apéritif (Horace *Satires* ii 2,15, Petronius 34,1).
It made you fat but you could live to a hundred on it (Pliny loc.cit). Apicius
has recipes for wine with additives: spiced mulled wine, vermouth, and
rose-petal wine and violet wine (i 1–4).

At the beginning of our period the finest wines came from various
Greek territories such as the offshore islands of Chios, Lesbos, and
Samos. The poetess Sappho's brother Charaxus was conveying Lesbian
wine to Egypt, never itself ideal for wine, around 600 B.C. (Strabo xvii
808). There is massive evidence of wine shipping: The study of stamps
on the handles of amphoras and thermoluminescent tests on amphora
pottery to indicate the provenance of the clay, will in due course clarify
the directions and extent of the trade. By Roman times the best wines
were produced in Italy, perhaps because of a favorable change of climate
(so states the agricultural writer Saserna of the first century B.C., quoted
by Columella i 1,7). Cato judged a vineyard of good quality to bring
more profit than any other crop (*RR* i 7). The arts of planting, propagat-
ing, pruning, and harvesting vines are explained in detail by the Roman
agricultural writers. Vines were cultivated for dessert grapes and raisins
as well as wine; but it was in connection with the wine trade that for-
tunes could be won and lost. Augustus' marshal, L. Tarius Rufus, had
risen from obscure origins to make a million gold pieces in the civil wars;
these he lost by producing wine, too fine to make a profit, in Picenum
(Pliny *NH* xviii 37). By contrast, the grammarian Remmius Palaemon
bought a farm ten miles from Rome for 6000 gold pieces, so improved
it that the vintage within eight years was sold for 4000, and the farm
bought up by the philosopher Seneca after ten years for four times its
original price (Pliny *NH* xiv 52). Some vintages were famous. The year
of Opimius' consulship, 121 B.C., produced a wine so good that even
after it had been reduced, two centuries later, to the consistency of
rough honey, it was still used in small quantities to improve other wines

(Pliny *NH* xiv 55). The Falernian wine celebrated by Horace and the Set-ine wine from near Naples, which was Augustus's favorite, must have been superb. Yet within a century Falernian had lost its reputation through being cultivated more for quantity than quality (Pliny *NH* xiv 62). Meanwhile, viticulture had spread to the north. Vergil, a northern Italian, praised the wine of the Valtelline (*Georgics* ii 95), still esteemed in modern Switzerland, as second only to Falernian. French wine had a bad reputation in Pliny's time (*NH* xiv 68) because it was colored by factory-induced smoke and adulterated with noxious drugs such as aloes (*NH* xiv 68). But the great wine-growing areas of Bordeaux and Burgundy were already active as such before the end of the Roman Em-pire; and the vine-clad slopes of the Moselle valley, to judge by Auso-nius's poem, looked in the fourth century A.D. much as they do now.

Next to grapes come *figs*. It makes sense to have a fig tree in a vine-yard (Luke 13:6), and the two fruits are often named together. "Do men gather grapes of thorns, or figs of thistles?" (Matt. 7:16). "The fig," said the Greek poet Hipponax, "is sister to the vine" (48 West). In the golden days of King Solomon, "Judah and Israel dwelt safely, every man under his vine and under his fig tree" (I Kings 4:25). The Bible is full of references to figs, beginning with the fig leaves with which Adam and Eve covered their nakedness after the Fall and ending with the vi-sion of the end of the world, when the stars shall tumble "even as a fig tree casteth her untimely figs, when she is shaken of a mighty wind" (Rev. 6:3). Abigail's two hundred cakes of figs and hundred clusters of raisins were a welcome present for David's men in the wilderness (I Sam. 24:18).

Athenaeus's discussion of figs is juicy. How succulent were the dif-ferent varieties of Greek figs, and how eagerly each region laid claim to produce the best of all! Their fleshiness and high sugar content recom-mended them: Here was a fruit that, more than any other, could assuage hunger. Figs were good dried. Their laxative qualities were valued. The range of fig products for medical use was astonishing, even in societies that missed no chance of pressing available fruits and vegetables into medical service (Pliny *NH* xvi 117–130). "Better than gold," the Ionic poet Ananius calls them (3,3 West). There are stories about their divine origin. Alongside the Sacred Way, outside the walls of Athens, stood the tombstone of the hero Phytalus; passers-by could read on it the story of how, long ago, he had entertained a visitor who proved to be the goddess of fruit and crops, Demeter; in gratitude she gave him the first fig tree (Pausanias i 37.2). A basket of figs was carried at the head of the procession during the annual festival of the washing of Athena's statue, called "leading" (ἡγητηρία) because the fig was believed to have been the first fruit ever cultivated (Hesychius *s.v.*, Athenaeus iii 74D). The

Athenians were proud of their figs. One Athenian comedy has two speakers discussing them (Antiphanes, Kock ii 43B, quoted by Athenaeus iii 74D-E):

> FIRST SPEAKER: . . . How our countryside brings forth better products, Hipponicus, than the whole wide world beside! Honey, loaves and figs—
>
> HIPPONICUS: Indeed, by Jove! the figs are excellent.

The poorest could afford a few figs in peace time. But when times were bad, some could not afford them. Aristophanes (*Wasps* 291-303) describes an old Athenian hurrying off to earn a small wage by serving on the jury-court, escorted by his small son. It is 422 B.C., during the Peloponnesian War, and there are scarcities because enemy action has ravaged the countryside.

> SON: Will you give me something, father if I ask you?
>
> FATHER: Indeed I will, my child. Tell me, what nice thing do you want me to buy you? I dare say you want some knuckle-bone-dice?
>
> SON: No, Papa, I want some dried figs; they're nicer.
>
> FATHER: Why, I couldn't do that to save you from hanging!
>
> SON: Right then, I won't go out with you any more.
>
> FATHER: Look, there are three of us, and I have to buy flour and firewood and a bit of relish from my pittance. Oh dear! And you ask me for figs!

Even in normal times, although the Athenians were happy to sell their surplus olive oil abroad, they forbade the export of figs so as not to deprive the home market. A man who denounced an exporter of figs to the courts was the archetypal sycophant, which literally means a fig-revealer (Plutarch, *Solon* 24).

The fourth of the quartet of indigenous Mediterranean fruits is the *pomegranate*; but it comes after the olive, grape, and fig in importance. The ancients would have valued this second-rate fruit less if they had been able to start with the full range of Mediterranean fruit that later became available. As it was, the pomegranate played a part in their religious symbolism. Moses was ordered to design an embroidered pomegranate at the bottom of the high priest's robe (Exod. 28:33–34); and carved pomegranates formed part of the ornament of Solomon's temple (I Kings 7:18). In Greek temples, too, carved pomegranates were to be found in the hands of statues of goddesses. Polyclitus's famous statue of Hera near Argos held one, and so did Athena of Victory in her shrine on the Athenian acropolis. Most celebrated is the Greek association of the pomegranate with Persephone, the daughter of the goddess Demeter, who was seized by Hades and dragged to the underworld. Demeter in her grief forbade the trees to bear fruit and the crops to grow; to save Nature from dying, Zeus, the Father of the Gods arranged for Persephone to be restored to her mother on condition of her having eaten nothing in the realm of the dead. And she had not: Out of protest, she had refused all food throughout her stay. Only at the last moment was it found that she had eaten a few pomegranate seeds; therefore she still has to return to the underworld for a few months every year.

Other Fruits and Nuts

Some less important fruits close our account. It comes as something of a surprise that the ancient Greeks valued the *quince*, so hard when raw, even in their sunny climate. Only one variety, according to Pliny (*NH* xv 37) could be eaten uncooked. The ancients will have stewed them, sweetening them with honey (since they had no sugar). They were a jamless people until late antiquity. It was only toward the end of the Roman Empire that the first attempts at jam were made from quinces and honey (Galen VI 603 Kühn). Quinces, in Greek, are κυδώνια μῆλα (*kydonia mēla*), after Cydonia in Crete, and honey is μέλι (*meli*). Hence the name *mēlomeli*, from which some derive our word *marmalade*, which in continental languages is used for any kind of jam.

What, before jam making, was the quince's attraction? Its fragrance could sweeten the breath or the bedroom (Pliny ad loc.) and also be imparted to wine or honey when quinces were steeped in them. And their appearance in love poetry is explained by an isolated surviving fragment from Comedy (Cantharus, Kock i 765, quoted by Athenaeus iii 81D): quinces are shaped like breasts. Hence their role in the marriage laws that Solon framed for Athens in 594 B.C. (Plutarch, *Solon* 20):

> To this legislation belongs the ruling that a bride should be shut up with her groom, eating a quince, and that he who marries an heiress should go in to her at least three times a month. For even in a childless marriage, this is an honour

that a husband should afford to a chaste wife; it engenders kindness, takes away the irritations of living together, and prevents differences from proceeding to a rupture.

The black *mulberry*, the first fruit in the year to ripen and so a joy for children (Nicander, quoted by Athenaeus ii 51E), needs to be eaten on the day it is picked; it could not be a trade staple. But it was liked and had additional odd uses: unripe mulberries were thought to expel intestinal worms, and the juice of ripe ones, mixed with oil of roses, was applied externally to cool the stomachs of fevered patients (Athenaeus ii 51B–52A). Poor people might eat the figlike fruit of the Egyptian *sycamore*, the handsome tree that little Zacchaeus climbed in Jericho to get a better view of Jesus (Luke 19:4); but it is inferior, and Amos in his poverty gathered it for lack of anything else (Amos 7:14).

Of the *berry fruits*, wild blackberries and raspberries were known, and the Romans also became acquainted with the little Alpine strawberry. But the ancients did not cultivate them and had no gooseberries or black currants, let alone the big modern strawberries that derive from South America.

No one could fail to delight in the *almond*, queen of nut trees, that grew in biblical Palestine and was valued in Greece and Italy. The Greeks and Romans also enjoyed *walnuts* and *chestnuts*—chestnuts are still a dietary staple in the Italian Apennines. Even *acorns* were eaten by primitive people such as the Arcadians and were a last resource for more advanced people when all else failed. The wheat farmer who does not fight the weeds in time will, says Vergil, envy his neighbor's store and himself ease his hunger by shaking oaks in the forest (*Georgics* i 155–159). Acorns, the Greeks believed, had been the diet of mankind before civilization began. They are edible if the bitter taste is first leached out of them.

REFERENCES

André, J. 1961. *L'Alimentation et la cuisine à Rome*. Paris: Librairie C. Klincksieck.

Blümner, H. 1912. *Technologie und Terminologie der Gewerbe und Künste bei den Griechen und Römern*, I, ed. 2. Leipzig: Teubner.

Crone, P. 1987. *Meccan Trade*. Oxford: Blackwell.

Davies, R. 1989. *Service in the Roman Army*. Edinburgh: Edinburgh University Press.

Edwards, J. 1984. *The Roman Cookery of Apicius*. London: Rider.

Flower, B., and E. Rosenbaum. 1958. *The Roman Cookery Book*. London: Harrap.

Garnsey, P. 1988. *Famine and Food Supply in the Graeco-Roman World*. Cambridge: Cambridge University Press.

Hehn, V. 1870. *Kulturpflanzen und Haustiere*, 7th ed. 1902. Berlin: Gebrüder Born-traeger.

Hopf, M. 1963. Die Untersuchung von Getreideresten und anderen Feldfrüch-ten aus Altkalkar, Kreis Kleve, und Xanten, Kreis Moers, *Bonner Jahrbücher* **163**:416–423.

Kock, F. 1880–1888. *Comicorum Atticorum Fragmenta*, I–III. Leipzig: Teubner.

McCrum, M., and A. G. Woodhead. 1961. *Select Documents of the Principates of the Flavian Emperors*. Cambridge: Cambridge University Press.

Mau, A. 1899. *Pompeii, Its Life and Art*, F. W. Kelsey, tr. New York: Macmillan.

Meiggs, R. 1960. *Roman Ostia*. Oxford: Clarendon Press.

Miller, J. I. 1969. *The Spice Trade of the Roman Empire*. Oxford: Clarendon Press.

Moritz, L. A. 1949. ἄλφιτα—a note, *CQ* **48**:113–117.

Moritz, L. A. 1955. Husked and 'naked' grain, *CQ* **5**:129–134.

Moritz, L. A. 1958. *Grain Mills and Flour in Classical Antiquity*. Oxford: Clarendon Press.

Pauly's *Real-Encyclopädie der classischen Alterumswissenschaft*, new ed. by G. Wis-sowa, 1894–1972 with 14 supplementary volumes.

Der Klein Pauly, Lexikon fur Antike I-V, 1964–1975. Stuttgart: Alfred Drucken-müller Verlag.

Renfrew, J. 1973. *Palaeoethnobotany—The Prehistoric Food Plants of the Near East and Europe*. London: Methuen.

Renfrew, J. 1985. *Food and Cooking in Roman Britain*. English Heritage: Historic Buildings and Monuments Commission for England.

Reynolds, P. 1979. *Iron Age Farm, the Butser Experiment*. London: British Museum Publications.

Reynolds, P. J., and J. K. Langley. 1979. Romano-British corn-drying ovens, an experiment, *Arch. J.* **136**:27–42.

Rickman, G. 1971. *Roman Granaries and Store Buildings*. Cambridge: Cambridge University Press.

Rickman, G. 1980. *The Corn Supply of Ancient Rome*. Oxford: Clarendon Press.

Schliemann, H. 1880. *Ilios*. London: John Murray.

Simmonds, N. W. 1976. *Evolution of Crop Plants*. Harlow, Essex: Longman.

Sparkes, B. A. 1962. The Greek kitchen, *J. Hellenic Studies* **82**:128–137.

Spurr, M. W. 1986. Arable cultivation in Roman Italy 200 B.C.—c. A.D. 100, *Jour. Roman Studies Monograph No. 3.*

Währen, M. 1963. *Brot und Gebäck im Leben und Glauben der alten Aegypter*. Berne: Schweizerisches Archiv für Brot und Gebäckkunde.

West, M. L., ed. 1978. *Hesiod's Works and Days*. Oxford: Clarendon Press.

White, K. D. 1970. *Roman Farming*. London: Thames and Hudson.

White, K. D. 1976. Food requirements and food supplies in classical times in relation to the diet of the various classes, *Prog. Food Nutr. Sci.* **2**:143–191.

White, K. D. 1984. *Greek and Roman Technology*. London: Thames and Hudson.

Wittmack, L. 1890. Samen aus den Ruinen von Hissarlik, *Verhandlungen der Ber-liner Gesellschaft für Anthropologie, Ethnologie und Urgeschichte*.

Wittmack, L. 1896. *Grabfunde des mittleren Reichs in den königlichen Museen zu Ber-lin, I. Das Grab des Mentu-hotep*, G. Steindorff, ed. Berlin: Kaiserliche Mu-seen.

Part II

TYPICAL MEDITERRANEAN
FOODS AND THEIR PHYSIOLOGY

3

Cereal Foods: Wheat, Corn, Rice, Barley, and Other Cereals and Their Products

Claudia Lintas
Aldo Mariani-Costantini

The role of cereals as a staple food in the history and evolution of Mediterranean peoples' lifestyles is well known and generally acknowledged. In ancient times *pulte autem, non pane, vixisse longo tempore Romanos menifestum* (on *puls* however not on bread the Romans were fed for a long period) (Pliny). The *puls* mentioned was a porridge made by boiling ground cereals in water or milk. At that time, *Triticum* species with naked caryopses (*T. turgidum, T. durum* Desp.) were not cultivated and not used in breadmaking. Only barley and, particularly in archaic Latium, emmer, named by the Romans "far" or "adoreum," and now identified as *T. dicoccum* Scrk., were available.

While barley gruel was common food in ancient Greece, the Romans used an emmer *farinata* (porridge). The specificity is innate in that Latin and Italian *farina* (flour) and *farinata* (porridge) have the common root *far.*

It was also customary to use flat wheat breads as a kind of table on which to place the food, to be eaten only if by the end of the meal people still felt hungry. Vergil mentions it when reporting that Aeneas and his followers once in Latium felt to have arrived to their new country since, according to the prophecy, for hunger they had eaten even the tables.

To limit the risk of insufficient crops, it was customary to cultivate various species of cereals together such as, in addition to emmer, millet, oats, and rye. The mixture was named *farrago* and was used first as human food, then with time became animal feed.

In the passage from scarcity to abundance, the diet mainly based on cereals, integrated with vegetable fats from olives (mostly consumed as such) was enriched with animal proteins. The *puls* was varied with the addition of fababean, lentils, and chick-pea and gradually was replaced by bread.

With evolution and society stratification according to wealth, a tendency emerged to consume diversified and richer foods such as meats (Neri 1986). As a consequence, luxury began to be recognized as a destabilizing element. *Holera et legumina* then acquired a reputation of being the ideal foods for a simple life.

In the ancient Mediterranean civilizations, vegetable food and particularly cereal foods had acquired a meaning beyond the alimentary function itself; for example, consider the offer of the emmer cake among Romans as a symbol of the wedding vows. At the oath that the ephebi pronounced to become citizens, they called as witnesses, in addition to the gods and the Country's border, the wheat and the barley with the grapevine, the olive tree, and the fig tree. The importance of cereals to contemporary nutrition and health has developed from the oldest roots of the Mediterranean culture.

GENERAL CHARACTERISTICS OF CEREALS

Cereals are characterized by relatively low protein and high carbohydrate content (Table 3-1); furthermore, cereal proteins are very high in biological value (Table 3-2). The carbohydrate fraction consists essentially of starch, dextrins, pentosans, and sugars, of which 90% or more is starch. The carbohydrate contents, including fiber, of various grains are shown in Table 3-3. The major portion of the carbohydrates, and consequently the main source of calories provided by the grains, is in the starchy endosperm.

Fatty acids in cereals occur in three main types: neutral lipids, glycolipids, and phospholipids. Total lipids and individual fatty acids in cereal grains and some of their products are shown in Table 3-4. The lipids in cereals are relatively rich in the essential fatty acid linoleic acid. Saturated fatty acids (mainly palmitic) represent less than 25% of the total fatty acids for most grains.

All cereals contain vitamins of the B group, but all are completely lacking in vitamin C (unless the grain is sprouted) and vitamin D (Table 3-5). Wheat also contains yellow pigments, almost entirely xanthophylls, which are not precursors of vitamin A. The oils of the embryos of cereal grains are rich sources of vitamin E. The relative distribution of vitamins in kernel structures is not uniform, although the endosperm invariably contains the least.

As a group, cereals are low in calcium, and the concentration of calcium and other ash constituents is greatly reduced by the milling proc-

TABLE 3-1. Composition of Important Cereal Grains (g/100 g, dry basis)

	Protein	Fat	Carbohydrates	Ash
Barley				
Whole grain	10.6	2.1	57.5	3.1
Pearled	10.4	1.4	62.2	1.2
Corn				
Grain	9.2	3.8	65.5	1.3
Flour	9.0	2.8	73.1	1.2
Oats				
Husked grain	12.6	7.1	61.2	2.9
Groats	13.9	5.8	ND	2.0
Rice				
Brown	7.4	2.2	74.6	1.2
Milled	7.2	0.7	78.4	0.5
Rye				
Grain	8.7	1.7	53.5	1.9
Flour	6.9	1.0	65.7	0.7
Wheat				
Hard red spring (HRS)	11.5	2.0	59.4	1.8
Durum	14.0	2.9	57.9	1.5
Flour	12.7	1.3	67.6	0.7

Source: Adapted from Pomeranz (1987).
Note: ND = no data.

esses used to prepare refined foods (Table 3–6). In these processes hulls, germ, and bran, which are the structures rich in minerals and vitamins, are more or less completely removed. The nutritional significance of this refining must be considered against the background of the diet. Whole grains are in fact devoid of vitamins A, D, and C and contain very little fat, present mainly in the germ. Germ is also rich in vitamin E.

WHEAT

Wheat is among the most important crops in the world and world wheat production in 1987–1988 was estimated at about 514 million tons (FAO 1989). There are 14 species, wild or cultivated, of the genus *Triticum;* however, only three species (*T. aestivum,* or bread wheat, *T. durum,* or macaroni bread, and *T. compactum,* club wheat) are grown to a significant extent today. Of these, *T. aestivum* comprises over 90% of the cultivated wheat, with some of the cultivars adapted to widely diverse climatic conditions.

Much research has been and continues to be conducted to produce new wheat varieties that have improved agronomic, morphologic, and

TABLE 3-2. Amino Acid Composition of Cereals (% by weight)

	Rice (brown)	Wheat (hard red spring)	Wheat (durum)	Corn	Barley	Oats	Rye
Tryptophan	1.16	1.19	1.2	0.68	1.25	1.30	1.12
Threonine	3.48	2.75	2.9	3.73	3.29	3.34	3.37
Isoleucine	4.10	3.88	3.6	4.10	3.88	4.05	3.83
Leucine	7.76	6.59	7.0	12.68	7.03	7.64	5.94
Lysine	3.66	2.70	2.2	2.92	3.44	3.90	4.16
Methionine	1.97	1.40	0.9	1.96	1.62	2.04	1.57
Cystine	1.88	2.15	—	1.73	2.11	1.63	2.01
Phenylalanine	5.03	4.59	4.1	4.55	5.13	4.94	4.46
Tyrosine	4.00	3.26	2.0	4.90	3.42	3.01	2.77
Valine	5.68	4.43	4.6	4.99	5.01	5.68	4.91
Arginine	5.38	4.63	3.5	4.13	5.08	6.31	4.76
Histidine	1.99	2.10	1.9	2.42	2.04	2.16	2.14
Alanine	4.30	3.40	4.8	8.69	4.35	5.48	4.56
Aspartic acid	6.36	5.12	4.7	9.42	5.63	8.43	6.81
Glutamic acid	18.12	30.82	32.3	18.29	23.28	21.59	22.40
Glycine	5.05	5.00	6.5	3.59	4.28	6.27	4.41
Proline	6.56	9.79	13.4	8.51	9.91	5.38	7.62
Serine	4.77	4.60	5.7	5.36	4.48	4.57	4.34
Total protein (%)	10.8	14.0	—	10.0	12.8	17.7	13.4
PER	1.7	1.5	—	1.2	—	1.9	1.6
NPU (%)	63.9	56.2	—	58.9	61.5	—	67.9

Source: Adapted from Pomeranz (1987).

TABLE 3-3. Carbohydrate Contents of Cereal Grains and Their Products (g/100 g)

| | Carbohydrates | | |
	Sugars	Starch	Dietary Fiber
Barley, grain	1.7	55.9	9.8
pearled	2.2	62.2	10.7
Corn, grain	1.4	63.8	9.2
Oats, grain	1.2	60.0	5.6
Rice, brown	1.9	72.7	4.0
white	tr	78.2	1.4
Rye, grain	0.9	52.6	13.2
flour	0.8	64.9	11.3
Wheat, grain	0.9	58.5	10.6
flour	0.8	66.9	2.4
bran	1.9	13.2	42.4

Note: tr = trace.

TABLE 3-4. Fatty Acid Composition of Cereal and Related Products (g/100 g food)

| | Saturated | | | Unsaturated | | | |
	Sum	16:0	18:0	Sum	18:1	18:2	18:3
Barley, whole grain	0.48	0.45	0.02	1.51	0.24	1.14	0.13
Corn							
Whole grain	0.47	0.40	0.06	3.07	0.91	2.12	0.03
Flour	0.30	0.25	0.04	2.00	0.64	1.34	0.02
Germ	3.93	3.30	0.54	25.53	7.58	17.70	0.25
Grits, degermed	0.09	0.08	0.01	0.60	0.18	0.41	0.01
Oatmeal or rolled oats	1.37	1.21	0.10	5.65	2.60	2.87	0.16
Rice							
Brown	0.62	0.54	0.04	1.36	0.54	0.78	0.03
White, polished	0.21	0.19	—	0.47	0.19	0.27	0.01
Rye, whole grain	0.27	0.25	0.02	1.30	0.22	0.95	0.12
Wheat, bread							
Whole grain	0.37	0.36	0.01	1.56	0.25	1.20	0.10
Flours	0.23	0.21	0.01	0.84	0.12	0.69	0.03
Bran	0.74	0.69	0.04	3.09	0.71	2.20	0.16
Germ	1.88	0.01	1.81	8.18	1.54	5.86	0.74
Wheat, durum							
Whole grain	0.54	0.51	0.03	1.88	0.40	1.36	0.11
Semolina	0.33	0.31	0.02	0.90	0.17	0.68	0.04

Source: Adapted, from Pomeranz (1987).
Note: Fatty acids include 16:0 = palmitic; 18:0 = stearic; 18:1 = oleic; 18:2 = linoleic; 18:3 = linolenic.

TABLE 3-5. Vitamin Content of Cereal Grains

	Thiamine (mg %)	Riboflavin (mg %)	Niacin (mg %)	Vit. B_6 (mg %)	Folic Acid (μg %)	Pantothenate (μg %)	Biotin (μg %)	Vit. E (mg %)
Barley	0.23	0.13	4.5	0.26	67	0.5	6	0.4
Corn	0.37	0.12	2.2	0.47	26	1	21	tr
Oats	0.67	0.14	1.0	0.21	104	1	13	1.7
Rice (brown)	0.34	0.05	4.7	0.62	20	2	12	0.8
Rice (polished)	0.07	0.03	1.6	0.04	16	1	5	0.1
Rye	0.44	0.18	1.5	0.33	34	1	2	1.6
Wheat	0.57	0.12	7.4	0.35	78	1	6	0.6
Wheat germ	2.01	0.68	4.2	0.92	328	2	22	22.0
Wheat bran	0.72	0.35	21.0	1.38	258	3	14	2.6
Wheat flour	0.14	0.04	1.8	0.05	22	1	1	0.3
Wheat durum	0.67	0.11	1.1	0.43	—	—	—	5.8
Wheat semolina	0.32	0.10	3.9	0.12	22	0.3	1	2.5
Wheat pasta	0.32	0.03	3.1	0.17	34	0.3	1	0.3

Source: Adapted from Pomeranz (1987).

TABLE 3-6. Mineral Content of Cereal Grains and Cereal Products (mg/100 g)

	Ca	Fe	Mg	P	K	Na	Cu	Mn	Zn
Barley	80	10	120	420	560	3	0.76	1.63	1.5
Corn, grain	30	2	120	270	280	1	0.21	0.51	1.7
Corn, bran	30	—	260	190	730	—	—	1.61	—
Corn, germ	90	90	280	560	130	—	1.10	0.90	—
Oats	100	10	170	350	370	2	0.59	3.82	3.4
Rice, brown	40	3	60	230	150	9	0.33	1.76	1.8
Rice, milled	30	1	20	120	130	5	0.29	1.09	1.3
Rye	60	10	120	340	460	1	0.78	6.69	3.1
Sorghum	40	4	170	310	340	—	0.96	1.45	1.4
Wheat, grain	50	10	160	360	520	3	0.72	4.88	3.4
Wheat, bran	140	70	550	1170	1240	9	1.23	11.57	9.8
Wheat, durum	34	4	186	370	494	—	0.89	3.20	3.0
Wheat, semolina	20	1	69	185	198	12	0.22	0.60	1.1

Source: Adapted from Pomeranz (1987).

technological characteristics. High-yielding dwarf or semidwarf wheats have resulted from crosses with Japanese wheats, and through selections and crosses, protein content of the grain has been increased without adversely affecting the biological value of the proteins and the total yield. New approaches are being explored to improve resistance to adverse climatic conditions and diseases and to improve overall quality through genetic engineering.

Structure and Composition

The wheat grain is a seed with the structure shown in Figure 3-1. The outer coverings are the pericarp and testa, rich in insoluble dietary fiber (DF) components (hemicelluloses, cellulose, and lignin). Beneath them is the aleurone layer, often considered as part of the bran, which is an envelope of cells rich in protein surrounding the endosperm. These outer layers form about 14% of the weight of the grain. Inside is the starchy endosperm, comprising about 83% of the weight of the grain. The germ (or embryo)—situated at the lower end of the grain—consists of the shoot and the root. The embryo is attached to the grain by a special structure, the scutellum. The embryo and scutellum, barely visible to the naked eye, comprise about 3% of the total weight of the grain.

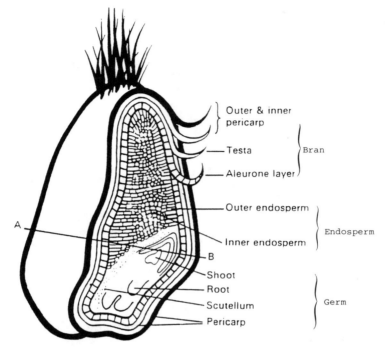

Figure 3–1.   Longitudinal section of the wheat grain.

Distribution of Nutrients

Much work has been done to determine the distribution of nutrients in the wheat kernel. Some of this work has been done by hand dissecting individual kernels and analyzing the various fractions.

The various components are not distributed uniformly in the different kernel structures (Table 3–7). The germ is high in lipid content and rich in protein, sugar, and ash constituents. The bran constituents, testa and pericarp, are high in DF (cellulose, pentosans) and minerals.

The starchy endosperm, containing virtually all the starch of the kernel, varies in composition from the outer portion, just beneath the aleurone layer, to the center. Clearly, both protein and mineral content decrease from the outer to the inner portion of the endosperm. The starchy endosperm contains only a small proportion of the thiamine, niacin, and pyridoxine of the kernel but an important proportion of the protein, riboflavin, and panthotenic acid, riboflavin being the most evenly distributed of the five vitamins.

TABLE 3-7. Nutrient Distribution in the Main Morphological Parts of the Wheat Kernel

Fraction	Function	Approximate % of kernel (by wt)	Nutrients Present (% of total)
Seed coats (bran layers)			Protein (12%), fat, ash (67%)
Pericarp ⎱ Testa ⎰	Protects the grain	7–8	Protein (4%), B vitamins (5–10%), dietary fiber (cellulose, hemicellulose, lignin), minerals (K, P, Mg, Ca)
Aleurone layer	Encases the endosperm	6–7	Niacin (80%), minerals (60%, espec. P) protein (15%), phytic acid, vit. B_6, thiamine, riboflavin, panthotenic acid
Endosperm	Stores food	81–84	Starch (100%), protein (72%), minerals (20%), panthotenic acid, riboflavin
Germ		3	
Embryo	Contains undeveloped root and shoot		Fat (30%), protein (30%), sugars
Scutellum	Stores food for embryo and transfers food from endosperm to embryo		B vitamins, phosphorus, thiamine (62%)

The aleurone layer contains high levels of minerals, total phosphorus, phytate phosphorus (87%), fat, and niacin. The thiamine and riboflavin contents are higher in the aleurone layer than in the other bran layers. The aleurone layer contains approximately 80% of the niacin, 60% of the pyridoxine, 60% of the total minerals, and an important proportion of each of the other three vitamins. Thiamine is virtually confined to the scutellum, containing about 60% of the total.

Not all the amino acids are distributed in the same manner as the total protein is. Of the essential amino acids, lysine is the only one that differs markedly, probably less than 30% being in the endosperm, with about 50% in the aleurone layer. The other essential amino acids appear to be distributed in much the same way as the total protein is. Of the nonessential amino acids, about 80% of the glutamic acid and proline is found in the endosperm and about 10% in the aleurone layer. The distribution of arginine is similar to that of lysine.

Similarly, the mineral elements are not distributed in the same way as the total minerals. About 50% of the calcium and copper is found in the endosperm, with 25–30% in the aleurone layer. About 40% of strontium and cobalt also is found in the endosperm, with 15–20% in the aleurone layer. On the other hand, no more than 10–20% of the magnesium, zinc, and manganese is found in the endosperm, 50–70% of the zinc, manganese, and copper being in the aleurone layer. It is significant that 87% of the phytate phosphorus is also found in this fraction (O'Dell et al. 1972).

Nutritional Value

Wheat has a relatively high content of thiamine and niacin. Like other cereals, it is a poor source of riboflavin and calcium. The composition of wheat is influenced by genetic variety and several environmental factors. Nitrogen fertilization may increase the protein content of the grains and change the amino acid composition of the protein. As an example, the lysine concentration is negatively correlated to the protein content (Chung and Pomeranz 1985a), but there is a positive correlation between the protein content of the whole grain and its content of thiamine, niacin, and iron.

Proteins

Based on solubility, the proteins of wheat can be divided into albumin 3–5%, globulin 6–10%, gliadin (prolamin) 40–50% and glutenin (glutelin) 30–40%. Although the storage proteins, gliadin and glutenin, make up most of the wheat protein (Table 3–8), the soluble proteins (albumin and globulin) are nutritionally important because about 45% of the total amino acids in these fractions are essential amino acids (Chung and Pomeranz 1985a). Gluten and its protein fractions are nutritionally inferior to whole wheat protein and to soluble proteins, primarily because of extremely low lysine scores.

The various proteins are not distributed uniformly in the kernel. Thus, proteins fractionated from the inner endosperm of wheat consist chiefly of gliadin (a prolamin) and glutelin, apparently in approximately equal amounts. The embryo proteins consist of nucleoproteins, an albu-

TABLE 3-8. Distribution of Cereal Endosperm Proteins According to Their Solubility (% total protein)

	Protein range (% dwb)	Albumin (water-soluble)	Globulins (salt-soluble)	Prolamin (alcohol-soluble)	Glutelin (alkali-soluble)
Barley	10–16	3–4	10–20	35–45	35–45
Corn	7–13	2–10	10–20	50–55	30–45
Oats	8–20	10–19	52–56	7–13	21–27
Rice	8–10	2–5	2–8	1–5	85–90
Rye	9–14	20–30	5–10	20–30	30–40
Wheat (HRS)	10–15	5–10	5–10	40–50	30–40
Wheat (Durum)	12–16	10–15	5–10	40–50	30–40

Source: Adapted from Pomeranz (1987).

min (leucosin), a globulin, and proteoses, whereas in wheat bran a prolamin predominates with smaller quantities of albumins and globulins. When water is added, the wheat endosperm proteins, gliadin and glutelin, form a tenacious colloidal complex known as gluten. Gluten is responsible for the superiority of wheat over the other cereals for the manufacture of leavened products, since it makes possible the formation of a dough network that retains the carbon dioxide produced by yeast, chemical, or other leavening agents.

In general, the protein content of wheat fractions is greatest in germ, followed by middlings, bran, whole wheat flour, and white flour, in decreasing order. Within types of wheat, the hard wheats are generally higher in protein than the soft wheats. When wheat is milled, the protein content decreases as the extraction rate decreases; the drop in protein from 14.2% for 100% extraction flour to 12.7% for 66% extraction flour reflects the removal of germ and the aleurone-containing bran, which are relatively rich in protein (Pedersen and Eggum 1983). In general, bread contains less protein than the flours from which it is made.

As a class, cereal proteins are not as high in biological value as those of certain legumes, nuts, or animal products. The limiting amino acid in wheat endosperm proteins is lysine. While biological values of the proteins of entire cereal grains are greater than those of the refined mill products, which consist chiefly of the endosperm, the North American and European diets normally include various cereals and legumes as well as animal products. Under those conditions, different proteins tend to supplement each other, and the cereals represent important and valuable sources of amino acids.

Minerals

Whole wheat flour contains amounts of calcium, iron, and zinc that would be nutritionally valuable if they were absorbed, but this absorption is greatly impeded by binding to dietary phytate.* A major proportion (50–80%) of the minerals in wheat is found in the aleurone layer; however, this fraction also contains nearly 90% of the phytate present in the whole kernel (O'Dell et al. 1972). Low extraction flours have lost much of these minerals (Table 3–9), but what remains may be better absorbed because of the loss of phytate.

Wheat bran from commercial flour mills is composed of the outer structures of the wheat kernel, from the aleurone layer outward, and contains major proportions of magnesium and trace elements, including iron, zinc, and copper. Thus, a significant fraction of these nutritionally essential inorganic nutrients are not retained in the refined flour (Pedersen et al. 1989).

Davis et al. (1984) studied the effect of growing conditions on mineral content of wheat. They examined the trace element content of one wheat variety (Centurk) grown in 13 different locations and noted large variations. The ranges they found (mg/kg) were: iron 35–133, zinc 24–61, copper 1–8, and manganese 35–65. Such differences were presumably due, at least in part, to soil mineral content and demonstrate that many factors related to growth conditions as well as wheat class affect trace element content of wheat. Mahoney (1982) presented a comprehensive compilation of the iron, zinc, copper, and manganese content of various wheat products.

Separate studies on selenium content of wheat clearly indicate that the availability of selenium in the soil is the major factor determining wheat selenium content (Lorenz 1978). The range of selenium wheat contents is much larger than ranges for other trace elements.

Information on the bioavailability of minerals in diets containing wheat foods is often conflicting and contradictory. The data obtained from studies on bioavailability of minerals are influenced by many variables. Furthermore, the difficulty in interpreting data on bioavailability of minerals in wheat is further complicated by differences of opinion on the role of the fiber:phytate interactions. Data presently available have not clarified the relative impact of fiber and phytate on the bioavailability of calcium, magnesium, iron, and zinc (Betschart 1988).

Editor's Note: The effect of phytates on mineral availability in humans is affected by many factors such as leavening of bread with yeast or other cultures and sprouting of grains, all of which seem to make minerals available.

TABLE 3-9. Mineral Content of Wheat and Wheat Products

	HRW (μg/g)	Flour (%)	Bread (%)	Durum (μg/g)	Semolina (%)	Pasta (%)	Soft Wheat (μg/g)	Patent Flour (%)	Cake (%)
Fe	44	19	35	40	35	41	37	21	11
Mn	38	12	12	32	19	19	35	14	5
Zn	24	26	32	30	37	35	5	18	11
Cu	5.1	39	46	4.8	2.2	53	4.5	36	17
Ni	0.5	32	155	0.3	0.2	52	0.3	58	26
Co	0.4	58	100	0.3	NA	87	0.4	78	89
Sn	5.6	73	173	6.8	6.0	75	7.9	47	408

Source: After Jones (1977).
Note: HRW = Hard red winter; NA = not available.

In general the minerals in cereal grains are not readily absorbed. According to Van Dokkum et al. (1982), the effect of wheat bran on mineral balance varied with the mineral and the particle size of the bran. The increased mineral absorption with fine wheat bran and whole wheat bread emphasizes the importance of particle size. Increased milling to produce smaller particles would be expected to increase the disruption of aleurone cell walls. The small particle size could increase the accessibility of nutrients contained in the aleurone cells as they pass through the gastrointestinal tract and improve their potential for being absorbed.

From results of several studies, Betschart (1988) concluded that there is selected interference in the percent of mineral absorption in the presence of whole wheat, although the absolute amount absorbed may be higher than in white bread. In circumstances in which wheat bran or fiber diminishes the bioavailability of minerals, there is considerable interest in the mechanisms involved. Two factors, dietary fiber and phytate, have received much attention and support for research.

Vitamins

According to Pomeranz (1987) significant differences in the vitamin content of wheat may occur because of diverse agronomical factors and cultural practices. Consequently, the average values found in tables of food composition probably do not reflect the actual amounts of vitamins in the wheat in a diet.

Vitamins are not distributed uniformly throughout the wheat kernel. Vitamin distribution in the endosperm, scutellum, embryo, aleurone layer, and other fractions differs more than the corresponding distribution of minerals. The endosperm contains less than 5% of the thiamine and more than 40% of the panthotenic acid. The aleurone layer contains 32% of the thiamine and more than 80% of the niacin.

In addition, vitamins vary enormously in their stability and sensitivity to light, temperature, and moisture. Therefore, altering the conditions of milling, processing, or storage of wheat and wheat products may have markedly different effects on the stability and bioavailability of specific vitamins (Betschart 1988).

Analysis of wheat has yielded relatively broad ranges of vitamin content (Davis et al. 1981). Some of the variations in the values are due to methodological differences but most of it is likely caused by effects of wheat class, growth location, and agronomic practices.

Fat soluble vitamins are influenced by some of the same factors and mechanisms of absorption as is dietary fat. Interest in fat soluble vitamins is due to their potential interference with bile salt reabsorption as well as the effect of various forms of fiber on bioavailability (Kasper et al. 1979). Data on the influence of wheat bran or whole wheat products on bioavailability of water soluble vitamins are somewhat limited.

Based on the evidence to date, there need be little concern about the negative effects of wheat bran or whole wheat foods on the bioavailability of vitamins in well-nourished populations. In populations with marginal intakes, especially of niacin and vitamin B_6, it would seem advisable not to consume excessive quantities of wheat bran.

Dietary Fiber

Although wheat is a rich source of DF, foods made from wheat show great differences in fiber content because the distribution of fiber within the cereal grain varies widely. DF components are present primarily in the outer tissues of the grain where they have structural and protective functions. Such tissues contain over 70% of the total DF, whereas the starchy endosperm contains relatively small amounts.

The DF content of wheat depends to a large extent on the degree of milling. Wheat flours of low extraction contain only small amounts of fiber (Table 3–3). That relatively low level is further reduced when the milled products are processed into foods such as bread, in which the water content reduces the effective DF content even more. Bread and baked goods produced from whole grains still have a relatively high fiber content. The levels of DF in bread can be increased by the addition of fiber concentrates from cereal grains (bran), legumes (guar, locust bean gum), or other sources. Addition of these DF concentrates creates relatively small problems in the production of breads consumed in some European countries. Furthermore, technological measures can be used to improve bread structure so that bread of acceptable quality is produced even with the addition of up to 16% concentrated DF.

The soluble fiber content of the flours is about 1.5% and independent of the degree of extraction. The content of insoluble fiber increases rapidly for extraction rates above 80%, which shows that soluble polysaccharides are derived essentially from the endosperm. The amount of soluble fiber is higher in rye, barley, and wheat than in other cereals.

The neutral sugar composition of DF was similar in wheat and rye and at low and high extraction rates of these cereals. Thus, glucose, xylose, and arabinose constituted 28–33%, 31–37%, and 24–25% of the total neutral sugars, respectively. In barley, glucose was the dominating sugar, especially at low extraction, reflecting the high beta-glucan content of the endosperm cell walls (Nyman et al. 1984).

The main dietary fiber components are noncellulosic polysaccharides, mainly arabinoxylans, beta-glucans, glucuronoarabinoxylans, cellulose, and lignin. There is little difference in fiber composition between whole wheat and the most refined flour, but refined flours do not contain lignin, in contrast to whole wheat, which contains about 2% of lignin. The DF content of cereal grains depends on the type of grain, variety, growth conditions, cultural practices, size of grain, and many other factors.

Phytic acid is associated with fiber and by binding minerals, especially divalent cations, may make them unavailable. Thus a high intake of wheat fiber has both advantages and disadvantages. The role of DF and its effects on health are now the subject of much discussion and research. Many nutritionists consider that moderate amounts of fiber are beneficial and wheat bran has impressive effects on colonic function.

Baking makes a starch fraction resistant to amylace, increasing the DF content by 1–2% (Englyst 1983). Dry heat treatment of wheat flour (180°C, 4 hours) gave a similar increase in DF (Theander 1983). On the other hand, extrusion cooking of wheat flour did not change significantly the DF content (Varo et al. 1983) but a solubilization of DF was observed (Bjorck et al. 1984). At severe conditions, total DF increased significantly.

Effect of Processing on the Nutritive Value of Wheat

Milling. Wheat is usually ground into flour before being prepared as food. Flour containing the whole grain may be used but usually the germ and a varying proportion of the outer layers are separated from the central portion of the grain and discarded as bran. The proportion of wheat recovered as flour is known as the extraction rate. Thus an 85%

extraction rate flour contains 85% by weight of the whole grain and 15% is discarded as bran. It is important to remember that the extraction rate refers to the proportion of the original grain in the flour and not in the bran. The flour of a "high extraction rate" has lost little of the aleurone layer and outer endosperm.

An extraction rate of 75% or less indicates a white flour. If it exceeds 80%, the flour will contain significant proportions of nonendosperm particles and when the flour extraction reaches 100%, a whole meal flour is indicated. In western countries, 70–75% flour is usually employed in breadmaking.

The milling of wheat reduces its nutrient content (Table 3–10). Lorenz et al. (1980) have carried out a study to assess nutrient losses in milling. The paper covers macronutrients as well as micronutrients and allows some important conclusions. Iron and zinc are markedly reduced by milling; the reduction is generally related to the extraction rate, especially for zinc. Selenium losses in milling are minor, only 15–20% and in most cases selenium is distributed evenly throughout the kernel of the grain (Ferretti and Levander 1974).

As shown in Table 3–11, the mineral content of wheat is greatly reduced by milling. In the refined flour minerals were reduced to about 30% of the original content, however, only traces of phytate were present.

The phytic acid content of cereals and cereal products is shown in Table 3–12. Phytic acid, a nutritionally undesirable metal-chelating agent, is located primarily in the mill by-products bran and dust and is present in relatively low levels in the major wheat products, semolina and flour.

The mean values of 63 commercially milled flours from the United States and Canada provide a meaningful base with which to compare other values (Keagy et al. 1980). In these samples, all vitamins except

TABLE 3-10. Chemical Composition of Wheat Flour of Different Extraction Rates (g/100 g)

	Water	Total N	Protein	Fat	Starch	Sugars	Dietary Fiber
Brown	14.0	2.20	12.6	1.8	66.8	1.7	6.4
Patent	14.1	1.89	10.8	1.3	76.6	1.4	3.1
White breadmaking	14.0	2.02	11.5	1.4	73.9	1.4	3.2
White plain	14.0	1.64	9.4	1.3	76.2	1.5	3.1
Whole meal	14.0	2.18	12.7	2.2	61.8	2.1	9.0
Bran	8.3	2.24	14.1	5.5	23.8	3.8	41.5

TABLE 3-11.   Protein, Ash, and Mineral Content of Wheat and Flour[a]

	Wheat		Flour		Flour as Percent of Wheat (Average)
	Average	CV	Average	CV	
Protein, %	15.8	4.0	14.7	4.4	93
Ash, %	1.91	3.1	0.48	4.2	25
P, %	0.443	4.1	0.118	7.9	27
K, %	0.465	6.3	0.109	9.9	23
Mg, %	0.146	2.5	0.030	6.4	21
Ca, ppm	487	7.1	319	8.2	66
Zn, ppm	27.9	7.5	6.53	15.2	23
Fe, ppm	49.9	6.2	13.7	19.2	28
Mn, ppm	56.0	7.1	6.93	9.0	12
Cu, ppm	5.14	8.1	1.49	15.0	29

Source: Pomeranz (1988).
Note: CV = Coefficient of variation.
[a]Dry matter basis of varietal composites from 23 locations.

TABLE 3-12.   Phytic Acid in Cereals and Cereal Products

Product	Phytate (% dry wt.)
Barley	0.97–1.16
Corn	0.89
Corn, bread	1.36
Oats	0.89–1.01
Rice, brown	0.52–0.89
Rice, polished	0.14–0.34
Rye	0.97
Rye, flour	0.33
Rye, bread	0.41
Wheat, hard red spring	0.62–1.43
Wheat, flour	0.45–0.72
Wheat, bread	0.03–0.12
Wheat, whole meal bread	0.36–0.61
Wheat, bran	2.33–4.32
Wheat, germ	4.14
Wheat, gluten	2.13
Wheat, durum	0.94
Wheat, semolina	0.16–0.34
Wheat, pasta	0.25

Source: Adapted from Reddy et al. (1982).

thiamine were present at slightly higher levels in the hard than in the soft wheats. Commercial milling removes about 68% of the thiamine, 58–65% of the riboflavin, and 85% of the pyridoxine contained in the whole wheat. Although removing wheat germ decreases the vitamin content of flour, the factor that accounts for the greatest loss of vitamins is removing the aleurone layer because of the high vitamin concentration in the aleurone layer. Nearly all the vitamin E present in whole wheat is removed by milling but other dietary sources usually produce adequate amounts. Data such as these are useful, along with other information, to develop guidelines or recommendations.

In low extraction flours large losses of water soluble vitamins occur during milling (Table 3–5). However, when white bread made from 70% extraction flour provides no more than 30% of the dietary energy and the other foods are varied and of good quality, requirements of all the known vitamins in this group are likely to be met. This situation exists in prosperous industrial countries where primary dietary deficiencies due to lack of any known vitamin are uncommon. Yet the loss of the vitamins in milling increases the risk of deficiency in individuals whose diets are otherwise poor and lacking in these vitamins. For this reason, in some countries, the United States, the United Kingdom, and Canada for example, white flours are often fortified with thiamine and nicotinic acid and sometimes with riboflavin.

Milling of wheat not only reduces the protein content of flours but also changes the amino acid composition of the protein. Milling of wheat results in a decrease in the concentration of lysine, present in larger amounts in the protein of the outer layers and germ than in the starchy endosperm. Thus this process potentially affects how much of the nutrients actually present in whole wheat are made available to the consumer. However, true digestibility, determined in rats, tends to be higher for lower extraction rates, with the net result that the overall utilization of ingested protein remains relatively constant. Similar results have been observed in metabolic studies with convalescent children. Thus, using whole wheat flour and 70% extraction white flour made from genetically high protein wheats, apparent nitrogen retention from whole wheat flour was not significantly different from that obtained with white flour (Graham 1977).

The whole wheat flour has significantly higher lysine content than the corresponding white flour; as a result, the percentage of absorbed nitrogen that was retained was higher. However, because there was less nitrogen absorbed, the apparent nitrogen retention was the same. Hence, by including 100% of the wheat grain a better amino acid composition is obtained but the digestibility is somewhat lower and the two factors balance each other out. Indeed, according to Graham (1977), through processing when whole wheat is converted to white flour, and particularly into pasta, this cereal becomes a high digestible food with high nitrogen retention because of the high digestibility of both the protein and carbohydrate components.

The nutritional quality of protein depends on the digestibility and availability of amino acids. Protein content and amino acid composition can be used, however, to assess potential protein quality. The protein content and amino acid composition of various wheat fractions and flours of several extraction rates have been extensively reviewed (Young and Pellett 1985). In addition, Pedersen and Eggum (1983) reported systematic studies of protein and lysine content, percentage of nitrogen digestibility, and net protein utilization (NPU) of hard and winter wheat flours ranging in extraction rate from 66% to 100%.

Amino acid composition indicates protein quality when compared with a given amino acid profile. Patterns such as the FAO provisional amino acid scoring pattern and suggested patterns of amino acid requirements for infants, children, and adults (FAO 1973) have been used to evaluate wheat protein quality (Bodwell 1985; Young and Pellett 1985). Table 3-13 summarizes the amino acid composition of various wheats and wheat fractions together with their amino acid scores and illustrates the high quality of germ, bran, and other milling by-products (red dog, shorts, middlings) and the relatively lower quality of whole wheat and white flours. Although wheat protein is limited in lysine when compared to the FAO reference pattern and suggested requirements for infants and children, it is adequate for adults, who require less lysine (Young and Pellett 1985).

Vitamins are largely present in wheat fractions removed during milling (Keagy et al. 1980). Commercial milling removes about 68% of the thiamine (Table 3-14), 58-65% of the riboflavin, and 85% of the pyridoxine contained in whole wheat. The content of thiamine, riboflavin, and pyridoxine were determined in whole wheat kernels and the various flours milled from it. Large average losses were noted for these vitamins. Higher extraction flours had generally higher vitamin content.

Since the outer layers of cereal grains have a much higher content of cell wall polysaccharides than the endosperm, the DF content of cereals is highly dependent upon the extraction rate. Wheat flour of low extraction rate contains only 2-3% DF, compared to about 12% in whole grain wheat (see Table 3-15). Soluble DF components remain constant, regardless of extraction rate, amounting to 3-4% in rye and barley and about 1% in wheat (Nyman et al. 1984).

Baking.   The baking process itself causes only a small loss of nutritive value with a moderate effect on protein quality. Small decreases in the

TABLE 3-13. Amino Acid Content of Whole Wheat and Milled fractions (g/16 g N)

	Whole Wheat	Milled Fractions			
		Patent Flour	Clear Flour	Bran	Germ
Isoleucine	3.8	3.9	4.0	3.5	3.5
Leucine	6.7	6.7	6.7	6.0	6.2
Lysine	2.7	1.9	2.0	4.0	5.4
Methionine	1.7	1.8	1.8	1.6	2.0
Cystine	2.2	2.3	2.1	2.0	1.7
Phenylalanine	4.6	4.9	5.0	3.9	3.8
Tyrosine	3.1	2.9	3.2	2.8	2.8
Threonine	2.9	2.7	2.7	3.3	3.7
Tryptophan	1.2	1.0	1.0	1.6	1.1
Valine	4.7	4.3	4.5	5.0	5.1
Total Essential Amino Acids	33.6	32.4	33.0	33.7	35.3
Arginine	4.6	3.6	4.0	7.0	7.4
Histidine	2.2	2.0	2.0	2.6	2.5
Alanine	3.5	2.8	2.9	4.9	5.7
Aspartic acid	5.0	3.9	4.0	7.2	7.9
Glutamic acid	30.6	34.3	35.0	18.6	16.4
Glycine	3.9	3.2	3.4	7.1	5.6
Proline	9.8	11.7	11.6	5.9	5.3
Serine	4.8	4.9	5.1	4.5	4.5
N (g/100g)	2.6	2.3	2.9	2.9	4.5

Source: After Chung and Pomeranz (1985*a*).

TABLE 3-14. Vitamin Concentration in Wheats and Flours

	Hard Red Wheat (dry weight) μg/g	Flour (% of wheat)	Durum Wheat (dry weight, μg/g)	Semolina (% of wheat)	Soft Wheat, (dry weight, μg/g)	Patent Flour (% of wheat)	Straight-Grade Flour (% of wheat)
Thiamine	5.7	23	6.7	48	5.4	23	39
Riboflavin	1.2	34	1.1	88	1.1	29	40
Niacin							
Total	74	28	111	35	72	14	17
Free	36	44	47	47	38	15	21
Vitamin B₆	3.5	15	4.3	28	3.3	10	14
Tocopherols	58	11	58	43	54	6	—

Source: Adapted from Toepfer et al. (1972).

**TABLE 3-15. Dietary Fiber Content of
Cereals and Cereals Products (g/100 g)**

	Extraction Rate (%)	
	66	100
Wheat	2.4	11.5
Rice	1.1	16.9
Corn	4.9	9.4
Barley	7.9	18.6
Oats	7.6	13.9
Rye	7.1	14.6

Source: Adapted from Nyman et al. (1984).
Note: Dietary fiber is expressed as the sum
of nonstarch polysaccharides and lignin.

crust are presumed to be a result of the Maillard reaction. The brown color of baked bread and of some breakfast cereals is caused by this reaction. An estimated loss of lysine from 10% to 30% occurs on baking bread and a slightly larger loss occurs when bread is toasted. Toasting leads to a greater loss in proteins and vitamins. Since the application of heat removes moisture, toast is a more concentrated source of calories than bread.

The composition of bread will vary depending on the type of flour from which it is baked as well as on the proportion of the original grain present. Table 3-16 shows the nutrient composition of white, brown, and whole meal breads. All breads contain nearly half their weight as starch, 40% as water, 8–10% as protein and 2% as fat. Protein provides about 13% of the energy value of white bread and about 16% of that of whole meal and brown bread. It can be seen that all types of bread are significant sources of protein with only minor differences between the three bread types. Therefore, bread should not be considered merely as a source of dietary energy. The fat content of white, brown, and whole meal bread is low, with brown and whole meal containing slightly more than white because most of the fat is concentrated in the germ. One difference between breads is in the amount of DF they contain. Whole meal bread provides more than three times the amount that white bread provides, but it should be noted that all types of bread, including white bread, provide useful amounts of DF. Because more white bread than brown or whole meal is eaten at present, white bread is an important source of DF.

Bread is an important source of some vitamins and minerals. The whole bread contains vitamins of the B group, particularly thiamine,

TABLE 3-16. Average Nutrient Composition of Bread
(g/100 g)

	Whole Meal	Brown	White
Water, g	40	40	39
Protein, g	8.8	8.9	7.8
Fat, g	2.7	2.2	1.7
Carbohydrate, g	41.8	44.7	49.7
DF, g	8.5	5.1	2.7
Total energy			
kcal	216	223	233
Kj	918	948	991
Calcium, mg	23	100	100
Iron, mg	2.5	2.5	1.7
Potassium, mg	220	210	100
Magnesium, mg	93	75	26
Phosphorus, mg	230	190	97
Copper, mg	0.27	0.23	0.15
Zinc, mg	2.0	1.6	0.8
Thiamine, mg	0.26	0.24	0.18
Riboflavin, mg	0.06	0.06	0.03
Niacin, mg	3.9	2.9	1.4
B_6, mg	0.14	0.08	0.04
Folic, μg (tot)	39	36	27
Pantothenic, mg	0.6	0.3	0.3
Biotin	6	3	1

and niacin. These vitamins are largely located in the outer layer of the endosperm and in the germ of wheat grains so that their content is higher in whole meal bread than in white. Bread also contributes certain minerals to our diet, notably iron.

There is a large difference in temperature between crumb and crust during baking (crust and crumb temperatures can reach 160°–180°C and 100°C, respectively). Since the stability of nutrients in the two parts of the bread is affected differently, such differences are of great nutritional significance.

Losses of 20–30% of thiamine and riboflavin have been reported in European-type breads (Pomeranz 1987). There is significantly less thiamine and riboflavin in the crust than in the crumb of whole wheat bread. On the other hand, niacin is fairly stable under normal baking conditions. Up to 75% of phytic acid in bread may be destroyed in converting dough to bread. The extent of destruction is affected by the pH of the dough, fermentation time, and baking conditions.

Protein digestibility tends to decrease as fiber content increases in wheat fractions, flours, and selected breads. Nitrogen digestibility is lowest for fractions containing the most fiber and highest for low-fiber fractions, such as white flour. Although whole wheat bread has a more favorable amino acid profile, the diminished protein digestibility of the bran protein is reflected in the fact that its protein efficiency ratio (PER) or quality is not significantly different from that of white bread (Table 3–17). A review of several rat studies showed, however, that the protein quality of white bread improves when the bread is supplemented with amino acids such as lysine and threonine (Betschart 1978).

A decrease in the limiting amino acids lysine, threonine, and methionine, especially in the crust, has been reported. Such decrease, substantially reducing the biological value of the proteins, was accompanied by a substantial reduction of polyunsaturated fatty acids of fat in the crust. Consequently, the biological value of proteins in the crust is considerably below that in the crumb. Apparently, less impairment in biological value of cereal proteins and less reduction in available lysine content occur in bread baked by high frequency than in conventional ovens.

Medical debate continues on the merits of DF, but there is now general agreement that cereal fiber is particularly effective in preventing constipation and of benefit in the treatment of the diseases aggravated by constipation. This experience may have contributed to the recent slight rise in the consumption of brown and whole meal breads recorded in the National Food Survey for the total sample and for different sections of the population.

Bread supplies a significant proportion of the nutrients required for growth and maintenance of health and well-being. Although not an outstandingly good source of any single nutrient, bread is a good source of most nutrients.

Extrusion.   Cereals can be processed into foods by extrusion; regular extrusion is used primarily for the production of pasta. More recently,

TABLE 3-17. Protein Content and Quality of Breads

	Nitrogen[a] (%)	Protein[a] (%)	PER (adjusted)
Enriched white	2.5	14.5	0.78
Whole wheat	2.9	16.3	0.72
Seven grains	2.6	14.8	0.98
Wheat germ	2.8	16.0	0.96

Source: After Betschart (1988).

[a] Percent moisture-free basis.

high-temperature short-time extrusion has been used extensively to produce instant and infant and baby food, breakfast cereals and snacks, pasta from nonwheat flours, crisp-bread products, dietetic foods, and modified starches.

Pasta manufacturing.   Manufacturing pasta from wheat is an ancient practice followed in many countries where wheat is grown. It is usually made from a dough consisting of coarse particles of endosperm (durum wheat semolina), which is shaped in various forms by forcing it under pressure through dies of an extrusion auger and then dried. The dried material is cooked in water and served with sauces and flavoring agents. Nutrients may be dissolved out of pasta during boiling, the loss depending on the quantity of water, the duration of boiling, and the kind of wheat used in making the pasta.

Because of its hardness and tenacity, durum wheat is the basic raw material for the production of high-quality pasta products that do not disintegrate readily on boiling. Semolina from durum wheat requires less water to form a dough and produces a translucent product of good cooking and eating properties. A variety of pasta products can be manufactured, however, from a wide range of wheats milled to various granulations without affecting the nutritive value (Mariani-Costantini 1988). The nutrient composition of pasta depends on the ingredients used in the preparation of the dough (eggs, gluten, cheese, vegetables).

Pasta production is accompanied by starch gelatinization. Protein quality and quantity are also significant factors affecting the cooking quality of spaghetti, particularly with respect to the maintenance of firmness and cooking quality (Grzybowski and Donnelly 1979). Various proteins (soy, pea, broad bean) can be used to produce high-protein pasta products with greatly improved nutritive value.

The nutrient concentration of common pasta does not reflect that of durum wheat, although pasta and semolina are similar in nutrient composition (Douglass and Matthews 1982). Although the differences between semolina and pasta are relatively small, it is important to note the large increase in reducing sugars during pasta manufacturing, reported by Lintas and D'Appolonia (1973) to be an index of the changes in carbohydrate composition during extrusion.

With regard to the protein quality, lysine is pasta's limiting amino acid. Data by Cubadda et al. (1968) show that the reduced bioavailability of lysine in pasta is related to drying temperatures. However, the pasta sauces or the variety of other ingredients in the diet might compensate for the reduced availability of the amino acid that was limiting in the raw product. Pasta, along with other cereal products may make a consistent contribution to total dietary fiber.

In relation to human gluten intolerance, recent research on wheat gliadin has demonstrated that peptides derived from durum (or tetraploid) wheat gliadin are less toxic than peptides from soft wheat (hexaploid) wheat. Such lack of toxicity seems to be related to intrinsic structural differences between durum and soft wheat gliadins (Mariani-Costantini 1988).

Extrusion cooking. As in other heat processes, protein nutritional value may be diminished due to the Maillard reaction, especially when reducing sugars are included in the ingredients or formed during the process. Lysine is by far the most reactive amino acid and is also a limiting amino acid in cereals. Thus, lysine retention in extruded products is especially important.

Processing in extruders can be performed with sufficient inactivation of protease inhibitors and while retaining good nutritional value. Under carefully selected and controlled process conditions, good retention of lysine and a good overall protein nutritional value can be obtained in extruded products.

By extrusion cooking starch can be completely gelatinized and made readily available for amylase degradation with depolimerization, a factor of importance for the glycemic and hormone response (Asp 1986). Enzyme inhibitors can be sufficiently inactivated to avoid blocking of enzymatic activities during digestion.

Cereals are an important source of B vitamins in the human diet, which makes the fate of these vitamins during extrusion cooking particularly important. Within the B complex, thiamine seems to be most sensitive to processing whereas the other vitamins are comparatively stable. Extrusion conditions that improve retention of one vitamin may increase destruction of another. Under extrusion conditions suitable for producing breakfast cereals, the loss of thiamine and riboflavin was 90% and 50%, respectively (Asp 1986).

Linko et al. (1981) reviewed the effect of extrusion cooking on protein digestibility and nutritional quality. Although moderate heat treatment improves enzymatic hydrolysis of protein, extremely high temperatures are likely to decrease cystine and diminish the availability of lysine. For example, pepsin hydrolysis of extruded corn and durum wheat semolina and of wheat flour increased with temperatures up to 225°C at 14% moisture and decreased at higher initial moisture levels. These data emphasize the importance of moisture-temperature interactions. In general, PER is not adversely affected by conventional extrusion cooking.

RICE

Characteristics and Composition

Rice is the staple food of about half of the human race. It provides over one fifth of the total food calories consumed by the people of the world. Most rice is produced in the Far East and is consumed primarily within the borders of the producing countries.

The caryopsis of rice is harvested with the hull or husk attached. This is called *paddy* or *rough rice*. The hulls, which represent about 20% of the weight of rough rice, are high in cellulose (30%), lignin (20%), pentosans (20%), and ash (21%) with smaller amounts of protein (3%) and fat (2%). In addition, they contain vitamins. The ash is about 95% silica.

Brown rice, rice after the hull is removed, has the same gross structure of that of the other cereals. Brown rice consists of a pericarp (about 2%), seed coat and aleurone (5%), germ (2–3%), and endosperm (89–94%). When brown rice is subjected to further milling, the bran, aleurone layer, and germ are removed, and the purified endosperms are marketed as *white rice* or *polished rice*.

Rice bran (8%) and polish (2%) are by-products from rice milling. The bran is the outer layers of the pericarp from brown rice; the polish is the inner layers, containing aleurone cells and small amounts of starchy endosperm. The general composition of the two fractions is shown in Table 3–18. In addition to the values shown, bran ash is high in magnesium, potassium, and phosphorus. The bran is also an excellent source of B vitamins (thiamine 10.6; riboflavin 5.7; niacin 309; and pyridoxine 19.2 $\mu g/g$) and vitamin E but contains little or no vitamins A, C, or D.

Starch, the major component of rice, is present in the starchy endosperm as compound granules 3–10 μm in size. Protein, the second major component, is present in the endosperm in the form of discrete protein

TABLE 3-18. Composition of Rice Milling Products (by percent)

	Bran	Polish
Protein	12.0	12.0
Fat	13.0	16.0
Ash	10.0	8.0
Carbohydrates	40.0	56.0
Crude fiber	12.0	7.3
Pentosans	10.0	—

Source: Hoseney (1986).

bodies that are 1–4 μm in size. The concentration of nonstarch polysaccharides is higher in the bran and germ fractions than in the starchy endosperm. Brown rice contains about 8% protein, 75% carbohydrates, and small amounts of fat, fiber, and ash. After milling, the protein content of rice is 7% and the carbohydrate content (mainly starch) about 78%. Starch is found primarily in the endosperm; fat, fiber, minerals, and vitamins are concentrated in the aleurone layers and in the germ.

Milling

The objective of rice milling is to remove the hull, bran, and germ with minimum breakage of the starchy endosperm. Rough rice is mechanically dehulled to brown rice which, in turn, is mechanically abrasively milled to remove its bran layers to yield milled rice and bran polish. The rough or paddy rice is cleaned and conveyed to shelling machines that loosen the hulls. The yield of white rice normally varies between 66–70%, based on the weight of rough rice. The effect of milling on the composition and nutritive value of rice is reported in Table 3–19.

Although the milling of rice results in a decrease in the concentration of most of the nutrients (except available carbohydrate), the energy content is only slightly reduced. The reduction in protein content is not reflected in changes in amino acid composition and the lysine content of milled rice is only slightly lower than that in the brown rice.

The commercial milling of rice comprises cleaning, shelling, or dehulling; it is a process in which a part or all of the bran and germ is removed by abrasive scouring or pearling. In brown rice only the hull has been removed. Undermilled rice or unpolished milled rice is rice from which the hulls and all or part of the germ and pericarp have been removed; little of the aleurone layer is removed.

Milling brings about changes in chemical composition, and the degree of milling dictates the amount of nutrients in the residual milled rice. Brown rice has a higher protein, fat, vitamin, and mineral content

TABLE 3-19. Effect of Milling on Rice Composition (by percent)

	Moisture	Protein	Fat	Ash
Brown rice	15.5	7.4	2.3	1.3
Rice bran	13.5	13.2	18.3	8.9
Polished rice	15.5	6.2	0.8	0.6

Source: Pomeranz (1987).

than milled rice and a higher lysine content in its protein. On the other hand, milling removes a large proportion of the phytate, which might adversely affect the utilization of some minerals and trace elements, notably zinc (House et al. 1982). Protein, vitamins, and minerals are present in greater quantities in the bran removed than in the remaining endosperm. However, fiber, which might interfere with mineral as well as protein utilization, is also removed (Resurreccion et al. 1979).

Among cereals, rice has a comparatively high content of essential amino acids and a fairly low content of glutamic acid and other nonessential amino acids (Table 3–2). Lysine, however, is still the first limiting amino acid followed by threonine. Because lysine is higher in the proteins of the bran, germ, and aleurone than in the proteins of the starchy endosperm, the protein in milled rice is nutritionally inferior to that in brown rice. However, milling improves palatability and digestibility of rice. Even though the proteins of milled rice contain less lysine than the protein of brown rice, they still contain more lysine than the proteins of most cereals.

Since the hulls are low in protein, fat, and starch, production of brown rice or milling of rough rice increases their content of those substances. Conversely, the fiber and ash content decreases. Conversion of brown rice to white or polish rice removes about 15% of the protein, 65% of the fat and fiber, and 55% of the minerals (Table 3–19).

Rough rice and brown rice differ little in vitamin content, but conversion of brown rice to white rice decreases the vitamin values considerably. Such losses have been the cause of much interest in the development of practical methods to retain more of the B vitamins in the milled rice kernel. The problem of improving the vitamin content of milled rice has been approached by processing the rice before milling to diffuse the vitamins and other water soluble nutrients from the outer portion of the grain into the endosperm. Processing of rough rice to increase vitamin retention involves parboiling or some similar modification (Bhattacharya and Ali 1985).

Parboiling

Parboiling, the process of heating paddy rice in water and then drying it, has been practiced since ancient times. Although probably started to aid in dehusking (or dehulling), its major advantage is nutritional. As mentioned previously, much of the vitamin and mineral content of rice is concentrated in the outer layers. Parboiling helps to move these nutrients into the kernel.

The process consists of three steps: steeping, steaming, and drying.

The main modifications are transfer of some vitamins and minerals from the aleurone and germ into the starchy endosperm, dispersion of lipids from the aleurone layer and germ, inactivation of enzymes, and destruction of molds and insects.

Parboiling results in inward diffusion of water soluble vitamins to the endosperm. Thus, parboiled milled rice tends to contain a higher amount of B vitamins than does raw milled rice, despite the partial thermal decomposition of thiamine during parboiling (Padua and Juliano 1974). Vitamin content, particularly thiamine, also decreases during grain storage (Pedersen et al. 1989).

The protein content appears on the whole unchanged after parboiling, although free amino acids may increase somewhat. According to Eggum (1979) the digestibility of protein is reduced after parboiling but the biological value is increased, with the result that total usable proteins remain unchanged. On the other hand, Benedito de Barber et al. (1977) found a small (lysine) to considerable (tryptophan and methionine) drop in available amino acids after parboiling.

Parboiling has also been reported to improve the digestibility of rice starch as evidenced by its increased susceptibility to in vitro enzymatic action (Bhattacharya and Ali 1985).

Nutritional Value

The main carbohydrate of rice is starch, comprising up to 90% of the rice solids. In common rice, amylose amounts to 12–35% of the total starch; waxy rices have a much lower amylose content.

Protein composition of milled rice is characteristic among cereals. Rice proteins in fact are low in prolamin and very rich in glutelins (Table 3–8) and have a relatively good amino acid balance (Table 3–2). The high lysine content of rice protein is due primarily to its low prolamin content. Proteins in milled rice are generally lower in lysine than proteins in brown rice. The proportions of albumin and globulin and the total protein are highest in the outer layers of the milled rice kernel and decrease toward the center; proportions of glutelin have an inverse distribution.

The subaleurone region, rich in protein, lies directly beneath the aleurone and is removed rather easily during milling. From a nutritional standpoint, it is therefore desirable to mill rice as lightly as possible to retain some of the protein.

Brown rice contains 2.4–4.0% lipids. The lipid content depends on the variety, degree of maturity, and growth and other conditions. The lipid content of bran is affected by the degree of milling and the milling procedure. The major proportion of the lipid in rice is removed with the bran, which contains the germ (10.1–23.5%) and the polish (9.1–11.5%). The main fatty acids in rice are oleic, linoleic, and palmitic.

Minerals are generally present in higher levels in brown than in milled rice. A considerable portion of the rice caryopsis ash is accounted for by phosphorus. Potassium, magnesium, and silicon are present also in large amounts in brown and milled rice. There is considerably higher concentration of ash and of individual minerals in outer layers of the milled rice kernel than toward the center. Phytate-phosphorus constitutes almost 90% of the total bran phosphorus and 40% of the milled rice phosphorus. From studies conducted by Masironi et al. (1977) milling results in loss of the essential elements zinc and copper but not of cadmium, a toxic pollutant.

Rice and its by-products contain little or no vitamin A, ascorbic acid, or vitamin D. Thiamine, riboflavin, pyridoxine, panthotenic acid, folic acid, and biotin are lower in milled than in brown rice. Vitamins are also present in higher levels in brown than in milled rice (Table 3–6).

The cooking of rice (and even more, the household washing of rice before cooking) leads to a considerable loss of water-soluble nutrients.

To increase the rate of water diffusion into the kernel during cooking, channels must be provided. Several techniques are used to produce quick-cooking rice. One is precooking to about 60% moisture followed by careful drying to 8% moisture. This process allows the rice to maintain a porous structure. Precooking followed by freezing, thawing, and drying or puffing by rapid changes in pressure have also been used to produce quick-cooking rice. In general, anything that opens the kernel and allows the water to penetrate readily decreases cooking time.

CORN

Composition

Corn, the second largest cereal crop in the world, is a staple food for large groups of people in Latin America, Asia, and Africa. In addition to human consumption, corn is used for animal feeding, for the manufacture of starch and is converted into syrups, sweeteners, and industrial spirits. The products of corn milling include grits, meal, flour (corn flour), germ and germ oil, hominy feed, starch, and protein. The breakfast cereal "corn flakes" is made from corn grits.

As human food, corn is prepared in several ways: (1) parched to be eaten whole; (2) ground to make hominy, corn meal, or corn flour; (3)

treated with alkali to remove the pericarp and germ to make lye hominy; and (4) converted to a variety of breakfast cereals and snacks.

Corn is milled by dry or wet processes. The first objective of both processes is to separate the germ from the remainder of the grain in order to extract and recover the germ oil; the oil is a valuable product but can lead to the development of rancidity in the meal.

After degermination, dry milling employs roller mills and plansifters in a process similar to wheat milling whereas wet milling involves steeping and the complete disintegration of the endosperm tissue to recover starch and protein as separate products.

Considerable efforts to develop high-lysine corn varieties with a hard endosperm have led to the development of high-quality protein corn lines with hard endosperm texture and significantly improved nutritional and agronomical properties (Rooney and Serna-Saldivar 1987).

On the basis of kernel characteristics corn is divided into five classes: flint, dent, flour, pop, and sweet. Flint corn has a hard kernel caused by the presence of a large volume of horny endosperm. Flint corn is common in Europe, Asia, and South America. Dent varieties, with significant differences in the ratio of horny to floury endosperm, are grown most widely in the United States and South Africa.

There are also considerable differences in the size, shape, and color of corn kernels as well as in hardness, correlated to differences in the ratio of horny to floury corn (Watson 1987). Hard, flinty corn is generally preferred in many areas of the world and the acceptance of the original high-lysine corn varieties (opaque-2), which have a soft floury endosperm and improved nutritional value, is poor.

The corn kernel contains about 75% starch, 10% protein, 5% fat, fiber, and minerals (Table 3–1). The ash content is around 1.4% and the level of total dietary fiber about 9%. Sugars, present mainly as sucrose, glucose, and fructose, amount to only 1–3% (Watson 1987). The endosperm contains 86–89% starch and about 8% protein. The cells are packed with starch granules embedded in a protein matrix. The starchy endosperm is of two types, floury and horny. The horny endosperm has a thicker protein matrix and thus a higher protein but lower starch content than the floury endosperm. The subaleurone layer contains very small starch granules surrounded by a thick protein matrix. The protein content of this layer is high. The outer layer of the endosperm, the aleurone layer, is a single layer of cells containing protein but no starch. In addition to high quality protein, these cells are rich in minerals and vitamins (Watson 1987).

The germ is high in fat (30–35%) and protein (18–20%). The germ contains about 83% of the total kernel lipids and about 25% of the kernel protein. The ash content is high and corn germ is rich in mineral and trace elements. Approximately 80% of the total kernel minerals are found in the germ as well as a major part of phytate, which may impair the utilization of protein and minerals, especially zinc.

Corn contains only low levels of antinutritional factors, such as trypsin and chymotrypsin inhibitors. Lectins have been shown to be present in corn endosperm and germ (Newberg and Concon 1985).

Dry Milling

Corn grits are equivalent to coarse semolina. The objective of dry milling is to remove the bran and germ and to recover the endosperm in the form of hominy or corn grits, coarse meal, fine meal, and corn flour. Relative yields of mill products depend on whether the main objective is to produce grits or meal and whether the corn was degermed before grinding. The composition of dry milled products is reported in Table 3-20. Grits and meal are largely produced from the horny or vitreous endosperm; they contain less than 1.0% and 1.5% fat, respectively. Flour produced by grinding the starchy endosperm contains more fat (2-3%) and fiber than the grits and meal from broken germ during processing. The large surface area and the relatively high fat content of corn flour lower its shelf life. Degermed products have a variety of uses because their fat and fiber contents are low and consequently have a better shelf life. However, their nutritional quality is inferior because protein content is lower in the milled products than in the whole kernels and the lysine (27-29%) and tryptophan (40%) scores are significantly low in corn grits and meals.

Modern dry milling is performed in tempering-degerming systems. After cleaning, the corn is adjusted to about 20% moisture and placed

TABLE 3-20. Chemical Composition of Corn and Milled Corn Products (% dry basis)

	Yield	Moisture	Protein	Fat	Ash
Corn, grain	100	15.5	9.0	4.5	1.3
Hominy grits	12	14.0	8.4	0.7	0.4
Grits	38	13.0	8.2	0.8	0.5
Cornmeal	6	12.0	7.6	1.1	0.6
Flour	4	12.0	6.6	2.0	0.7
Hominy feed	35	13.0	12.5	6.3	3.3
Germ meal	10	15.0	14.9	18.0	4.7

Source: After Pomeranz (1987).

in a tempering bin. The product is then processed in a degerminator in which the bran (pericarp) and germ are removed from the endosperm by an abrasive action.

The protein content of corn is similar to that of other cereals (10%). Based on the FAO/WHO scoring protein pattern, lysine is the first limiting amino acid followed by tryptophan and threonine. Compared to other cereals, the protein score for corn is fairly low (Table 3–2). About 50% of the protein in the endosperm is represented by zein, lacking lysine and tryptophan and also low in threonine, valine, and sulphur amino acids. On the other hand, corn germ protein has a higher nutritional value than the endosperm because of a much better balance of essential amino acids.

The mutant opaque-2 discovered by Mertz et al. (1964) has a reduced level of zein, elevated quantities of other fractions, and hence increased levels of lysine and tryptophan and a better nutritional quality.

The nutrient composition of different types of corn flour is strongly affected by the extent to which bran and germ have been removed and is determined by the relative proportion of the different grain tissues.

To study the effect of milling on composition and nutritive value of corn, whole meal and corn flour from degermed grits were compared (Pedersen et al. 1989). Relevant differences in nutrients and DF content were observed (Table 3–1). In degermed flour the content of fat and minerals was reduced to about 28% of corresponding levels in whole corn. The content of DF was also greatly reduced, from 9.3% in wholemeal to 3.9% in degermed flour. The soluble DF fraction was small (0.5%) in all products. The protein content of degermed corn was reduced to 88% of the level in the whole corn kernel.

Milling also alters protein content and quality. In comparing whole meal and corn flour, a pronounced reduction in lysine and tryptophan, caused by degerming, was observed.

The concentration of minerals and trace elements is lower in corn than in other cereals (Table 3–6). A major proportion of the nutritionally important minerals as well as phytate is present in the germ and the content of minerals and phytate in corn products is largely determined by the extent to which the germ is retained. Like other cereals, corn is low in calcium and about 80% of the phosphorus in corn is in the form of phytate. Iron absorption has been reported to be low in corn and cornmeal seems to be a relatively poor source of available iron. Zinc availability in whole corn also appears to be relatively low, while zinc from raw endosperm seems to be highly available.

With respect to the effect of milling on the content of minerals in corn products, degerming strongly reduces the mineral content of corn (the content of zinc was reduced to one-fifth and that of calcium, iron, and copper more than halved). Phytate-phosphorus represented 80% of the total phosphorus in whole corn; in degermed corn only traces were left.

Nutritional Value

Even without milling, corn is deficient in a number of essential nutrients; removing bran and germ fractions enhances such deficiencies. The deficiency disease pellagra is commonly found in areas heavily dependent on corn as a staple food. The bound niacin in corn is liberated during alkali cooking. In Central and South America, where legumes are consumed along with lime-treated corn, pellagra is not a common problem.

Yellow corn is the only grain that contains useful quantities of carotenes. Carotenoid pigments are mostly concentrated in the horny and floury endosperm of yellow corn while they are nearly absent in white corn. They are easily destroyed and are reduced during prolonged storage. In addition to vitamin A, corn contains some or all of the important B vitamins, with the exception of vitamin B_{12}. Corn is also a good source of vitamin E. The degree of milling has a pronounced effect on the vitamin content of corn flours and degerming strongly reduces its vitamin content.

Interpretation of data on vitamin content is complicated by the fact that some of the vitamins are present in a bound form that may not be completely available and adequate information on the availability of vitamins is lacking.

Alkali cooking improves flavor, starch gelatinization, and water uptake and partially removes the germ and pericarp of the corn kernel. Dry matter losses during traditional tortilla processing are estimated at 8–17% of the original grain. A considerable variation in the composition and content of nutrients in tortillas has been reported (Ranhotra 1985).

Corn processing using a lime cooking step, as in the preparation of tortillas in Mexico and other Latin American countries, has been shown to improve niacin availability (Rooney and Serna Saldivar 1987). However, losses of vitamins during alkali cooking are considerable (up to 60%, 52%, and 32% for thiamine, riboflavin, and niacin, respectively).

The alkali peeled corn is made into a dough by grinding on a metate. The dough, *masa*, is made into bread by frying or baking on both sides on a hot griddle; the thin, leathery corn cakes are known as tortillas. Alkaline treatment of foods induces the hydrolysis of arginine and guanido groups to give ornithine residues, destruction of some amino acids, elimination of certain side chains to give olefinic compounds, and formation of unusual amino acids such as lysinoalanine.

The calcium content is significantly increased during processing and such increase is of considerable interest in diets. However, calcium hydroxide residues remaining from the lime treatment may negatively affect the utilization of other nutrients (e.g., iron) (Pedersen et al. 1989).

Khan and Eggum (1978) have shown that baking had no effect on true protein digestibility, but lysine was slightly reduced and the biological value of the protein lowered when corn flour was baked into unleavened bread.

Processing increases the rate of starch digestion and new methods of processing, such as extrusion cooking, have been shown to increase the rate of corn starch digestion. Resistant starch, formed in small amounts during processing, largely escapes digestion (Englyst and Cummings 1985).

Corn has received particular interest because of its potential as a source of DF that shows a high resistance to digestion in the small intestine and colon.

BARLEY

Barley is principally used as feed for animals, as barley meal, for malting and brewing beer, and for distilling whisky. Most barley for human consumption is pot barley or pearl barley. Pot and pearl barley are both manufactured by carefully removing the hull and outer portions of the barley kernel by abrasive action. The pearling or decortication process used to produce pot barley is merely carried out further to produce pearl barley; barley flour is a secondary product, used in baby foods and breakfast cereals. The composition of barley products obtained in pearling barley is compared in Table 3–21.

TABLE 3-21. Composition of Barley Milling Products (by percent)

	Moisture	Protein	Fat	NFE[a]	Ash
Dehulled barley	12.5	10.6	1.7	72.1	1.5
Pearls	12.5	7.8	1.0	76.2	1.1
Pearling dust	12.5	9.5	1.4	74.3	1.5
Feedmeal	12.0	12.5	2.0	64.0	3.5
Bran	10.5	14.0	3.5	57.1	4.9
Husks	10.4	3.6	1.0	49.2	7.2

Source: Pomeranz (1987).

[a] Nitrogen-free extract.

Composition

Barley is surrounded by a husk, which is not separated during thresh-ing. The hull fraction (husk, pericarp, and testa) comprises 7–25% of the kernel by weight and varies in accordance with morphological and agricultural characteristics.

Starch is the major constituent of barley followed by dietary fiber, protein, fat, free sugars, and ash (Table 3–1). In barley varieties suitable for malting, starch is higher and dietary fiber lower, consequently di-gestible energy is higher than in conventional barley varieties. Starch comprises about 50–68% of kernel dry matter. Starch, located in the en-dosperm, consists of two types of glucose polymers: amylose, a linear polymer, and amylopectin, a branched polymer in the proportions of amylose 22–30% and amylopectin 70–78%. In high-amylose types, amy-lose contents of 41–47% have been found whereas for the waxy (high amylopectin) types amylose contents as low as 2–8% have been found. The amylose/amylopectin ratio determines the uptake of water and consistency after cooking. A high amylopectin content gives rise to soft and gelatinous products with a high water content, whereas a high amy-lose content results in a drier, harder product.

Mature barley may contain over 2% of fructosans. Unlike starch, which is restricted to the starchy endosperm, fructosans are distributed throughout the grain. Sucrose is virtually restricted to the embryo and aleurone layer; it represents 12–15% of the embryo but only 1–2% of the whole grain. Raffinose is also a major embryo constituent, about 5% of the dry weight.

In the fiber fraction of whole grain, hemicelluloses (arabinoxylans) amount to 40%, cellulose to 27% and beta-glucans to 25%. Mixed linked beta-glucans are an important constituent of endosperm and aleurone cell walls. The beta-glucans account for approximately 75% of the endo-sperm wall.

Lysine is the limiting factor for an optimal utilization of barley pro-teins (Table 3–2). Most barley is harvested with the husk (about 10% of the kernel) intact. In general, the husk is low in protein but its proteins are relatively high in lysine. The endosperm is relatively high in glu-tamic acid (35%) and proline (12%), with about 3.2% lysine, higher than in most cereals.

Protein content is highest in the germ (35%) and lowest in the husk (2–3%) with aleurone and starchy endosperm having intermediate con-tents (16%). However, husk, germ, and aleurone tissue have a higher lysine and threonine and a lower glutamic acid and proline content than the starchy endosperm.

Barley lipid content accounts for about 2–4% of dry matter and is composed mainly of triglycerides with a high proportion of palmitic, oleic, and linoleic acids and with the unsaturated components accounting for nearly 80% of the total fat. In the embryo the lipid content might amount to 15–20% (Bhatty and Rossnagel 1980).

The main minerals in barley are phosphorus and potassium, with relatively less calcium, sodium, and magnesium (Lin et al. 1974). The mineral concentration in germ and aleurone cell tissues are substantially higher than in the endosperm (Weaver et al. 1981).

Milling

Barley may be blocked, pearled, flaked, or milled into different flours for human consumption. Blocking removes the husk (palea and lemma) and pearling is an extension of this process proceeding until pericarp, testa, and aleurone layer have been removed. The husk, pericarp, and testa are relatively easy to remove by pearling, but it is more difficult to separate the aleurone cells from the endosperm.

Hemicelluloses (arabinoxylans), cellulose, and lignin are concentrated in the external layers of the kernel and beta-glucans in the low extraction, endosperm rich flour (64.5%).

When barley is milled to flour, protein, dietary fiber, fat, and minerals are reduced while starch and sugars increase (Table 3–22). In the most refined flours (70% extraction) protein content is reduced to 82% of that of the whole grain flour, minerals to 50% and dietary fiber to 44% (Pedersen et al. 1989). The reduction in dietary fiber is significant, particularly of the insoluble fraction, while soluble DF is kept constant, irrespective of extraction rate. Since soluble DF in barley primarily contains soluble beta-glucans, their level is considerable as the endosperm cell walls contribute most of the beta-glucans in the grain. Compared to the concentration in the whole barley kernel, phosphorus, potassium, magnesium, calcium, sodium, iron, manganese, copper, aluminum, and

TABLE 3-22. Chemical Composition of Milled Barley Products (% dry matter)

	Moisture	Protein	Fat	Ash
Pearl barley	10.8	8.7	1.0	1.2
Barley flour	10.0	10.2	1.7	1.2
Barley husk	10.4	1.4	0.3	5.6
Barley bran	10.0	14.9	3.6	5.0
Barley dust	13.0	11.8	2.2	3.2

Source: After Kent (1966).

molybdenum are all low in the endosperm and fractionated flours produced either by milling or by hand dissection (Lin et al. 1974). The phytate content decreases strongly with a low rate of extraction and in the most refined flours only traces of phytate are left.

Pearl barley contains about 1.2, 0.35, and 25 μg/g of thiamine, riboflavin, and nicotinic acid, respectively.

The importance of barley as a food grain has declined during the last century, particularly when compared with wheat. However, because of the renewed interest in DF as an important factor in health and disease, the future of barley might look brighter than in the past. With respect to wheat, DF levels, irrespective of extraction rate, are higher in barley than in wheat.

OATS

Composition

Oat products are milled to provide oatmeal for porridge and oatcake, rolled oats for porridge, oat flour for baby foods and ready-to-eat breakfast cereals.

Oats are harvested with their hulls on. The hulls represent about 25% of the total weight. After they are removed, the oats are called groats. Oat groats are higher in fat and protein than are most other cereals. They are also a good source of several enzymes. The most troublesome of these is a very active lipase system; unless the lipase system is denatured, milled products have a very short shelf life.

Oat milling is a major industry for the production of breakfast cereals. Rolled oats and oatmeal are high in protein, fat, and energy value and are rich sources of calcium, phosphorus, iron, and thiamine. They have a high nutritive value because they are made from oat groats, which are obtained by removing the fibrous hull and adhering portions from oat grain. Groats correspond to the caryopsis of wheat; the bulk of the bran, the aleurone layer, and the germ, which are rich in proteins, vitamins, and minerals, remain with the portion used as food. Hence, rolled oats and oatmeal, like brown rice, are essentially whole grain products from a nutritional standpoint. Typical composition of oats and oat products are given in Table 3–1.

Oat proteins are nutritionally superior to the other cereal proteins because of their relatively high lysine content. Even though lysine is the first limiting amino acid in oat proteins, the lysine score is still higher in oat endosperm than in that of wheat, corn, or barley (Table 3–2).

Antinutritional factors in oats are either unknown or of little consequence. A trypsin inhibitor found in oat flour was inactivated by heat and by treatment with pepsin and is of little nutritional significance (Chung and Pomeranz 1985*b*).

Nutritional Value

Results of human studies indicate that oat protein has a higher nutritive value than most other cereal proteins. The protein of oats is uniquely different from that of other cereals in that the major protein fraction is represented by the salt soluble globulin fraction (Table 3–8). The alcohol soluble prolamins are only 10–15% of the total protein, with the glutelins making up about 20–25%. The high percentage of globulin is probably the primary reason for the better protein nutritive value of oats. This higher nutritive value is believed to be the result of the higher level of lysine in the globulin fraction than in the glutelin and prolamine fractions. Oats are unique among cereals in that their amino acid balance is quite good from a nutritional standpoint (Table 3–2). In addition, the protein content of oat groats is much higher than that found for other cereals.

A comparison of the biological value of oat protein and the protein of other cereal grains is given in Table 3–2. The protein quality of oats is second only to that of the genetically modified opaque-2 corn. Oats also have the highest protein level of any of the grains.

The lipid content of oats is generally higher than that of other cereals but also varies widely. Values as low as 3% and as high as 12% have been reported. Most lines contain 5–9% lipids. Oats are also unique in that most of the groat lipid (80%) is in the endosperm instead of the germ and bran. Oat lipids have more oleic acid than most other cereals (Table 3–4). Oats contain only about 2–3 mg of tocopherols per 100 g of grain, somewhat lower than the levels in wheat and barley. However, oats are known for their antioxidant activity, which appears to be the result of a series of phenolic compounds. The antioxidant activity, related to the content of caffeic acid, is of the same order as that of the synthetic antioxidants BHT and prophyl gallate.

Although there have been few nutritional studies on the value of oat lipid, the high content of oleic and linoleic acid, the resulting favorable polyunsaturated/saturated fatty acid ratio of 2.2/1, and the accompanying lipid-soluble antioxidant properties all stress the importance of oats in the diet.

The nutritional focal point of oat carbohydrates rests primarily with the high beta-glucan or gum content.

Oats are a good source of manganese, magnesium, and iron, as well

TABLE 3-23.   Mineral Distribution Within the Groats

	Bran	Endosperm
Phosphorus (%)	1.02	0.26
Calcium (%)	0.11	0.10
Potassium (%)	1.00	0.16
Magnesium (%)	0.38	0.07
Manganese (mg/kg)	88	31
Iron (mg/kg)	90	18
Zinc (mg/kg)	58	24

as calcium, zinc, and copper. The micronutrient content of oats is not evenly distributed throughout the groat. To determine the relative distribution of these constituents, Peterson et al. (1975) hand dissected samples of groats into their component parts and assayed each part for its mineral content. Their results (Table 3–23) demonstrate that the mineral components of the groat are concentrated in the outer bran fraction. Since oats are generally consumed as whole grains, including the bran fraction, milling does not alter the relative content of the mineral components (Lockhart and Hurt 1986).

In mature grains, phytate accounts for 60–80% of the total phosphorus. Furthermore, phytase has a much lower activity in oats than in rye or wheat.

The vitamin content of groats and rolled oats are presented in Table 3–5. As noted, they contribute a small but significant amount of vitamins to the diet. Little research has been done on the relative distribution of vitamins in the oat kernel. It has been observed that the hull and endosperm of oats contain little thiamine, whereas the major portion of the vitamin content is located in the outer bran fraction. Since oats are generally eaten as a whole grain, the consumer gets the benefits of the nutrients in the bran.

REFERENCES

Asp, N.-G. 1986. Effects of extrusion-cooking on the nutritional value of foods. In *Pasta and Extrusion-Cooked Foods,* Chr. Mercier and C. Cantarelli, eds., pp. 9–13. Tecnoalimenti Food and Nutrition Technology Series 1.

Benedito de Barber, C., J. Martinez, and S. Barber. 1977. Effects of parboiling on the chemical and nutritional characteristics of rice bran. In *Rice By-Products Utilization,* vol. IV, S. Barber and E. Tortosa, eds., pp. 121–130. Valencia, Spain: Int. Agroquimica Tecnol. Alimentos.

Betschart, A. A. 1978. Improving protein quality in bread. Nutritional benefits and realities. *Adv. Exp. Med. Biol.* **105**:703-734.

Betschart, A. A. 1988. Nutritional quality of wheat and wheat foods. In *Wheat: Chemistry and Technology,* vol. II, Y. Pomeranz, ed., pp. 91-130. St. Paul, Minn.: AACC.

Bhattacharya, K. R., and S. Z. Ali. 1985. Changes in rice during parboiling and properties of parboiled rice. *Adv. Cereal Sci. Technol.* **7**:105-167.

Bhatty, R. S., and B. G. Rossnagel. 1980. Lipid and fatty acid composition of Riso 1508 and normal barley. *Cereal Chem.* **57**:382-386.

Bjorck, I., M. Nyman, and N.-G. Asp. 1984. Extrusion cooking and DF: effects on DF content and on degradation in the rat intestinal tract. *Cereal Chem.* **61**:174-179.

Bodwell, C. E. 1985. Aminoacid content as an estimate of protein quality for humans. In *Digestibility and Aminoacid Availability in Cereals and Oilseeds,* J. W. Finley and D. T. Hopkins, eds., pp. 1-14. St. Paul, MN: AACC.

Chung, O. K., and Y. Pomeranz. 1985a. Aminoacids in cereal proteins and protein fractions. In *Digestibility and Aminoacid Availability in Cereals and Oilseeds,* J. W. Finley and D. T. Hopkins, eds., pp. 65-108. St. Paul, MN: AACC.

Chung, O. K., and Y. Pomeranz. 1985b. Functional and nutritional characteristics of cereal proteins. In *Digestibility and Aminoacid Availability in Cereals and Oilseeds,* J. W. Finley and D. T. Hopkins, eds., pp. 169-231. St. Paul, MN: AACC.

Cubadda, R., G. Fabriani, and P. Resmini. 1968. Variazioni della lisina utilizzabile nelle paste alimentari indotte dai processi tecnologici di essiccamento. *Quad. Nutr.* **28**:199-208.

Davis, K. R., R. F. Cain, L. J. Peters, D. LeTourneau, and J. McGinnis. 1981. Evaluation of the nutrient composition of wheat. II. Proximate analysis, thiamine, riboflavin, niacin and pyridoxine. *Cereal Chem.* **58**:116-120.

Davis, K. R., L. J. Peters, R. F. Cain, D. LeTourneau, and J. McGinnis. 1984. Evaluation of the nutrient composition of wheat. III. Minerals. *Cereal Foods World* **29**:246-248.

Douglass, J. S., and R. H. Matthews. 1982. Nutrient content of pasta products. *Cereals Food World* **27**:558-561.

Eggum, B. O. 1979. The nutritional value of rice in comparison with other cereals. In *Chemical Aspects of Rice Grain Quality,* pp. 91-111. Los Banos, Philippines: Int. Rice Res. Inst.

Englyst, H. N., and J. H. Cummings. 1985. Digestion of the polysaccharides of some cereal foods in the human small intestine. *Am. J. Clin. Nutr.* **42**:778-787.

Englyst, H. N., V. Anderson, and J. H. Cummings. 1983. Starch and non-starch polysaccharides in some cereal foods. *J. Sci. Food Agric.* **34**:1434-1440.

FAO 1987-89. *FAO Production Yearbooks.* Rome: Food and Agriculture Organization.

Ferretti, R. J., and D. A. Levander. 1974. Effect of milling and processing on the selenium content of grains and cereal products. *J. Agr. Food Chem.* **22**:1049-1051.

Graham, G. G. 1977. Factors affecting the human nutritional value of cereals grains. In *Nutritional Evaluation of Cereal Mutants,* pp. 1-12. Vienna: IAEA.

Grzybowski, R. A., and B. J. Donnelly. 1979. Cooking properties of spaghetti: factors affecting cooking quality. *J. Agric. Food Chem.* **27**:380.

Hoseney, R. Carl. 1986. Rice, oat, and barley processing. In *Principles of Cereal Science and Technology*, pp. 167–183, St. Paul, MN: AACC.

House, W. A., R. M. Welch, and D. R. van Campen. 1982. Effect of phytic acid on the absorption, contribution and endogenous excretion of zinc in rats. *J. Nutr.* **112**:941–953.

Jones, J. M. 1971. Trace elements in human nutrition: The contribution cereals. *Cereal Foods World* **22**:573–574.

Kasper, H., V. Rabast, H. Fassel, and F. Fehle. 1979. The effect of DF on post-prandial serum vitamin A concentration in man. *Am. J. Clin. Nutr.* **32**:1847–1849.

Keagy, P. M., B. Borenstein, P. Ranum, M. A. Connor, K. Lorenz, W. E. Hobbs, G. Hill, A. L. Bachman, W. A. Boyd, and K. Kulp. 1980. Natural levels of nutrients in commercially milled wheat flours. II. Vitamin analysis. *Cereal Chem.* **57**:59–65.

Kent, N. L. 1966. Barley: Processing, nutritional attributes, technological uses. In *Technology of Cereals*, pp. 198–210. London: Pergamon Press.

Khan, M. K., and B. O. Eggum. 1978. Effect of baking on the nutritive value of Pakistani bread. *J. Sci. Food Agric.* **29**:1069–1075.

Lin, D. J., G. S. Robbins, and Y. Pomeranz. 1974. Composition and utilization of milled barley products. 4: Mineral composition. *Cereal Chem.* **51**:309–316.

Linko, P., P. Colonna, and C. Mercier. 1981. HTST extrusion cooking. In *Advances in Cereal Science and Technology*, vol. IV, Y. Pomeranz, ed., pp. 145–235. St. Paul, MN.: AACC.

Lintas, C., and B. L. D'Appolonia. 1973. Effect of spaghetti processing on semolina carbohydrate. *Cereal Chem.* **50**:563–570.

Lockhart, H. B., and H. D. Hurt. 1986. Nutrition of oats. In *Oats: Chemistry and Technology*, F. H. Webster, ed., pp. 297–308, St. Paul, Minn.: AACC.

Lorenz, K. 1978. Selenium in wheats and commercial wheat flour. *Cereal Chem.* **55**:287–294.

Lorenz, K., R. Loewe, D. Weadon, and W. Wolf. 1980. Natural levels of nutrients in commercially milled wheat flours. III. Mineral analysis. *Cereal Chem.* **57**:65–69.

Mahoney, A. W. 1982. Mineral contents of selected cereals and baked products. *Cereal Foods World* **27**:147–150.

Mariani-Costantini, A. 1988. Image and nutritional role of pasta in changing food patterns. In *Durum Wheat: Chemistry and Technology*, G. Fabriani and C. Lintas, eds., pp. 283–302. St. Paul, MN: AACC.

Masironi, R., S. R. Koirtyohann, and T. O. Pierce. 1977. Zinc, copper, cadmium, and chromium in polished and unpolished rice. *Sci. Total Environment* **7**:27–43.

Mertz, E. T., L. S. Bates, and O. E. Nelson. 1964. Mutant gene that changes protein composition and increases lysine content of maize endosperm. *Science* **145**:279–280.

Neri, V. 1986. L'alimentazione povera nell'Italia romana. In *Atti del Convegno l'Alimentazione nell'antichita*. Parma.

Newberg, D. S., and J. M. Concon. 1985. Lectins in rice and corn endosperm. *J. Agric. Food Chem.* **33**:685–687.

Nyman, M., M. Siljestrom, B. Pedersen, K. E. Bach Knudsen, N.-G. Asp, C.-G. Johansson, and B. O. Eggum. 1984. DF content and composition of six cereals at different extraction rates. *Cereal Chem.* **61**:14–19.

O'Dell, B. L., A. R. de Boland, and S. R. Koirtyohann. 1972. Distribution of phytate and nutritionally important elements among the morphological components of cereal grains. *J. Agric. Food Chem.* **20**(3):718–721.

Padua, A. B., and B. O. Juliano. 1974. Effect of parboiling on thiamine, protein and fat of rice. *J. Sci. Food Agric.* **25**:697–701.

Pedersen, B., and B. O. Eggum. 1983. The influence of milling on the nutritive value of flour from cereal grains. 2. Wheat. *Qual. Plant. Plant Foods Human Nutrition* **33**:51–61.

Pedersen, B., E. B. Knudsen, and B. O. Eggum. 1989. Nutritive value of cereal products with emphasis on the effect of milling. In *Nutritional value of cereal products, beans and starches*, G. H. Bourne, ed. World Rev. Nutr. Diet. vol. 60, pp. 1–91. Basel: Karger.

Peterson, D. M., J. Senturia, V. L. Youngs, and L. E. Schrader. 1975. Elemental composition of oat groats. *J. Agric. Food Chem.* **23**:9–13.

Pomeranz, Y. 1987. Bread in health and disease. In *Modern Cereal Science and Technology*, pp. 350–370. St. Paul, MN: AACC.

Pomeranz, Y. 1988. Chemical composition of kernel structure. In *Wheat: Chemistry and Technology*, vol. I, Y. Pomeranz, ed., pp. 97–158. St. Paul, MN: AACC.

Ranhotra, G. S. 1985. Nutritional profile of corn and flour tortillas. *Cereal Foods World* **30**:703–704.

Reddy, N. R., S. K. Sathe, and D. K. Salunkhe. 1982. Phytates in legumes and cereals. *Adv. Food Res.* **28**:1–92.

Resurreccion, A. P., B. O. Juliano, and Y. Tanaka. 1979. Nutrient content and distribution in milling fractions of rice grain. *J. Sci. Food Agric.* **30**:475–481.

Rooney, L. W., and S. O. Serna-Saldivar. 1987. Food uses of whole corn and dry-milled fractions. In *Corn: Cereal chemistry and technology*, pp. 399–429. St. Paul, MN: AACC.

Selvendran, R. R. 1984. The plant cell wall as a source of DF: Chemistry and structure. *Am. J. Clin. Nutr.* **39**:320–337.

Theander, O. 1983. Advances in the chemical characterization and analytical determination of DF components. In *Dietary Fibre*, G. G. Birch and K. J. Parker, eds., pp. 77–93. London: Applied Science Publ.

Toepfer, E. W., M. M. Polansky, J. F. Eheart, H. T. Slover, E. R. Morris, F. N. Hepburn, and F. W. Quackenbush. 1972. Nutrient composition of selected wheats and wheat products. XI Summary. *Cereal Chem.* **49**:173.

Van Dokkum, W., A. Wesstra, and F. A. Schippers. 1982. Physiological effects of fiber-rich types of bread. I. The effect of DF from bread on the mineral balance of young men. *Brit. J. Nutr.* **47**:451–460.

Varo, P., R. Laine, and P. Koivistoinen. 1983. The effect of heat treatment on DF: a collaborative study. *J. Assoc. Anal. Chem.* **66**:933–935.

Watson, S. A. 1987. Structure and composition. In *Corn: Chemistry and Technology*, pp. 53–82. St. Paul, MN: AACC.

Weaver, C. M., P. H. Chen, and S. L. Ryneavson. 1981. Effect of milling on trace element and protein content of barley and oats. *Cereal Chem.* **58**:120–124.

Young, V. R., and P. L. Pellett. 1985. Wheat proteins in relation to protein requirements and availability of aminoacids. *Am. J. Clin. Nutr.* **41**:1077–1090.

4

Legumes

Flaminio Fidanza

The edible seeds of leguminous plants (family of Leguminosae) hold an important place in the Mediterranean diet. Of more than 13,000 species, only about twenty of the subfamily Papilionoideae are consumed by humans and even fewer by European Mediterranean people.

Aykroyd and Doughty (1964) produced an excellent history of legumes and we regard it as definitive. In ancient Europe, the only legumes available were the pea (*Pisum* sp.), chick-pea (*Cicer arietinum*), lentil (*Lens esculenta*), broad bean (*Vicia faba*), cowpea (*Vigna unguiculata*), and lathyrus pea (*Lathyrus sativus*). Others such as the kidney bean (*Phaseolus vulgaris*), lima bean (*Phaseolus lunatus*), horse gram (*Dolichos uniflorus*), soybean (*Glycine max*), and groundnut (*Arachis hypogaea*) originated in Asia and the New World and became available much later.

In some parts of the world, legumes are popularly called pulse, from the Latin *puls*. In ancient Rome, however, puls was a pottage made of cereals (mostly spelt, a hardy European wheat, *Triticum spelta*) and legumes, generally broad beans. Also etymologically derived from *puls* was the Italian word *polenta* for a mush made of corn, also imported from the Western Hemisphere.

In the past, dry legumes have been called the "poor man's meat" because, having a high protein content, they were consumed instead of meat, which was much more costly. In addition to this socioeconomic connotation, legumes were considered, erroneously, a second-class food. It is true that the protein of legumes is not of very high quality; however, in combination with cereals, the resulting quality of protein approaches that of meat.

PRODUCTION AND CONSUMPTION

World production of dry legumes increased markedly after 1985, with a progressive increase in the yield (see Table 4–1). A similar trend in yield can be seen in most of the European countries considered. Going from France to Spain a remarkable decrease in yield is evident. In addition, production in many cases does not meet market demand, and imported dry legumes ranges between 20% and 40%, mostly from the Middle East and Asian countries.

Soybean production is not considered because it was only recently begun in the Mediterranean countries; there it has met with great success. After oil extraction, soybeans are used most often to produce protein concentrate or isolate to enhance the protein content of cereal products or to provide a substitute or additive for meat products.

A dramatic decrease in the consumption of dry legumes during the last few years has occurred in the four countries considered (see Table 4–2); consumption in Spain and Greece is greater than in France and Italy (Alberti, 1990). The values reported refer to entire countries, but differences exist regarding regionality and socioeconomic status. For instance, in Italy legume consumption is higher in the south, and in Spain rural people consume more legumes than those in cities. On the other hand, in most of the countries, a remarkable increase occurred in the consumption of green legumes. This increase can be attributed to the availability of frozen legumes, particularly peas.

CHEMICAL COMPOSITION AND NUTRITIVE VALUE

Table 4–3 presents the chemical and nutritional composition of green, frozen, dry, and canned legumes available in Italy (Carnovale and Miuccio 1989; Fidanza and Versiglioni 1987). They show a high protein content, particularly the dry form; the protein content of soybeans is even higher although soybeans are not often consumed as such. The quality of the protein in legumes and their digestibility are reported in Table 4–4 (page 108), where they are compared with egg. The protein quality is not very high but higher than that of cereals; because of the high lysine content of legumes, they can complement the deficiency of this amino acid in cereals. The content of sulfur-containing amino acids is low, but Indian researchers have been able to breed a chick-pea with 50% more methionine, with a parallel increase of lysine (Fidanza 1979). The fat content is low, with the exception of the soybean and, to a lesser degree, the chick-pea. Of great nutritional interest is the high percentage of polyunsaturated fatty acids.

Legumes have a very high carbohydrate content, mainly starch. Raffinose and particularly verbascose and stachyose are present in the soluble fraction; these seem to be responsible for flatulence, as also are starch and hemicelluloses, according to El Faki et al. (1983).

TABLE 4-1. Production and Yield of Some Dry Legumes

	1952–56		1961–65	
	Prd (1000 metric tons)	Yield (kg/ha)	Prd (1000 metric tons)	Yield (kg/ha)
Total				
World	—	—	42,395	626
Beans, dry				
France	102	930	72	954
Greece	42	940	43	624
Italy	148	340	184	569
Spain	94	950	129	1,295
Broad beans, dry				
France	74	1,220	47	1,523
Greece	25	810	23	881
Italy	433	780	432	887
Spain	105	780	127	868
Chick-peas				
Greece	16	710	15	720
Italy	52	520	41	620
Spain	137	450	124	523
Lentils				
France	10	820	10	821
Greece	11	670	9	567
Italy	15	570	14	684
Spain	22	550	29	618

Source: FAO production yearbook, Vol. 23, 29, 36, 41.

Dietary fiber is well represented, particularly hemicelluloses. In addition, the presence of saponins can induce a reduction of serum cholesterol by absorption of bile acids to unavailable carbohydrates (Fidanza 1979). This cholesterol-lowering effect seems to be associated with an increase in the prevalence of gallstones (Nervi, 1989). Of the minerals, calcium reaches values of some interest, particularly in the kidney bean, lentil, and chick-pea, but the presence of phytates reduces its availability. The presence of iron is relevant, but its bioavailability is rather low also because of phytates. All the other minerals are present in satisfactory amounts; the sodium content is low. Among the vitamins, thiamine and niacin are well represented; values for vitamins A and C are rather low.

The higher content of water in green beans dilutes nutrients. Of some interest is the composition of frozen peas and canned legumes. As Fidanza (1979) has shown, processing lowers the value of some nutrients and, in addition, seems to cause less flatulence.

TABLE 4-1. *Continued*

1974–76		1979–81		1985		1987	
Prd (1000 metric tons)	Yield (kg/ha)	Prd (1000 metric tons)	Yield (kg/ha)	Prd (1000 metric tons)	Yield (kg/ha)	Prd (1000 metric tons)	Yield (kg/ha)
42,234	664	40,809	676	51,366	774	53,345	777
25	1,090	30	1,699	17	1,910	14	1,750
43	1,103	41	1,230	31	1,476	27	1,559
109	1,508	78	1,609	61	1,573	55	1,647
107	643	86	641	71	687	69	697
44	2,039	70	3,063	130	3,283	138	3,730
13	1,410	11	2,048	7	2,000	6	1,627
253	1,207	205	1,277	174	1,341	175	1,359
118	1,005	78	972	61	1,158	50	1,020
14	913	15	1,044	6	1,209	5	1,164
18	1,080	16	1,181	12	1,257	12	1,281
63	544	53	565	57	634	64	703
12	1,255	15	1,695	20	2,000	20	2,000
6	1,063	6	1,313	5	1,101	2	1,333
3	920	1	909	1	820	1	956
47	642	42	576	49	797	49	538

TABLE 4-2. **Consumption of Dry Legumes**

	Year	Consumption (kg/capita/yr)
France	1925	7.3
	1970	2.3
	1978	1.7
	1980	1.4
Greece	1961–65	8.0
	1971–75	8.0
	1981–85	5.0
Italy	1926	14.9
	1951–55	5.3
	1961–65	5.5
	1971–75	4.5
	1981–85	3.6
Spain	1964–65	15.0
	1980–81	8.8
	1986	9.3

TABLE 4-3. Chemical Composition of Legumes/100 g of Edible Portion

	Edible portion (%)	H_2O (g)	Protein (g)	Fat (g)	Carbohydrates Available[a] (g)	Starch (g)	Soluble (g)	Cellulose (g)	Dietary Fiber (g)	Energy (kcal)	(kj)
Green											
Broad bean (*Vicia faba*)	30	81	5.4	0.2	4.2	3.4	0.4	—	5.1	37	155
Kidney bean (*Phaseolus vulgaris*)	41	62	6.4	0.6	19.4	16.5	1.3	3.0	10.6	104	435
Pea (*Pisum sativum*)	47	76	7.0	0.2	12.4	7.3	4.4	1.0	5.2	76	318
Frozen											
Pea	100	79	5.7	0.4	7.5	3.4	4.1	—	7.8	54	228
Dry											
Broad bean	100	13	27.2	3.0	55.3	45.4	4.9	2.8	7.0	342	1,432
Chick-pea (*Cicer arietinum*)	100	13	21.8	4.9	54.3	46.0	3.7	5.7	13.8	334	1,398
Kidney bean	100	11	23.6	2.5	51.7	43.2	4.0	6.9	17.0	311	1,302
Lentil (*Lens esculenta*)	100	12	25.0	2.5	54.0	46.5	2.4	2.8	13.7	325	1,360
Lupin treated (*Lupinus albus*)	76	69	16.4	2.4	7.2	6.0	0.5	—	—	114	477
Pea	100	13	21.7	2.0	53.6	45.7	2.9	5.0	15.7	306	1,281
Soybean (*Glycine max*)	100	8	36.9	18.1	23.3	11.1	11.0	—	11.9	398	1,665
Canned											
Chick-pea	100	78	4.7	1.4	6.7	4.8	1.4	2.1	7.0	56	236
Kidney bean	100	82	4.0	0.5	6.3	4.7	1.1	2.1	6.8	44	184
Lentil	100	80	5.1	0.4	10.7	8.6	1.1	2.5	5.3	64	268
Pea	100	76	5.8	0.8	6.8	4.3	2.0	4.7	9.7	56	234

[a]Expressed as monosaccharides.

Most of these values can vary, because in cultivars, cultural conditions and other environmental factors can induce changes in nutrient content, particularly vitamins and minerals; also, some studies may not have considered this aspect in sufficient detail.

In the past few years, the breeding of different species of legumes has contributed to improvements in yield and nutritional value. Of particular interest is improvement in protein quality and the decrease in toxic factors and the flatus effect.

For an in-depth review of the composition and nutritive value of beans the paper by Sgarbieri is recommended (Sgarbieri, 1989).

TOXIC SUBSTANCES

Among the toxic substances present in some legumes are the trypsin inhibitor, cyanogenetic glucosides, saponins, alkaloids, goitrogenic fac-

TABLE 4-3. *Continued*

	Ca (mg)	Fe (mg)	Cu (mg)	Na (mg)	K (mg)	P (mg)	Thiamin (mg)	Ribo-flavin (mg)	Niacin Equiv. (mg)	Vitamin A Retinol Equiv. (μg)	Carotenes (μg)	Vitamin C (mg)
Green												
Broad bean (*Vicia faba*)	23	1.8	—	18	210	98	0.20	0.10	1.9	11	64	24
Kidney bean (*Phaseolus vulgaris*)	44	3.0	—	2	650	180	0.44	0.10	2.1	18	(108)	10
Pea (*Pisum sativum*)	47	1.8	—	1	202	101	0.42	0.18	2.2	49	294	28
Frozen												
Pea	33	1.5	0.2	3	190	90	0.32	0.10	3.0	50	300	17
Dry												
Broad bean	90	5.0	1.9	—	1,028	420	0.50	0.28	6.5	10	(60)	4
Chick-pea (*Cicer arietinum*)	117	6.1	3.0	6	800	299	0.36	0.14	4.1	30	(180)	5
Kidney bean	137	6.7	4.2	4	1,445	437	0.40	0.17	5.1	3	(18)	3
Lentil (*Lens esculenta*)	127	5.1	3.0	8	980	347	0.57	0.20	5.2	10	(60)	3
Lupin, treated (*Lupinus albus*)	45	5.5	—	—	—	100	0.10	0.01	5.4	—	—	—
Pea	48	4.5	0.5	38	990	320	0.58	0.15	5.8	10	(60)	4
Soybean (*Glycine max*)	257	6.9	—	4	1,740	591	0.99	0.52	11.4	—	—	—
Canned												
Chick-pea	40	1.5	0.4	336	96	—	—	—	—	—	—	—
Kidney bean	40	1.9	0.4	305	232	—	—	—	—	—	—	—
Lentil	19	1.2	0.2	399	208	77	0.11	0.04	1.1	3	20	tr.
Pea	30	1.7	0.3	306	128	73	0.13	0.10	2.9	50	300	8

tors, hemagglutinins, polyphenols, and the factor responsible for lathyrism.

These have been fully described in *Toxic Constituents of Plant Foodstuffs* by Liener (1980). Most of these substances are eliminated by common methods of preparation. Of some concern is favism, which is still present in some Mediterranean areas. Favism is due to a selective toxicity of broad beans in individuals with an inherited biochemical abnormality.

LEGUMES IN THE DIET

Dry legumes are usually soaked in water to soften the skin and to reduce the cooking time. If they are soaked in cold water for a long time and the water is changed several times, many toxic substances can be eliminated, particularly the trypsin inhibitor. In addition, prolonged soaking induces germination of the seeds, which increases the content of some

TABLE 4-4. Essential Amino Acid Content (mg/g N) and Protein Quality of Some Dry Legumes and Egg

	Chick-pea	Kidney Bean	Broad Bean	Lentil	Soybean	Egg
Phenylalanine	358	326	270	327	309	358
Isoleucine	277	262	250	270	284	393
Leucine	468	476	443	477	486	551
Lysine	428	450	404	449	399	436
Methionine	65	66	46	50	79	210
Cystine	74	53	50	57	83	152
Threonine	235	248	210	248	241	320
Tryptophan	54	63	54	60	80	93
Valine	284	287	275	313	300	428
BV	68	58	55	45	73	94
NPU	—	38	48	30	61	94
PER	1.7	1.5	—	0.9	2.3	3.9
EUD	60	*62	51	55	62	100
Digestibility	86	73	87	85	90	97
Protein score	40	34	28	31	47	—

nutrients (e.g., vitamin C, niacin) and improves the bioavailability of others because of a decrease in phytic acid. Also, a rearrangement of carbohydrates, particularly starch, has been observed. According to El Faki et al. (1983), fermentation seems to further reduce flatulence. Decortication removes most of the tannins.

As shown by Keys and Keys (1967), legumes can be used at every meal; their publication contains about 200 excellent recipes. Because legumes provide a high level of energy from carbohydrates and protein and a low level of energy from fats, they can contribute to the correct proportion of the three energy nutrients in the diet.

Legume proteins combined with other proteins in mixed diets help substantially to fulfill amino acid requirements.

There is no doubt that scientific evidence has demonstrated the important and beneficial effects of legumes in the Mediterranean diet.

REFERENCES

Alberti, F. 1990. Mediterranean meal patterns. *Biblthca Nutr. Dieta.* **45**:59, 1190.
Aykroyd, W. R., and J. Doughty. 1964. *Legumes in Human Nutrition.* Rome: FAO Nutritional Studies, No. 19.
Carnovale, E., and F. Miuccio. 1989. *Tabelle di Composizione degli Alimenti.* Rome: Istituto Nazionale della Nutrizione.

El Faki, H. A., T. N. Bhavanishanger, R. N. Tharanathan, and H. S. R. Desikachar. 1983. Flatus effect of chick-pea (*Cicer arietinum*), cow pea (*Vigna sinensis*) and horse gram (*Dolichos biflarus*) and their isolated carbohydrate fractions. *Nutr. Reports Intern* **27**:921.

FAO Production Yearbook 1968, Vol. 23. Rome: FAO, 1969.

FAO Production Yearbook 1975, Vol. 29. Rome: FAO, 1976.

FAO Production Yearbook 1982, Vol. 36. Rome: FAO, 1983.

FAO Production Yearbook 1987, Vol. 41. Rome: FAO, 1988.

Fidanza, F. 1979. Ruolo e importanza delle lguminose nella nutrizione umana. In *Prospettive delle proteaginose in Italia*, C. Pompei, ed., p. 9. Rome: CNR.

Fidanza, F., and N. Versiglioni. 1987. *Tabelle di Composizione degli Alimenti*. Naples: Idelson.

Keys, M., and A. Keys. 1967. *The Benevolent Bean*. Garden City, N.Y.: Doubleday.

Liener, I. E., 1980. *Toxic Constituents of Plant Foodstuffs*. New York: Academic Press.

Nervi, F., C. Covarrubias, P. Bravo, N. Velasco, N. Ulloa, F. Cruz, M. Fava, C. Severin, R. Del Pozzo, C. Antezana, V. Valdivieso, A. Arteaga. 1989. Influence of legume intake on biliary lipids and cholesterol saturation in young Chilean men. *Gastroenterology* **96**:825.

Sgarbieri, V. C. 1989. Composition and nutritive value of beans. *World Rev. Nut. Diet* **60**:132.

5

Vegetables and Fruits

Giulio Testolin
Ambrogina Alberio
Ernestina Casiraghi

A characteristic of the Mediterranean diet is the high intake of fruit and vegetables. From the nutritional point of view, the diet is rich in elements such as minerals, fiber, and optimally bioavailable vitamins, plus minor organic substances. Several of these (mineral salts, vitamins, and other organic substances) have pharmacological or protective functions that contribute to maintaining health (Burr and Sveetnam 1982; Acheson and Williams 1983; Gey 1986; Ames 1983). It is interesting to determine how the Mediterranean diet differs from diets typical of other populations, such as those of northern Europeans, who have a high incidence of chronic degenerative diseases. The most noticeable differences between the diets are in fruit and vegetable intake.

FRUIT AND VEGETABLE CONSUMPTION

The consumption of fruit and vegetables in Europe is shown in Table 5-1. The table draws attention to the different dietary models with respect to the traditional Mediterranean model, considered to be the Italian diet of the 1950s. The differences between the various countries in the consumption of fruit and vegetables in the 1955 to 1960 period do not change over the considered time span. It is worthwhile to note the greater quantity of vegetables consumed in Italy.

Contrary to the general trend, the consumption of vegetables in France has diminished, dropping to levels much lower than in Italy and nearer to those of the other European countries. The French diet seems to be moving away from the Mediterranean pattern toward models more typically north and central European.

TABLE 5-1. European Consumption of Fruit and Vegetables

	Ger.	Fra.	It.	Neth.	UEBL[a]	U.K.	Irl.	Den.
Total vegetables and fresh fruit								
1955–60	118	168	165	103	123	—	—	—
1968–69	154	186	270	140	139	96	103	91
1976–77	155	165	249	143	149	107	110	88
1984–85	151	173	256	155	135	123	114	101
Total vegetables								
1955–60	49	133	111	67	79	—	—	—
1968–69	59	129	162	77	85	61	61	41
1976–77	71	111	151	80	94	77	82	52
1984–85	72	118	147	91	85	85	84	63
Tomatoes								
1955–60	12	15	28	11	—	—	—	—
1968–69	9	15	43	8	18	—	—	—
1976–77	14	19	39	13	25	14	10	11
1984–85	14	21	56	16	21	14	11	14
Total fresh fruit								
1955–60	69	35	64	36	44	—	—	—
1968–69	93	57	108	63	54	35	44	50
1976–77	84	54	98	73	55	30	28	36
1984–85	79	55	108	64	50	38	30	38
Apples								
1955–60	20	9	10	22	17	—	—	—
1968–69	27	19	11	33	25	—	—	—
1976–77	23	16	19	34	23	12	11	17
1984–85	22	16	20	33	20	12	18	19
Pears								
1955–60	5	4	6	7	8	—	—	—
1968–69	6	6	16	7	6	—	—	—
1976–77	5	6	14	6	6	2	2	3
1984–85	4	6	14	5	6	2	2	3
Citrus fruit								
1955–60	14	13	12	19	15	—	—	—
1968–69	20	16	30	25	16	—	—	—
1976–77	23	19	36	52	18	13	11	13
1984–85	28	13	39	82	21	14	15	11
Potatoes								
1955–60	141	121	42	92	139	—	—	—
1968–69	109	97	45	89	119	100	127	80
1976–77	80	83	37	79	101	86	114	58
1984–85	73	75	37	85	97	107	126	66

Source: Eurostat (1970–1985).

Note: Annual average consumption for the considered years (kg/person)

[a]UEBL = Union Economic Belgium–Luxemburg.

Obviously, the consumption of particular products varies from country to country; for example, greater quantities of tomatoes are consumed in Italy, whereas potatoes are more popular in northern Europe.

The data show that apples are consumed in more or less equal quantities throughout all the European countries, whereas Italy has the highest consumption of pears. In addition, there has been a much greater increase in the consumption of citrus fruit in Italy than in the other countries, the only exception being the Netherlands, where the huge increase is due, in part, to the use of industrially processed citrus products.

Within the Mediterranean region, there are no great differences regarding vegetables as can be seen in Table 5–2, but it does emerge that Spain's consumption of potatoes is in line with that of the northern countries.

From 1950 to 1965 the overall vegetable and fruit consumption in-

TABLE 5-2. Consumption of Fruit and Vegetables in the Mediterranean Regions

	Italy	Spain	Turkey	Portugal
Garden vegetables				
1958–60	116	—	—	—
1973–75	149	131	154	142[a]
1983–85	148	127	186	—
Tomatoes				
1958–60	27	—	—	—
1973–75	42	32	33	—
1983–85	55	26	43	—
Fresh fruit				
1958–60	66	—	—	—
1973–75	103	129	76	78
1983–85	116	147	90	55
Citrus fruit				
1958–60	13	—	—	—
1973–75	36	23	16	—
1983–85	38	38	17	—
Potatoes				
1958–60	42	—	—	—
1973–75	39	116	45	107
1983–85	42	109	56	90

Source: OCDE (1985).

Note: Annual average consumption for the considered years (kg/person).

[a]Including tomatoes.

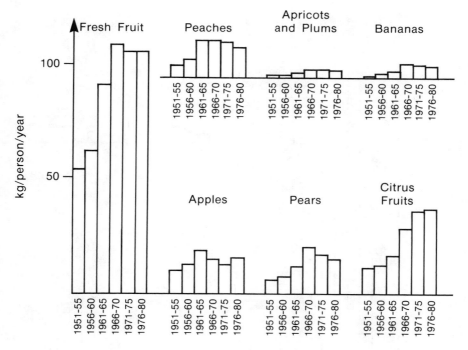

Figure 5–1A.   Fruit consumption in Italy, 1951–1980.

creased in Italy; the levels reached at that time were then maintained in the following years (Fig. 5–1) (Istituto Centrale di Statistica 1960–1985). The consumption of fresh fruit doubled, rising from about 53 kg/person/year in 1951 to 1955 to around 105 kg in the 5-year period from 1975 to 1980. Also, the vegetable intake increased markedly from 75 kg/person/year in the period 1951–1955 to around 140 kg in 1975–1980; the consumption of tomatoes more than doubled. Among the vegetables, those such as cabbage, cauliflower, onions, artichokes, and fennel, all typical of the Mediterranean diet, are eaten in quantities equal to or only slightly greater than those consumed in the 1950s, whereas there has been a marked increase in the consumption of other garden vegetables such as salad greens and zucchini.

CLASSIFICATION AND TECHNOLOGY
OF FRUITS AND VEGETABLES

Most of the fruits and vegetables cultivated or consumed in Mediterranean area belong to the seven botanical families that appear in Table

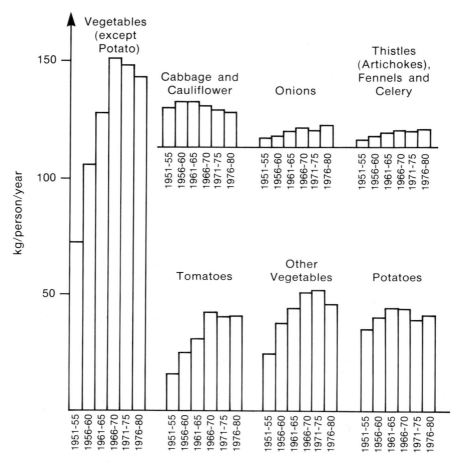

Figure 5-1B.   Vegetable consumption in Italy, 1951-1980.

5-3. Table 5-4 classifies the vegetables according to their edible parts and indicates their principal nutritional components, their characteristics, and growing seasons.

For several groups of fruits and vegetables, the commercial season extends all year because of either the keeping qualities of the vegetables, as in the case of root vegetables and nuts, or different seasonal varieties, such as the salad greens, which are grown throughout the year.

Beginning in ancient times, a number of preservation techniques have been developed to make fruits and vegetables available year-round. Among the oldest are sun-drying of fruits and preservation of

TABLE 5-3. Botanical Families

Order: Family:	Rheodales Cruciferae	Rosales Rosaceae Pomidee	Prunoidee	Terbintales Rutacea	Rhamnales Umbrelliflorae
	Cabbage	Apple	Peach	Orange	Fennel
	Turnip	Pear	Apricot	Mandarin	Celery
	Radish	Quince	Plum	Citron	Carrot
	Cress	Medlar	Almond	Grapefruit	
	Cole		Cherry	Lemon	
			Walnut		
			Strawberry		

Order: Family:	Tubiflorae Solanaceae	Ligustrales Compositae	Liliflorae Liliaceae
	Potato	Chicory (endive)	Asparagus
	Tomato	Lettuce	Garlic
	Capsicum	Artichoke	Onion
	Eggplant		Leek

Source: Tonzing (1986).

vegetables in brine, vinegar, and oil. All technological treatments, especially when the product is heated, reduce the nutritional value of the fruit or vegetable, mainly because of the deactivation of vitamins.

Regarding both the Mediterranean diet and the loss of nutrients, two considerations are useful. The first is that processing techniques have evolved, bringing about lower nutrient losses: for example, the trend in fruit drying has progressed from sun drying to air drying to vacuum drying and then to freeze drying. The second point is that in the Mediterranean region, fresh fruit and vegetables are much preferred to preserved products.

DIET AND NUTRITION

Since the 1950s, dietary habits in the Mediterranean area have changed dramatically following socioeconomic developments such as urbanization, increased buying power, and the entry of women into the work force. Also, the development of new food producing and handling technology has led to more consumption of new products and has made foodstuffs more readily available both over greater distances and for longer periods.

In Italy, such changes have emphasized the differences in lifestyles,

TABLE 5-4. Fruit and Vegetable Classification

	Products	Interesting Compounds	Season
Roots	Carrot, turnip, beetroot, radish	Retinol, simple sugars	May–September[a]
Fruits	Tomatoes, cucumbers, eggplant, pumpkin	Vitamin C, retinol	April–September[a]
Stems and sprouts	Artichokes, brussel sprouts, asparagus	Fiber	December–May[a]
Leafy vegetables	Salad greens, cress, spinach, leeks, celery	Vitamin C, fiber	All year
Tubers	Jerusalem artichoke, potato	Starch, fiber	All year
Bulbs	Onion, garlic, shallot	Vitamin C, trace elements, active compounds	All year
Vegetables for seasoning	Parsley, basil, chervil, tarragon	Vitamin C, trace elements, active compounds	May–September[a]
Citrus fruits	Orange, grapefruit, mandarin, lemon, tangerine	Vitamin C	November–April[a]
Pulpy fruits with seeds	Apple, pear, grape, quince	Simple sugars, fiber	August–November[a]
Stone fruits	Apricot, peach, plum, cherry	Vitamin C, retinol	May–August
Berry fruits	Strawberry, raspberry, red and black currants	Vitamin C, retinol	May–July[a]
Dried fruits	Figs, prunes, dates	Simple sugars	August–October
Nuts	Walnuts, hazelnuts, almonds, peanuts, pine nuts	Unsaturated fatty acids	September–December

[a] Season extends all year for products grown in greenhouses or imported.

already quite substantial, between the north and the south. In the south, the consumption of vegetables, olive oil, and cereals has remained high or has increased compared to that in the north (Table 5-5) (Agradi 1988).

Vegetables in the Italian Diet

In Italy, vegetables are generally eaten as a side dish to the main course of meat, fish, eggs, or cheese and, more often than not, are eaten raw. These include salad greens, tomatoes, cucumbers, peppers, onions, and carrots. As shown in Table 5-6, most vegetables are also used for the preparation of pasta and rice dishes and of vegetable soups. Typical dishes are pasta with tomato sauce, eggplants, artichokes, peppers, or broccoli. Less often, vegetables are used for the preparation of rice dishes. Soups are made of a great variety of vegetables including legumes, and rice or pasta is usually added.

In Mediterranean cuisine, the same vegetable can be prepared with

TABLE 5-5. Annual Consumption of Animal and Vegetable Foodstuffs in Italy: Comparison of Different Areas and Periods

	North		South	
	1953–54	1983	1953–54	1983
Animal source				
Meat	34.4	61.3	19.0	51.9
Cheese	8.3	14.8	7.2	11.9
Milk	88.3	87.0	39.3	68.4
Fish	7.1	4.5	15.8	11.4
Eggs	6.6	8.1	5.3	8.4
Butter	4.4	5.2	0.8	1.5
Total	149.1	180.9	87.4	153.5
Vegetable source				
Cereal	151.9	111.7	185.7	151.4
Dry pulses	3.2	a	7.3	a
Potato	28.7	30.0	26.8	36.3
Vegetables	52.4	50.1	77.8	67.6
Fresh fruit and nuts	60.0	84.0	52.8	78.1
Oil	10.6	25.8	13.2	30.0
Margarine	—	1.3	—	0.7
Total	306.8	302.6	363.6	361.1

Source: Agradi (1988).
a Included in vegetables.

TABLE 5-6. Combinations of Vegetables and Fruits with Other Foods

	Tomatoes	Leafy Vegetables	Cauliflower, Carrots, Eggplant, Peppers, Squash	Potatoes	Spices	Fresh Fruit
Milk	—	—	—	o	—	o/+
Cheese	o/+	o/+	o	o/+	o	o
Pulses	+	—	—	o	+	—
Cereals						
bread	+	+	—	—	o	o/+
rice	+	+	+	—	+	—
pasta	+	o	+	—	+	—
Eggs	+	+	+	o	o	—
Fish	+	+	+	+	+	—
Meat	+	+	+	+	+	—

Note: — = Not combined; o = seldom combined; + = frequently combined.

different seasonings, herbs, and spices. The tomato is an example. It can be eaten with any other food. Raw, it is an ingredient in salads; cooked and concentrated, it is the basis of many sauces used in the preparation of meat, fish, pasta, and pizza. In the preparation of typical Mediterranean dishes, especially sauces, small quantities of vegetables such as celery, parsley, basil, garlic, and hot peppers are used, as are such herbs as rosemary, sage, bay leaves, oregano, mint, marjoram, and fennel seeds. These ingredients, which impart a characteristic flavor and aroma, often contain active compounds, for example, garlic, which contains ajoiene and diallyl trisulfide, both active in inhibiting platelet aggregation (Carson 1987).

Table 5-7 lists aromatic herbs together with their most common uses and active components.

Fruit in the Italian Diet

Fresh fruit represents the classic final course of every meal, particularly in Italy, and often is the dessert. The fruit in season is usually chosen and is eaten raw. As indicated in Table 5-6, fruit is directly associated with milk only in the preparation of yogurts, milk shakes, and ice cream; it is eaten with bread primarily as jam. In Italy, fresh fruit is seldom eaten with cheese or cured meat. Dried fruit (figs, dates) and several varieties of nut (almonds, walnuts, hazelnuts, chestnuts) are commonly served with the fruit course, especially in winter. Also, nuts and dried

TABLE 5-7. Aromatic Herbs: Uses and Active Principles

	Uses	Active Principles
Garlic	Raw and cooked for pasta, meat, sauces, salami	Sulphorate glucoside, mixture of sulphide and allyl oxide, allicin, garlicine, allistatine
Basil	Mainly raw in salads and in meat and sauces	O-cimene, cineol, esdragol
Capers	Fresh or preserved in salt or vinegar	Biflavones, resins, glucosides, pectins
Laurel (bay leaves)	Mostly for meat	Tannins, resins
Fennel seeds leaves	Certain types of bread and meat	Phenol, esdragol, anethol, chlorogenic and caffeic acids
Mint	Broths, sauces, vegetables, soups Meat, soups	Menthol, cineol, menthoruran, several terpenes (menthene, phellandrene, limonene)
Marjoram	Meat, vegetables	Terpineol, camphene, borneol, rosmarinic acid, mineral salts
Hot red peppers	Fresh and dried for sauces, meat, cheese, salami	Vitamins C and B, capsaicin
Parsley	Pasta, vegetables, meat, fish	Vitamins A, B, C; Fe, K, Ca, P, Mg, Na, I, Cu, Mn, S; apoil, pinene, terpenes, apiin (components of essential oil)
Thyme	First courses and meat	Thymol, carnarole, tannins, terpenes
Oregano	Pizzas, vegetables, soups, salads, sauces	Thymol, carnarole, terpenes
Rosemary	Meat, fish	Pinene, camphene, borneol, bornyl acetate, organic acids
Sage	First course, meat	Borneol, camphor, cineol, tuyone, tannis

fruit are traditionally used in the preparation of sweets such as marzipan and sultana (raisin) bread.

Nutritional Content of Fruits and Vegetables

Vegetables and fruit, important for their macronutrient content, are even more important as sources of fiber, vitamins, mineral salts, and particular organic substances. Among these organic compounds are citric, malic, and tartaric acids, which have an alkalizing effect in the intestine and contribute to the buffering power of the stomach. Other organic substances present in fruit and vegetables are polyphenols, which favorably affect cholesterol metabolism and might have a bacteriostatic effect; tannins, which regulate plasma cholesterol; and flavonoids. In addition, fruits' phenols have other not completely understood pharmacological properties that seem to play a significant role in preventing degenerative diseases.

Particular importance has recently been ascribed to omega-3 fatty acids. Such acids inhibit platelet aggregation and act as a precursor of prostaglandin synthesis. They are present in grape and raspberry seeds and in a few vegetables, particularly in purslane, which is often consumed in southern European countries (Simopulos and Salem 1986, 1989).

Fruits and Vegetables as Sources of Fiber.   A characteristic of fruit and vegetable fiber is that it contains mostly pectin and cellulose, whereas cereals and legumes contain hemicellulose and polysaccharides (glycomannan and galactomannan) in greater quantities. A daily intake of about 20 g of fiber from fruits and vegetables (Lewis et al. 1981; Lewis, Mancini, and Puska 1987) that are particularly rich in the insoluble fiber fraction plus about 15 g from other sources, helps regulate both the metabolism of fat and the intestinal function.

In 1960, a European Atomic Energy Community (EURATOM) investigation (Cresta et al. 1969) in Italy and other European countries revealed (Table 5–8) that the amount of fiber in the Mediterranean diet is no different from that in the diets of other countries. An analysis of the vegetables consumed shows that in northern European countries the potato contributes significantly to the fiber intake, whereas in Italy potato consumption is low and the intake of fiber from other vegetables is much higher.

In fiber intake, in addition to regional diversity, there is also a notable individual and seasonal variation. Among the rural population of southern Italy, such variation ranges from an average of 32.4 g (minimum,

TABLE 5-8. Daily Dietary Fiber Intake and Principal Fiber Sources

	S. It.	N. It.	Neth.	Lux.	Bel.	Fra.	Ger.
Dietary Fiber (g)	28.0	21.1	23.4	28.1	26.0	25.5	24.3
Source (% of total)							
Cereals	55	61	54	45	49	50	33
Cooked potatoes	2	8	12	21	19	11	15
Cooked and raw garden vegetables	29	21	24	21	20	24	21
Cooked legumes	4	2	1	5	2	3	1
Fresh fruit	8	6	9	9	8	7	10
Dried fruit and nuts	2	2	0.4	—	0.8	4	—

Source: Cresta et al. (1969).

15.1 g to maximum, 45.3 g) to 49.6 g (28.9 g to 73.1 g) in winter and spring, respectively (Lintas 1985).

Table 5-9 shows the daily intake of dietary fiber from fruit and vegetables in Italy. Data have been computed from the fiber content of the edible part of various vegetables (Fidanza and Liguori 1984) and the daily consumption per person of each product. As a consequence, such data must be considered as indicative only.

Fiber, although indispensable for good intestinal function, renders minerals, vitamins, and other organic substances less bioavailable. Apparently, however, fiber from fruit and vegetables has a less negative effect than fiber from cereals (Cook et al. 1983).

Fruits and Vegetables as Sources of Vitamins. A diet rich in fruit and vegetables contains a notable quantity of vitamins, particularly vitamins A and C. The vitamin content of food, however, especially fruit and vegetables, varies greatly and depends on freshness (vitamins tend to

TABLE 5-9. Daily Per-Person Intake of Dietary Fiber from Fruit and Vegetables in Italy (g/day)

	Vegetables and Potatoes	Vegetables	Potatoes	% Potatoes Veg. and Pot.	Fruits	Total	% Potatoes Total
1951–55	4.9	3.2	1.7	34.7	3.7	8.6	20.0
1956–60	6.6	4.7	1.9	28.8	4.3	10.9	17.4
1961–65	7.7	5.6	2.1	27.3	5.3	13.0	16.1
1966–70	8.8	6.7	2.1	23.9	6.0	14.8	14.2
1971–75	8.4	6.5	1.9	22.6	5.6	14.0	13.6
1976–80	8.2	6.2	2.0	24.4	5.7	13.9	14.4

deteriorate with time), genetic characteristics, growing techniques, and soil composition (Machlin 1984). Furthermore, the preparation and preservation treatments of vegetables, especially if high temperatures are used, bring about vitamin losses that are almost total for water soluble vitamins (C) and partial for those that are fat soluble (A, E).

The vitamin content of vegetables consumed in Mediterranean countries such as Italy is, nevertheless, elevated because places of production are near those of consumption, and the vegetables are used raw shortly after harvest; in addition, stored products are not consumed in large quantities.

Vitamin C levels are high in fruit, especially citrus fruit, variable in leafy vegetables, and rather modest in roots and tubers. It emerges from the investigation of the 1960s that in southern Italy, vitamin C is supplied primarily by fruit and vegetables (Table 5–10) that are mainly eaten raw. In other European countries, a substantial part of the vitamin C comes from vegetables (potatoes, spinach) that are cooked before consumption.

Vitamin A is present in green, leafy vegetables, carrots, peppers, melons, apricots, and persimmons. It can be assumed that this vitamin is either retinol or the precursor β-carotene. The main sources of retinol are products of animal origin, whereas β-carotene is found predominantly in vegetables (carrot, pumpkin, spinach, cabbage) and in the pigment of certain fruit (apricot, orange). It should be noted that epidemiological studies (Peto et al. 1981; Shekelle et al. 1981) have shown that β-carotene is more effectively associated with a lower incidence of cancer caused by chemical agents than is retinol.

Some vegetables (broccoli, tomatoes, carrots, potatoes, cabbage, green salad vegetables) also supply some vitamin E to the diet. Considering the trends of fruit and vegetable consumption from 1951 to 1980,

TABLE 5-10. Principal Sources of Vitamin C in the Average Daily Ration (% of total)

	S. It.	N. It.	Neth.	Lux.	Bel.	Fra.	Ger.
Fresh fruit	33.0	15.5	17.6	12.5	15.0	23.0	40.0
Leafy vegetables	43.5	37.3	38.0	31.3	26.4	41.5	22.3
Tomatoes	14.0	2.0	1.2	—	2.0	1.5	2.0
Tomato concentrate	0.1	0.4	—	—	—	—	—
Potatoes	4.0	31.0	26.4	44.0	44.3	23.0	26.5

Source: Agradi (1988).

**TABLE 5-11. Daily Intake
of Vitamin E from Fruits
and Vegetables in Italy**

	Intake (mg/day)
1951–55	1.26
1956–60	1.83
1961–65	2.17
1966–70	2.62
1971–75	2.52
1976–80	2.44

the vitamin E intake has been evaluated with the assumption that the products are eaten raw. As Vitamin E becomes inactive with heat treatment, though to a lesser extent than vitamin C, the values reported are not the true values. It is possible, however, to hypothesize that an increase in the consumption of vitamin E assumes a proportional increase in the consumption of the active form.

The data reported in Table 5-11 were based on consumption of the edible part of fruits and vegetables and the vitamin E content therein.

Vitamin E prevents the oxidation of polyunsaturated fatty acids (PUFA) deposited in the fatty tissues or incorporated in the phospholipids of cell membranes. European-type diets contain a greater quantity of foodstuffs in which vitamin E is associated with PUFA than do the diets consumed in the Mediterranean area, where there is, instead, a high consumption of foods in which the vitamin E is not associated with PUFA. It can, therefore, be hypothesized that, in a diet rich in fruit and vegetables, there is a greater availability of alphatocopherol for the protection of the lipidic quota.

REFERENCES

Acheson, R. M., and D. R. R. Williams. 1983. Does consumption of fruits and vegetables protect against stroke? *Lancet* **2:**1191–1193.

Agradi, E. 1988. Le basi scientifiche della dieta Mediterranean. *Nutrizione e salute.* Rome: Verducci.

Ames, B. N. 1983. Dietary carcinogens and anticarcinogens: Oxygen radicals and degenerative disease. *Science* **221:**1256–1264.

Burr, M. C., and P. M. Sveetnam. 1982. Vegetarianism, dietary fiber, and mortality. *Am. J. Clin. Nutr.* **36:**673–677.

Carson, J. F. 1987. Chemistry and biological properties of onions and garlic. *Food Rev. Internat.* **3**:71–103.

Cook, J. D., N. C. Noble, T. A. Moveek, S. R. Lynch, and S. J. Petersburg. 1983. Effect of fiber on nonheme iron absorption. *Gastroenterology* **85**:1354–1358.

Cresta, M., S. Ledermann, A. Garnier, E. Lombardo, and G. Lacourly. 1969. *Etude des consommations alimentaires des populations de onze régions de la communauté européenne en vue de la détermination des niveaux de contamination radioactive.* Rapport établi au Centre d'Etude Nucléaire de Fontenay-Aux-Roses, France: EURATOM, Commissariat à l'énergie atomique (CEA).

Eurostat. 1970–1985. Rapporti agricoli. In *Yearbooks of Agricultural Statistic.* Luxemburg: Office for Official Publications of the European Communities.

Fidanza, F., and G. Liguori. 1984. *Nutrizione Umana.* Naples: Idelson.

Gey, H. F. 1986. On the antioxidant hypothesis with regard to arteriosclerosis. *Bibl. Nutr. Dieta* **37**:53–91.

Istituto Centrale di Statistica. 1960–1985. *Annuari statistici italiani.* Rome.

Lewis, B., F. Hammett, M. Katan, R. M. Kay, I. Merkz, A. Nobles, N. E. Miller, and A. V. Swan. 1981. Towards an improved lipid-lowering diet: additive effects of changes in nutrient intake. *Lancet* **2**:1310–1313.

Lewis, B., M. Mancini, and P. Puska. 1987. Dietary measures for control of lipoprotein risk factors. In *Atherosclerosis Biology and Clinical Science,* A. G. Olsson, ed., pp. 409–417. New York: Churchill Livingstone.

Lintas, C. 1985. Document presented to the meeting of SINU (Italian Society of Human Nutrition), Pisa.

Machlin, L. J., ed. 1984. *Handbook of Vitamins—Nutritional, Biochemical and Clinical Aspects.* New York: Marcel Dekker, Inc.

OCDE. 1985. Food Consumption Statistics. Paris.

Peto, R., R. Doll, J. D. Buckley, and M. B. Sporn. 1981. Can dietary β-carotene materially reduce human cancer rates? *Nature* **290**:201–208.

Shekelle, R. B., M. Lepper, et al. 1981. Dietary vitamin A and risk of cancer in the Western Elective Study. *Lancet* **2**:1189–1190.

Simopulos, A. P., and N. Salem. 1986. Purslane: a terrestrial source of omega-3 fatty acids. *New Eng. J. Med.* **313**:833.

Simopulos, A. P., and N. Salem. 1989. Omega-3 fatty acids in eggs from range-fed Greek chickens. *New Eng. J. Med.* **320**:1412.

Tonzing, S. 1986. In *Botanica,* vol. 2. Milan: Ambrosiana.

6

Edible Fats and Oils

Enzo Fedeli
Giulio Testolin

Traditionally, olive oil has been the fat of choice in the Mediterranean basin, that is, in the regions where the olive tree can be grown; since ancient times, however, fats other than olive oil have been locally used when available (Fedeli and Jacini 1971). The pattern in the region is similar, in general, to that in Italy. In the peninsular regions situated between the three Mediterranean seas, Tyrrhenian, Aegean, and Adriatic (except in the northern part, around Venice, Ravenna, and Trieste), olive oil was traditionally the principal dietary fat while the continental part of Italy consumed mostly seed oils or animal fats. Around the major Italian lakes, Como, Garda, and Iseo, although they are situated in the north, olive oil still was the major fat consumed because it was produced locally.

The same situation existed in most of the Mediterranean countries, so that olive oil consumption followed the coastlines, in a band of varying width, greater in the south and sometimes interrupted, as has occurred in Italy around the arch of the Adriatic sea, from Ravenna to the Trieste region.

We refer to this pattern in the past tense because the situation has changed drastically in the last forty years. Greater opportunities for travel and new trading activity have brought olive oil to populations traditionally consuming other fats and, conversely, seed oils to those who at one time depended primarily on olive oil for most of their dietary fat.

The band of olive oil consumers has widened and weakened. In effect, the amount of olive oil produced in the world, as a percentage of total oil production, is a constant except for yearly fluctuations (Table 6–1).

In the past, in addition to olive oil in the "olive oil strip," several other fats have had a place in local consumption. Seeds from regional

TABLE 6-1. Yearly Production of Edible Oils (kT)

	Olive Oil	Total Oils	% Olive Oil
1980–81	1,850	40,257	4.60
1981–82	1,495	41,868	3.57
1982–83	2,029	44,215	4.59
1983–84	1,576	43,152	3.65
1984–85	1,908	46,749	4.08
1985–86	1,480	49,480	2.99

agricultural products have been used to produce edible oils, for instance: cottonseed oil has been an alternative fat in Spain, Sicily, and Morocco; sunflower seed oil in Italy and Spain; rapeseed oil in Italy; tobacco seed oil in Italy and Turkey; grape seed oil in Italy and France; and sesame seed oil in Egypt.

Animal fats have also been traditionally used: butter fat from cows and goats, pork fat, tallow from several animals, and so forth, but undoubtedly olive oil of various qualities has accounted for at least 75% to 85% of the visible fat in the diet.

As noted, in the past forty years, the situation has changed markedly, and massive importations of untraditional crops have occurred. Because of the need for animal feed, soy beans have become the chief trade commodity. Oil obtained as a by-product of milling has replaced olive oil in increasing proportions. Growing soy beans has become a part of the agricultural industry in a number of Mediterranean countries such as Italy, Turkey, Egypt, and Spain. A similar situation is developing with rapeseed, while sunflower cultivation, one time a local activity, is now widespread in Italy, Greece, Turkey, Egypt, and Spain.

Fat is still consumed mostly as a liquid instead of being manufactured into solid products; for instance, margarine consumption in most of the Mediterranean countries has shown very little increase (Table 6-2).

Because of the introduction of the various seed oils, the overall fatty acid composition of the diet has changed in the past forty years, and the trend is toward a higher proportion of unsaturated fat. Meanwhile, the overall quantity of fats has increased greatly in diet and in commerce in Italy and is steadily increasing in the other Mediterranean countries (Table 6-3).

Olive oil can be consumed without refining, in which case it is known as virgin oil quality (VOQ), or as a refined product. The refined product is made from virgin oil and is called refined virgin oil (RVO) or from solvent-extracted oil called refined husk oil (RHO) (Fedeli 1977).

TABLE 6-2. Production and Consumption of Margarine (kT)

	1979			1984		
	Prod.	Cons.	Cons./Cap.	Prod.	Cons.	Cons./Cap.
France	159	189	3.4	156	209	3.8
Greece	23	21	2.1	23	26	2.6
Italy	68	74	1.3	64	71	1.2
Portugal	45	45	4.5	57	57	5.7
Spain	40	40	1.1	46	47	1.2
Europe (mean)			5.9			6.3

In fatty acid composition, no differences exist between virgin and re-fined oil; the main fatty acid in olive oil is oleic, with palmitic and linoleic acids a distant second and third (see Table 6–4).

The proportion of linoleic acid in oils from the more southerly, warmer regions of the Mediterranean tends to be higher than in the others. In addition to the nutritionally important monounsaturated oleic acid, olive oil supplies the consumer with a significant amount of essential linoleic acid.

VOQ, RVO, and RHO differ slightly in composition if we consider the minor components that account for 1% of VOQ to 3% of RHO. These minor components, several hundred chemical substances, can be grouped in classes (Mariani and Fedeli 1989; Morchio et al. 1987; Mariani and Fedeli 1986; Cortesi et al. 1985; Fedeli 1983):

- Hydrocarbons (saturated, unsaturated, linear, branched)
- Esters (fatty acid derivatives of short-chain alcohols, long-chain alcohols, sterols, triterpenic alcohols, monoterpenic alcohols, phenols)
- Aldehydes (medium- and long-chain, monoterpenic)
- Ketones (medium- and long-chain, monoterpenic)
- Alcohols (medium- and long-chain, monoterpenic, triterpenic)

TABLE 6-3. Production Import and Export of Oils and Fats in Italy (kT)

	1981	1982	1983	1984	1985
Production	1,179	1,213	1,137	1,268	1,235
Import	320	447	556	485	637
Export	106	95	126	209	224
Consumption	1,393	1,565	1,567	1,544	1,648
Cons/capita (kg)	25	28	28	27	29

TABLE 6-4. Fatty Acid Composition of Olive Oils

	VOQ %	RVO %	RHO %
Oleic	63.0–83.0	63.0–83.0	63.0–83.0
Palmitic	7.0–17.0	7.0–17.0	7.0–17.0
Linoleic	max 13.5	max 13.5	max 13.5
Stearic	1.5–4.0	1.5–4.0	1.5–4.0
Palmitoleic	0.3–3.0	0.3–3.0	0.3–3.0
Linolenic	max 1.5	max 1.5	max 1.5
Arachidic	max 0.7	max 0.7	max 0.7
Eicosenoic	max 0.5	max 0.5	max 0.5
Eptadecanoic	max 0.5	max 0.5	max 0.5
Eptadecenoic	max 0.5	max 0.5	max 0.5
Lignoceric	max 0.5	max 0.5	max 0.5
Beenic	max 0.3	max 0.3	max 0.3

• Phenols (tocopherols, etoxyphenols)
• Acids (in addition to free fatty acids, triterpenic acids, phenoxy acids)
• Chlorophyll

The higher absolute amount of RHO minor components, compared to those of VOQ and RVO, is chiefly due to fatty acid derivatives of long-chain alcohols (waxes) and to triterpenic alcohols.

Many of these compounds contribute to the classical flavor of the oil; some are related to the taste, imparting bitterness or a burning taste (Flat et al. 1973; Fedeli et al. 1973; Fedeli and Jacini 1970; Yoo et al. 1988; Cortesi and Fedeli 1983). The high keeping property of olive oil is partly due to its oleic acid content, since oleic oxidizes less than linoleic and linolenic acids, but a strong contribution comes from the simple and complex phenolic compounds present in the oil, plus tocopherols (Yoo et al. 1988; Cortesi and Fedeli 1983).

Since refining causes a partial loss of the preservative action of antioxidants in virgin oil, as happens with any refined oil, RVO and RHO are mixed with a portion of VOQ; this mixing restores some of the flavor and storage characteristics.

FATS AND OILS CONSUMED IN ITALY
AND IN OTHER MEDITERRANEAN COUNTRIES

It is difficult to report on fat and oil consumption on a quantitative basis in the Mediterranean countries because of lack of statistics and because of the variations in practice among the heterogeneous populations. It must also be considered that most of these countries are in a preindustrialized stage.

It is, however, evident from the fragmentary data available that the total consumption/capita/year is increasing, mostly because more seed oils are consumed. The gain in individual use of oils is due mostly to the increased availability of untraditional seed oils, chiefly soy bean, rapeseed, and sunflower seed oils, some imported and some locally grown (Table 6–5).

The consumption of solid fats of animal origin and the use of margarine remain relatively constant. In regard to content in the balance of oils consumed, the tendency is toward more unsaturated fat.

TECHNOLOGIES

A distinction must be made between extraction technologies used for olive oil and those used for seed oils because they are very different. Refining technologies for raw oils can be similar or different for the two categories of oils; therefore, extraction technologies will be considered separately, while refining of olive and seed oils will generally be discussed together.

Olive Oil Extraction

The ripening period for olives is very long—three months—in comparison to seeds. Since the fruit has a high water content (mean: 50%), olives cannot be stored and traded as seeds are but must be processed promptly because of the damage that the enzymes can cause in the presence of such a high water content. Hence, the industrial apparatus must be available for processing the oil immediately.

In addition to water, olives contain 20% oil (mean value) and 30% solid material (mean value), consisting of pulp and pit.

TABLE 6-5. Seed Oils Other Than Olive Sold in Italy (MI)

	Total	Peanut	Sunflower	Corn	Mixed Seed
1980	340	37	41	78	184
1981	353	31	46	88	187
1982	360	28	50	94	187
1983	365	25	51	95	193

Before extraction, the olives are first cleansed of dirt and then washed with water; this also removes any trace of agricultural contaminants present on the skin (Fedeli 1987, 1988).

The washed olives are coarsely ground to make a paste; this operation is extremely important to both the amount and the quality of the final product, because enzymes can cause intensive hydrolysis in the oil, which will also affect the flavor and keeping quality if the particles are very fine. If the particles are too big, impressive losses can also occur.

The choice of a correct grinding system depends on the variety of the olives, among other variables; olives differ greatly in size and in the ratio between the pulp, in which most of the oil is contained, and the woody pit. The old-fashioned grinder built of siliceous stone is still considered the best tool for the size-reduction operation, though hammer mills are sometimes used.

After grinding, the paste is thoroughly mixed and again ground during the mixing process. The apparatus used for the mixing operation is very similar to that previously described, the preferred siliceous stone mill. After this preliminary process, several options are open for the extraction of the oil.

In the past, the discontinuous hydraulic press was the most widely used tool. Dimensions, final pressure attained, and operating modalities can differ but basically, several round layers of paste are formed, 2 cm to 3 cm thick, around a nylon-net divider (Fedeli 1987). Between every three or four layers, a steel disk is interposed; an assembly of about 60 layers is formed and placed in the hydraulic press. The press has a perforated axis so that the liquor expressed by the pressure can percolate both through the sides and into the center of the assembly. Pressure is applied gradually, reaching a maximum of 400 atm in the most modern extraction plants.

Although many extraction units still use hydraulic presses (Fig. 6–1), because of the large manpower requirement, the tendency is toward replacement by other systems.

By one of the most generally used methods, the paste is mixed with warm water (30–60°C), strained to remove solid particles and then centrifuged in a horizontal system to separate the oil from the water (Fig. 6–2). A less commonly used extraction system is based on the adherence of the oil to stainless steel blades repeatedly immersed in the paste. In ancient times, the separation depended on spontaneous settling.

Even in the simple operation of separating water from oil, both old and new procedures have advantages and disadvantages. Undoubtedly, the rapid removal of the natural water content of the olive is very beneficial in preventing further enzymatic action, but it sometimes does not allow enough time for equilibrium to be reached between essential sub-

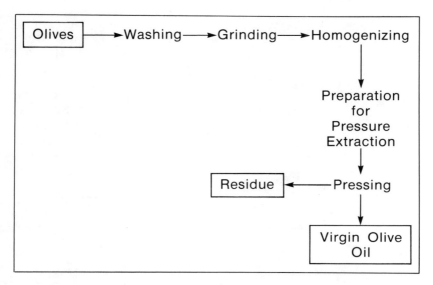

Figure 6-1.   Pressure extraction of virgin olive oil.

stances, such as the phenolic and aromatic components that are evenly distributed in water and oil.

If the oil is to be consumed immediately, it is filtered in a precoated filter-press before bottling. If not, it is sent to the refinery.

Any of the extraction procedures leave a certain amount of oil in the solid residue. To recover it, the fiber remnants are dried and extracted by the solvent hexane using semicontinuous equipment (Fig. 6-3).

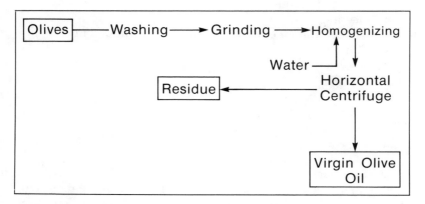

Figure 6-2.   Centrifuge extraction of virgin olive oil.

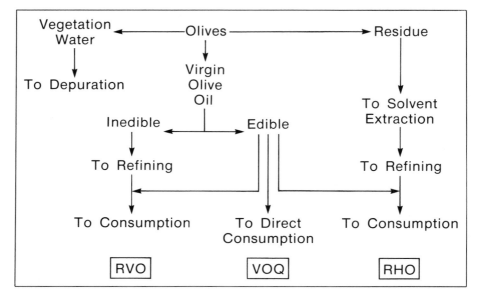

Figure 6-3.   Types of olive oils.

Seed Oil Extraction

In the Mediterranean area, seed extraction is usually done in large instal-
lations equipped with continuous presses and solvent extraction units.
Most factories proceed by the following steps:

1. Seed storage in large facilities
2. Seed cleaning
3. Internal seed transportation by continuous equipment
4. Seed dehulling
5. Seed crushing
6. Seed conditioning
7. Continuous expelling
8. Seed laminating
9. Solvent extraction with hexane
10. Solvent removal

Most of the factories in the Mediterranean basin are not devoted to
extraction of a specific seed but adjust the sequence to the requirements
of the raw material; for instance, the sequence 1, 2, 3, 4, 5, 6, 8, 9, 10
is followed for soy beans. In the underdeveloped countries, extraction

methods are less flexible, and plants generally process a specific seed; normally, their capacity is also lower.

In addition to providing the principal fat for the Mediterranean human diet, the processing plants produce a residue that meets the need for animal feed in all the countries of the region.

Refining

Refineries in Mediterranean countries use several up-to-date technologies to refine vegetable oil, according to its kind and quality.

At the present time, the most generally employed refining systems are (1) the classical, comprising the following steps:

a. Degumming
b. Alkaline neutralizing, washing, and drying
c. Bleaching
d. Physical neutralizing and deodorizing
e. Winterizing

Many refiners, however, use (2) the following sequence for olive oil: a, c, d, eliminating the b stage or (3) rearrange the steps: a, c, d, b, e.

Refineries in developed countries of the Mediterranean region usually are equipped to use both schemes enabling them to process any type of oil and to use mostly continuous systems. Refineries in the underdeveloped countries tend to be more specialized and smaller in size and more often use discontinuous systems.

High-acidity oils, such as those obtained from olive oil residue, are usually refined by employing the third procedure or by neutralizing with alkali in the presence of solvents. Hexane is the solvent for the oil fraction, isopropanol or acetone for the polar materials, that is, neutralizing agents and soapstock. Seed oils, which comprise most of the polyunsaturated oils, are refined according to the a, b, c, d, e procedure or by the a, c, d, b sequence, which is used to refine palm oil.

Oil Preservation

Seed oils are usually canned after refining. Olive oil of any grade is sometimes stored, before refining if the oil is of the grade that must be refined. Part of the production is purchased and stored by the governments or by the European Economic Community. Furthermore, since the quantity produced fluctuates widely, sometimes part of the product is stored for as much as one year. The storage units must meet established standards to preserve the quality of the product; normally, storage by private enterprise is less efficient. In any instance, long-term storage tends to lower the quality of virgin olive oil that is to be consumed without refining.

REFERENCES

Cortesi, N., and E. Fedeli. 1983. I composti polari di oli di oliva vergini. *Riv. Ital. Sost. Grasse* **60:**341.

Cortesi, N., E. Fedeli, and E. Tiscornia. 1985. I componenti polari degli oli di oliva. *Riv. Ital. Sost. Grasse* **62:**281.

Fedeli, E. 1977. Lipids of olives. In *Progress in the Chemistry of Fats and Other Lipids*, vol. 15, R. T. Homan, ed. New York: Pergamon Press.

Fedeli, E. 1983. Compasants mineurs des lipides. *Rev. Franc. des Corps Gras* **30:**51.

Fedeli, E. 1987. The impact of conventional technologies on the chemical composition of fats. In *Fat Production and Consumption*, NATO ASI series, E. Fedeli and C. Galli, eds., p. 185. New York: Plenum Press.

Fedeli, E. 1988. L'industria delle Sostanze Grasse. *Riv. Ital. Sost. Grasse* **65:**415.

Fedeli, E., and G. Jacini. 1970. Sui componenti odorosi dell'olio di oliva. *Chim. e Ind.* **52:**161.

Fedeli, E., and G. Jacini. 1971. Lipid composition of vegetable oils. In *Advances in Lipid Research* vol. 9, R. Paoletti and D. Kritchews, eds. New York: Academic Press.

Fedeli, E., D. Baroni, and G. Jacini. 1973. Componenti odorosi dello olio d'oliva. *Riv. Ital. Sost. Grasse* **50:**38.

Flat, R. A., R. R. Forrey, and D. G. Guadagni. 1973. Olive oil flavor. *J. Agric. Food Chem.* **21:**948.

Mariani, C., and E. Fedeli. 1986. Individuazione di oli di estrazione in quelli di pressione. *Riv. Ital. Sost. Grasse* **63:**3.

Mariani, C., and E. Fedeli. 1989. Minor components of vegetable oils: nonglyceridic esters. *Riv. Ital. Sost. Grasse* **63:**397.

Morchio, G., R. De Andreis, and E. Fedeli. 1987. Indagini sul contenuto di steroli totali in oli di oliva. *Riv. Ital. Sost. Grasse* **64:**185.

Yoo, Y. J., E. Fedeli, and W. W. Nawar. 1988. The volatile components produced from olive oil by heating. *Riv. Ital. Sost. Grasse* **65:**415.

7

Dairy Products

Giorgio Ottogalli
Giulio Testolin

Information concerning production and consumption of dairy products in the Mediterranean area in ancient times has come mainly from Greece, Rome, and Etruria (Istituto Poligrafico e Zecca dello Stato 1987; Erkahof-Stork 1976).

As concerns Greece, Homer on Odysseus in the cave of Polyphemus wrote:

> There were racks heavily laden with cheese. In the stable the lambs and rams were pushed against each other. . . . The casks were overflowing with whey. . . . He sat down and he milked the sheep and the bleating goats, everything according to the rules of the art. . . . After that, he curdled half of the white milk and stacked it in plaited baskets; the other parts he put away in barrels to drink from.

This description is not only charming poetry but also scientifically correct; it constitutes a realistic picture of a normal scene that for centuries has remained unchanged in many Mediterranean regions. A less famous Greek writer, Ateneo, making a survey of the kitchen utensils, described a tool for grating hard cheese; this is in line with the practice in Mediterranean countries of using a sprinkle of grated hard cheese as a dressing for a number of foods.

Archeological explorations of Etruscan civilization have produced earthenware filters and milk-boiling pots, offering proof that even these enthusiastic meat eaters consumed dairy products.

Dairying in ancient Rome is well documented. Cato, Varo, Columella, Suetonius, Pliny, Martial, Apicius, Vergil, and many others give more or less detailed instructions for making special varieties of cheese and for cooking with cheese. Oxygala was an acid curd aromatized with herbs such as marjoram, thyme, and coriander. Moretum was a dry cheese marinated in oil, vinegar, and herbs. Savillum was made with meal, cheese, honey, and beaten eggs, sprinkled with poppy seeds, and baked in an oven. Librum was a cheese cake. The consumption of milk was probably not very popular if we consider that Pliny in his *Naturalis historia* wrote of the two fluids most salutary for the human body: wine and oil, making no mention of milk.

In the Middle Ages, the art of cheese making was frequently confined to monasteries and abbeys. The consumption of dairy products was certainly widespread judging by the frequency with which cheese is mentioned in literature. *Regimen sanitatis,* in which the rules of the famous medical "Scuola salernitana" are collected in Latin verses, contains favorable mention of milk, whey, and cheese (*Caseus et panis bonus est cibus:* Cheese and bread is good food). Boccaccio's description in a story from the *Decameron* is worth quoting: "There was a mountain made entirely of grated Parmesan cheese, and on top of it people were making macaroni and noodles."

The discoveries of the last few centuries have only recently begun to change the dietary habits of Mediterranean peoples, including the use of dairy products.

Pasteur discovered the process for killing the pathogenic bacteria in wine and milk, but pasteurization is feasible only with refrigeration. Refrigerated storage of raw and pasteurized milk has been widespread only since World War II, changing not only technology but also social life. More recent important discoveries such as the application of ultra-pasteurization (UHT), coupled with aseptic packaging, have been determinants in increasing milk consumption in hot climates, as this new kind of product retains freshness and palatability.

STATISTICAL DATA

Some statistics on dairy product consumption in several countries selected as following the typical Mediterranean diet are given in Tables 7-1, 7-2, and 7-3 (ASSOLATTE 1987; International Dairy Federation [IDF] 1982, 1989).

TECHNOLOGY

For further reading on the technology of dairy products in the Mediterranean countries, see Robinson 1986, Battistotti et al. 1983, Scott 1986, Davies and Law 1984; IDF 1988, Burton 1983, and Alais 1984.

For the purpose of this discussion we have divided dairy products

TABLE 7-1. Milk Production in Five Mediterranean Countries in 1986 (thousand tons)

	Source			
	Sheep	Goat	Cow	Totals
France	1,087	454	33,700	35,241
Greece	600	400	642	1,642
Italy	483	119	10,270	10,772
Yugoslavia	140	—	4,600	4,740
Spain	232	360	6,702	7,394

Source: FAO (1986) data elaborated by ASSOLATTE.

into five main groups: fluid milks, concentrated and dried milks, fermented milks, cream and butter, and cheese and related products.

Fluid Milks

Raw Milk. Until recently in many places around the Mediterranean, raw milk was often bought in cans or directly from the farm. Bottled and certified raw milk was permitted by law in some countries but was rarely found in stores. In all cases, raw milk should be boiled as a safety precaution.

Pasteurized Milk. In the pasteurization process, milk is treated in a plate exchange heater to inactivate the pathogenic microorganisms present. Choices of the most frequently used time and temperature parameters are: 62.7°C × 30 min for low pasteurization, 71.7°C × 15 sec for high temperature, short time (HTST) and 88.4°C × 1 sec for HTST. After pasteurization, milk is packaged in cardboard containers or in glass or plastic bottles and cooled at 5°C or below. Average shelf life is four or five days. This relatively mild treatment preserves practically unchanged the nutritive value of the milk. It is estimated that, in Mediterranean countries, pasteurized milk usually constitutes less than half the total milk market.

Ultrapasteurized Milk. In ultrapasteurizing, milk is heat treated at an ultrahigh temperature (138°C) for 2 to 3 seconds. Steam is injected into milk, and this operation is followed by a vacuum treatment to flash off excess water. Sterile cardboard containers are aseptically filled with the milk, which can then be distributed without refrigeration. Average shelf

TABLE 7-2. Per-Capita Annual Consumption of Dairy Products in Seven Mediterranean Countries

	Product	1966	1986
France	Liquid milk	103.0 l	79.7 l
	Fermented milk	4.2 l	13.0 l
	Butter	9.0 kg	7.5 kg
	Cheese	12.1 kg	21.1 kg
Greece	Liquid milk	—	54.0 l
	Fermented milk	—	6.0 l
	Butter	—	0.9 kg
	Cheese	—	22.2 kg
Israel	Liquid milk	60.0 l	72.5 l
	Fermented milk	8.0 l	16.8 l
	Butter	1.2 kg	0.7 kg
	Cheese	8.8 kg	15.4 kg
Italy	Liquid milk	66.8 l	78.0 l
	Fermented milk	0.5 l	3.2 l
	Butter	1.6 kg	2.2 kg
	Cheese	9.1 kg	17.3 kg
Yugoslavia	Liquid milk	—	100.7 l
	Fermented milk	—	—
	Butter	—	0.5 kg
	Cheese	—	17.0 kg
Malta	Liquid milk	—	53.3 l
	Fermented milk	—	—
	Butter	—	0.7 kg
	Cheese	—	7.6 kg
Spain	Liquid milk	71.0 l	108.1 l
	Fermented milk	1.2 l	6.9 l
	Butter	0.3 kg	0.5 kg
	Cheese	2.1 kg	5.1 kg

Source: FAO (1985).

Note: The data, when available, are referred at a distance of 20 years (IDF 1982, 1989).

life is considered to be three months. Flavored milks and desserts are treated in the same way. The nutritive value is only slightly diminished.

Sterile Milks. Milk is preheated by the HTST method and placed in bottles, which are capped and then autoclaved. Shelf life is around six months, but nutritive value is severely diminished. UHT and sterile milk, particularly the UHT, are very widely used in Mediterranean coun-

TABLE 7-3. Per Capita Human Consumption of Calories, Proteins, and Lipids (General and from Dairy Products) in Seven Mediterranean Countries

	Population (thousand)	Calories number/day		Proteins (g/day)		Lipids (g/day)	
		Total	Milk	Total	Milk	Total	Milk
France	55,162	3,359	347	104.2	24.0	146.2	21.4
Greece	9,970	3,637	311	103.9	18.9	150.1	21.1
Israel	4,289	3,019	264	97.1	18.9	11.6	15.0
Yugoslavia	23,120	3,499	240	98.9	13.7	104.5	15.0
Italy	57,128	3,493	337	103.3	19.7	142.7	21.1
Malta	383	2,565	255	81.0	15.5	77.9	15.1
Spain	38,356	3,303	269	88.7	14.5	137.8	15.6

Source: FAO (1985); data elaborated by ASSOLATTE.

tries, especially in hot climates, because of their good keeping quality at room temperature.

Modified Milks. A category of milks modified to meet special dietary requirements includes the following products: milks with reduced fat, lactose, or sodium chloride and "filled" and "sweet acidophilus milk."

Fat-reduced milks, with low (1–1.8%) or very low (<0.5%) fat content, are available in most Mediterranean countries.

Lactose-reduced milk is prepared by adding the lactase enzyme directly to milk or pretreating milk by a lactase immobilized in a variety of carriers. By these methods, hydrolysis of lactose to glucose and galactose is partially induced, producing a sweeter and more digestible drink for people affected by lactase deficiency (see Lactose section).

A lactose-reduced milk produced by the second method is distributed in Italy by the Centrale del Latte di Milano, which has patented it.

Sodium-chloride-reduced milk (5 mg salt/l instead of 500 mg/l) is obtained through a dialysis process; this product is recommended for low-sodium diets.

In filled milks, natural butter is replaced by fats of vegetable origin to obtain a product lower in cholesterol and higher in unsaturated fatty acids. In Mediterranean countries, these milks are obtainable only in dry form as baby food.

Sweet acidophilus milk is prepared by adding a suspension of *Lactobacillus acidophilus* to pasteurized milk prior to final packaging. The taste and pH of the milk are not altered and the product supposedly has a probiotic effect (see section on probiotic microflora). This product has only recently appeared on the market in Mediterranean countries.

Some milks are modified by the addition of vitamins and fluoride, although this practice is rare in Mediterranean countries.

Concentrated and Dried Milks

The long keeping quality of these commodities is due to the low water activity, which inhibits microbial growth. These milks, which include evaporated, sweetened condensed, and dried and which were once quite popular in hot climates, have been partially or fully replaced by ultrapasteurized and sterile milks.

Evaporated Milk. Unsweetened evaporated milk is a whole milk from which about 60% of the water has been removed by evaporation.

Sweetened Condensed Milk. Condensed milk is produced by the evaporation of a considerable portion of the water from whole milk and the addition of sugar and/or dextrose.

Dried Milk Powders. Several dairy products, such as whole milk, skim milk, whey, buttermilk, and cream, may be prepared in dry form by the roller or by the spry-dry system. These milks are usually not produced in Mediterranean countries but are imported from nations having a milk surplus.

Powdered skim milk has a wide variety of uses, including for the preparation of starter cultures, as a basis for baby foods, and for fortifying milk for yogurt and cheese making, where allowed by law.

Fermented Milks

Table 7–4 presents a classification of the main groups and types of fermented milks produced and consumed in Mediterranean countries.

Fermented milks are obtained from heat-treated milk inoculated with starters and allowed to acidify until coagulation occurs. Normally, they should not be drained off. Microorganisms must be alive until the time of sale.

Yogurt. Because of its unique flavor and relatively long keeping quality, the most popular fermented milk in Mediterranean countries today is yogurt. Yogurt is manufactured with pure, lactic, thermophilic cultures, which are incubated at 45°C and then cooled to 5°C. The inability

TABLE 7-4. Classification of Fermented Milks, with Special Reference to Mediterranean Countries

Group	Micro-organisms			Type	Characteristic Compounds
Acid	Thermophilic	a	Str. thermophilus / Lact. bulgaricus	Yogurt	Lactic acid, acetaldehyde
		b	Lact. acidophilus	Acidophilus milk	Lactic acid
		c	Bifidobacterium	Bifidus milk	Lactic acid, acetic acid
	Mesophilic	d	Str. lactis or / Str. cremoris	Sour milk (esp. leben)	Lactic acid
		e	Str. lactis + / diacetylactis + / Leuconostoc sp.	Buttermilk	Lactic acid, diacetyl
Acid-alcoholic	Mesophilic	f	Lactic acid bacteria + yeasts	Kefir Gioddu	Lactic acid, ethanol, CO_2

Note: The letters *a* through *f* refer to mentions in the text.

of the lactic acid cultures of yogurt to grow at temperatures below 15°C produces reliable stability in the refrigerated product.

In the past, raw sheep milk was the principal base for making fermented milks; at present, it has been replaced by cow's milk. Only in some countries (e.g., Greece) and some other regions is sheep milk still employed, alone or in combination. When sheep milk is used, a product of thick consistency results. The same effect is obtainable by previously concentrating milk by vacuum evaporation or by ultrafiltration. Strained yogurt in Greece or *labneh* in the Middle East are products of this type that differ from the usual yogurt in their higher viscosity. The great increase in yogurt consumption in some Mediterranean countries (see Table 7–4) can be ascribed mainly to the appearance on the market of fruit yogurts. These are prepared by the addition of various kinds of fruit (cherry, strawberry, apricot, apple, banana, etc.) cut into pieces or in the form of jam, with or without flavorings.

Other Acid Thermophilic Products.   Acidophilus milk and bifidus milk (see Table 7–4 b and c) or analogous products contain microorganisms that are considered highly probiotic because of their supposed capacity to colonize the human bowel. Only recently have these products appeared on the market of some Mediterranean countries, such as France and Italy, but their consumption is still limited.

Acid and Acid-Alcoholic Mesophilic Products.   In the past, when such products were prepared only at home or on the farm, acid and acid-alcoholic mesophilic products (Table 7–4 d and f) were commonly available; hence, the terms *leben* and *gioddu*, which today are applied to yogurt, indicated different kinds of products containing mesophilic lactic acid bacteria and yeasts. At present, these fermented milks are not widely used except in France, where limited amounts of sour milk, or leben (type d), and buttermilk (type e) are produced, and in Israel, where a large quantity of type e is consumed. Buttermilk is the by-product of butter but can also be prepared by fermenting milk with aromatic cultures, which are used for maturing the cream prior to butter churning.

Kefir is a foamy, acid-alcoholic drink that utilizes "grains" as starters; these granules consist of a rubbery matrix of polysaccharidic origin in which are embedded lactic acid bacteria and yeasts. In the Mediterranean region, kefir grains are imported from Middle Eastern countries, and kefir is usually prepared in the home.

Other Products.   Some products are made by adding cereals to fermented milks. In Greece, dried yogurt is mixed with cereal flour in the form of a biscuit and is called *trahanas*. *Kishk* is a yogurt-wheat mixture, shaped into balls and sun dried, produced in Lebanon, Syria, and Jordan; similar products are found in Egypt and Israel.

Pasteurized fermented milks cannot be considered yogurts, as no living bacteria are present: such preparations must be labeled "dessert," with a fancy name.

Cream and Butter

Cream.   Cream is classified according to its fat content with at least three main grades, sometimes differing from country to country: 10% for coffee, 20% for other home uses, and 30% for whipping and bakery use. Cream is either pasteurized or, more frequently, UHT treated. Cream is not commonly used in Mediterranean countries and is mainly limited to confectionery and bakery use. Its use in home cooking is recent and not in line with Mediterranean tradition.

Butter.   Butter is produced by churning the cream obtained either by spontaneous creaming of milk or by centrifuging milk or whey. The cream can be previously ripened by adding cultures of *Streptococcus lactis, Streptococcus lactis var. diacetylactis* and *Leuconostoc cremoris.* These cultures produce, as principal metabolites, lactic acid and diacetyl, which impart the distinctive flavor to butter. Unripened butter is improperly called "sweet."

Butter can be salted with the addition of sodium chloride; originally this practice was justified to improve the keeping quality of the product, but now salt is added only for the sake of flavor, and preponderantly in northern Europe. Butter quality in Mediterranean countries is not exceptional, at least if judged by fastidious experts, partly because of the difficulty in keeping it fresh in hot climates and partly because of the traditional use of olive oil as a fat and seasoning. In tropical countries, butter is largely replaced by *ghee,* which is made by melting butter and boiling away the water, or by analogous products.

Cream and Butter Derivates.   Cream acidified with lemon or vinegar results in mascarpone, a typical product of northern Italy. In the south of Italy, butter is inserted into openings in mozzarella or similar types of cheese; these products are known as *burrata* or *burrini* or *manteca,* which is the Spanish word for butter.

Cheese and Related Products

In Mediterranean countries, cheese making has always been the preferred means for preserving the nutritional value of milk. Cheese making includes many raw materials and processes that differ among varieties and countries of manufacture. Table 7–5 lists the principal types of cheese and related products in four countries or regions, which we have selected as representative of the Mediterranean diet. The following paragraphs are numerically keyed to the products listed in the table.

1. Milk Species.   At the present time, cow's milk is the most common raw material; sheep and goat milk were formerly predominant, and their use is still important for making particular types of cheese. In Italy, buffalo milk is also used for the typical mozzarella.

2. Curdling Agents.   Most cheeses are made with animal, some with microbial, a few with vegetable, enzymes. On the other hand, cheeses obtained by simple acidification are not very popular in Mediterranean countries. In the table, (2) refers to cheeses made with vegetable coagulant.

TABLE 7-5. Examples of Typical Cheeses of Four Mediterranean Countries

Technological Features		Country of Manufacture			
Age Ripening	Consistency	Spain	Italy	France (south and Corsica)	Greece
Fresh or Short-Ripened (<1 month)	Soft	Burgos Manchego (fresh) Cabra	Stracchino Robiola (6) Mozzarella (4) Caprino (10) Ricotta (8) Cacioricotta (8)	Banon Cachat Buccio Niolo	Feta (7) Mitzitria (8)
Medium-Ripened (1–3 months)	Semisoft	Mahon Tetilla Aragon Cabrales (5)	Caciotta Provola (4) (9) Caciocavallo (4) Gorgonzola (5) Caciofiore (2)	Roquefort (5) Blu de Corse (5)	Kasseri (4) Kopanist (5)
Long-Ripened (3–12 months)	Hard (3)	Manchego (aged) Iditiobal (9) St. Simon Pedroches (2)	Grana Pecorino Fiore sardo		Kefalxotyri

Note: Numbers in parentheses refer to the numbered paragraphs in the text.

3. Hard Grating Cheeses. These cheeses are the most important. The curd is cooked in a vat, then pressed and left to ripen for a long period until it acquires a very firm consistency suitable for grating. It is used directly as grated cheese and in cooking.

4. Pasta Filata. Curd is warmed at approximately 45°C, left to acidify, and then immersed in hot water. It acquires a plastic consistency so that it can be kneaded and sculpted into balls, salami shapes, and so forth.

5. Blue-Veined Cheeses. These cheeses are characterized by the presence of molds of *Penicillium* grown inside the curd after it has been pierced by needles to attain relatively aerobic conditions. In two to three months, blue cheeses undergo a strong proteolysis and lipolysis process.

6. Rind Microflora. Surface microflora is frequently present on many Mediterranean cheeses, but the classical white mold flora and orange red smear cheeses are not typical, with few exceptions, of the Mediterranean tradition.

7. White-Brined Cheeses. These rindless, highly salted, drained curd cheeses have a high acidity. They are stored in brine at a low temperature in airtight packages such as tinned steel or plastic boxes. The presence of a high percentage of salt, formerly a device for preserving quality over time, imparts a flavor that is highly appreciated in many countries of the Mediterranean area, especially in the east and southeast.

8. Whey and Albumin Cheeses. Whey cheeses are typical of, if not exclusive to, Mediterranean countries. Whey is acidified and heated to produce the curd recooked cheese called in Italy ricotta and in Greece mitzitria. When milk is acidified and heated, an albumin cheese known as cacioricotta is obtained. Ricotta is usually considered a low-fat product, but its fat content varies (from 5% to 20%) and is higher when sheep milk is the base.

Whey cheeses actually should not be considered as true cheeses not only because of their composition but also because they do not contain lactic acid bacteria. Due to the absence of competition between lactic acid bacteria and the bacteria that cause spoilage, these cheeses are highly perishable.

9. Smoked Cheeses. Some cheeses, especially of the pasta filata type, after salting are left in a smoke-charged atmosphere. The smoke has a preservative effect and imparts a distinctive flavor to the cheese that is highly appreciated in some Mediterranean countries.

10. Under Oil. Some cheeses, particularly those made from goat milk, are immersed in olive oil, with or without herbs and aromatics, to increase their keeping properties or their flavor.

DAIRY MICROBIOLOGY AND HYGIENE

Microflora

The functions of microflora in dairy products are summarized in Table 7–6.

TABLE 7-6. Classification of Microorganisms According to Behavior and Effects

Types			Effects
Useful	Typical	Naturally present Inoculated as starters	Producing useful effects on the organoleptic properties
	Probiotic	Naturally present Inoculated as starters	Producing beneficial effects on human health
Harmful	Alterative	Modificatory Spoilage	Making the products atypical Making the product inedible
	Pathogenic	Infectious Toxinfectious	Producing harmful effects on human health

Source: Ottogalli and Caserio (1989).

Typical Microflora. Starters and natural flora (lactic acid bacteria, yeasts, *Penicillia*, etc.) perform a useful function for the liberation of favorable substances to obtain a typical product. In Mediterranean countries, the thermophilic lactic acid bacteria are more generally used than the mesophilic, and the natural starters are often preferred to the industrial (Lawrence et al. 1976; Blanc 1983).

Probiotic Microflora. Microorganisms can exert a beneficial influence on human health by modifying the equilibrium of the intestinal microflora and by producing useful substances such as vitamins, organic acids, and bacteriocins. Lactic acid bacteria are considered probiotic microorganisms, but Bifidobacteria, Propionibacteria and possibly many others could also be included in this list. Fermented milks and cheeses can be considered as effective carriers of probiotic microflora. The use of raw milk for making cheese, especially the medium- and long-ripened cheeses, is common in Mediterranean countries and helps to produce cheeses rich in probiotic microflora (Ottogalli and Galli 1988; IDF 1983; Hentges 1983).

Pathogenic Microorganisms and Toxins. Pathogenic bacteria, that is, *Brucella, Listeria, Salmonella, Shigella, Yersinia* and *Escherichia coli* EEC; food-borne viruses; bacterial toxins, for example, *Staphylcoccus aureus* enterotoxins; and mycotoxins, for example, aflatoxins, can be found in improperly processed dairy products. When the consumption of raw liquid milk and of cheeses made with unpasteurized milk was extremely common in Mediterranean countries, melitensis fever, tuberculosis, and gastrointestinal disorders were frequent. In this regulated era, milk, yogurt-milk and cheese-milk are submitted to pasteurization according to governmental regulations (Thatcher and Clark 1986; Bryan 1982; IDF 1980).

Alterative Microflora.   This microflora is directly responsible for a series of alterative processes that either change the character of the product or cause it to spoil. *Pseudomonas,* coliforms, *Bacillus, Clostridium,* some yeasts and some molds are considered particularly harmful in this respect.

Health Hazards

We have already seen that microorganisms and their toxins can cause health hazards, but other problems can be caused by chemical residues in milk and milk products and by biogenic amines.

Chemical Residues.   Antibiotics are used in the treatment of udder infections. Milk from the affected animals should not be consumed for 72 to 96 hours after administration of the medications.

Residuals of disinfectants derived from incorrectly cleaned equipment may contaminate milk. Very low concentrations of some heavy metals (arsenic, cadmium, copper, iron, lead, mercury) reach milk via fodder or through contamination during or after milking (IDF 1979, 1978).

Biogenic Amines.   During cheese ripening, some aromatic amines such as histamine and tyramine sometimes are released in many cheeses (Table 7–7). In most cases, consumption of such cheeses does not lead to physiological problems because amino-destroying enzymes in the digestive tract prevent the uptake of these compounds by the bloodstream. However, when amine degradation is impaired, food poisoning can occur, producing migraine and neurological disturbances. Toxicity is greatly increased by the contemporary intake of monoamino oxydase (MAO) inhibiting drugs or by drinking amine-containing wines (Joosten and Northolt 1987; Edwards and Sandine 1981; Cerutti et al. 1971).

Additives

Some additives are permitted in Mediterranean countries, at defined concentration, to improve the rheological properties or the keeping quality (see Table 7–8) (Cerutti 1989).

TABLE 7-7. Histamine and Tyramine in Some Italian Cheeses

Variety	Istamine (mg/kg)	Tyramine (mg/kg)
Pecorino (2–4 mo)	0–trace	35–100
Pecorino (9–14 mo)	0–50	40–300
Grana, aged	0	0–traces
Gorgonzola, fresh	0	0–traces
Gorgonzola, aged	20–30	100–1,000

Source: Cerutti et al. (1971).

NUTRITION AND DIET

Nutritional Aspects

Different species of mammals produce milk with different characteristics (Table 7–9). Human milk is a complete and ideal food for the newborn baby. Goat milk is considered very similar to it; being easily digestible by humans, it has frequently been used in nutrition of the young and old in Mediterranean countries. Sheep milk is rich in fat and is used mainly for making yogurt and cheese. Cow's milk is a nearly complete food for the newborn human baby but has some drawbacks. To make it more suitable, it is advisable to modify it both physically by reducing the size of the fat globules and casein mycelles and chemically by adding unsaturated fatty acids. Cow's milk is used for the preparation of many dairy products whose compositions are reported in Table 7–10 (Renner 1982).

Consumption of dairy products is considered very important in Mediterranean countries primarily because of their lactose, protein and mineral salt content and secondarily for their fat and vitamin content.

TABLE 7-8. Additives Permitted by Italian Legislation

E-System	Additives	Product
E200	Sorbic acid	Fruit for yogurt and cheeses
E235	Pimaricin	Cheese
E240	Formic aldeid	Milk for Grana Padano
E239	Exametilentetramine	Provolone
E280	Propionic acid	Cheese (surface)
E234	Nisin	Cheese
E400	Alginates	Cheese (quark or cottage type)
E331	Citrates	Melted cheeses
E450	Polyphosphates	Melted cheeses

TABLE 7-9. Milk Composition of Different Species (average g per 100)

	Water	Total Solids	Lactose	Fat	Nitrog. Matter	Mineral Salts	Calories
Human	89.3	11.7	6.5	3.5	1.5	0.2	66
Cow	87.5	12.5	4.7	3.5	3.5	0.8	66
Goat	86.4	13.6	4.5	4.3	4.0	0.8	74
Sheep	80.9	19.1	4.5	7.5	6.0	1.1	112
Buffalo	82.2	17.8	4.7	7.5	4.8	0.8	108

Lactose.   Lactose is the substrate of many kinds of microbial fermentation activity, producing lactic acid, which is antagonistic to putrefactive bacteria. In humans, the presence of the enzyme lactase in the cells of the small intestine enables the assimilation of lactose (Dahlquist 1983 and Costet et al. 1983). Various types and grades of lactose intolerance are caused by the absence of lactase. These are distinguished as follows:

- Congenital lactase deficiency, beginning at birth, causes a complete intolerance of any kind of milk.
- Adult lactase deficiency, or isolated hypolactasia, appears at 3 to 6 years of age and is distributed differently among ethnic groups: A large proportion occurs among non-Caucasian people, who are generally lactase deficient (LD), and a smaller proportion among white and Hamite (North African) populations, who are prevalently lactose persistent (LP), as shown in Table 7–11.

TABLE 7-10. Chemical Composition of Some Dairy Products Obtained from Cow's Milk (average g per 100)

	Water	Total Solids	Lactose	Lactic Acid	Fat	Proteins	Mineral Salts	Calories
Milk	87.5	12.5	4.7	tr	3.5	3.5	0.8	66
Dried Skimmed Milk	5.0	95.0	50.0	tr	1.5	34.0	8.0	358
Cream (35% Fat)	60.0	40.0	2.5	tr	35.0	2.0	0.5	343
Yogurt	86.0	14.0	3.5	1	3.7	3.8	0.9	68
Butter	16.0	84.0	0.8	tr	82.0	1.0	0.2	770
Cheese:								
Stracchino	60.0	40.0	3.0	1	20.0	15.0	2.0	260
Grana	32.0	68.0	tr	2	23.0	39.0	6.0	380

Note: tr = trace.

**TABLE 7-11. Adult Lactase Deficiency
in Different Populations**

	Percent Affected
Sweden	3
Denmark	3
Finland	16
Switzerland	17
England	20–30
France	42
USA (Whites)	6
(Negroes)	73
Africa (Hamites)	10
(Negroids)	100
Japan and Far East Populations	100

Source: Dahlquist (1983).

- Secondary lactase deficiency is acquired as a result of a primary disease: toxi-infection, gastric disorders, or severe malnutrition. The use of lactase preparations or low-lactose milk has been proposed for lactose-intolerant subjects. An only partial hydrolysis (30–70%) seems sufficient in most cases to solve the intolerance problem (Repelins 1983). In some countries, of which France is one, products of this kind are not authorized because of adverse effects of the even rarer galactosemia and the consequent possibility of causing cataracts in galactouridase-deficient subjects (MacDonald and Williams 1983).

Fat and Cholesterol.   Fat content is highly variable in milk from different mammal species and also in milk from the same source. Fat is composed of glycerin and fatty acids, the proportions of which determine its properties and type.

Milk fat is not always easily digested. It can cause dyspepsia and can retard the emptying of the stomach. Mediterranean people, who seem to suffer from these disturbances, refer to some of these symptoms as liver upsets. According to some authors, about 10% of these cases can be attributed to intolerance to milk lipids. Whole milk and derivative products are high-fat foods: hence the cholesterol content in butter and full-cream cheese is relatively high (see Table 7–12). To render milk more digestible, the diameter of the fat globule is reduced by homogenization, a useful technological practice. It is also possible to standardize and lower the fat content by centrifuging or even by natural creaming. In

**TABLE 7-12. Average Cholesterol
Content of Milk and Dairy Products**

	Cholesterol (mg/100 g)
Cow's milk	13
Skim milk	2
Human milk	20
Goat's milk	10
Sheep milk	11
Condensed milk	30
Skim milk powder	20
Whole milk powder	100
Cream	90
Butter	230
Buttermilk	2
Cheese (depending on type)	0–100

Source: Renner (1982).

Mediterranean countries, yogurt and fluid milk with reduced fat content are now readily available.

Butter must have a minimum fat content, which in most countries is around 82%.

Finding low-fat or low-cholesterol cheese is more complicated for technical and legal reasons. While it is easy to obtain defatted fresh and soft cheese, medium- and long-ripened cheeses need a quota of fat to develop the proper texture and flavor. Apart from this technical problem, not all the countries allow the sale of low-fat cheese as such; in Italy, most cheeses must contain more than 45–48% fat in dry matter. Otherwise, they cannot be called cheeses but must have a fictitious name (Gurr 1983, 1988a; Van der Merr 1988).

Proteins. Milk proteins can be subdivided into casein and whey proteins. Casein is curdled at pH 4.5 or by enzymes such as chimase in the human stomach or rennin, which is used for milk curdling. Whey proteins, lactoalbumin and lactoglobulin, are denaturated by heat; whey milk, acidified and heat treated, becomes ricotta cheese.

Milk proteins contain all the essential amino acids. When added to other proteinaceous foods, particularly those of vegetable origin, they improve the nutritional value of the diet, for example, when bread or cereals are eaten with milk or cheese as is customary in the Mediterranean diet. Milk proteins are very digestible: 96% in comparison to 74–84% of plant proteins (Hambreaeus 1981). Milk proteins also are an effective buffer and are recommended for preventing gastric hyperacidity in the treatment of stomach ulcers.

The immunoglobulins (mainly IgA) of milk play a role not only in defending the gut mucosa against the invasion of pathogenic microorganisms but also in preventing the absorption of foreign proteins. Intolerance of cow's milk protein is relatively rare and can be due either to enzyme (tripsine or enterotoxinase deficiency) or to allergy. The latter can appear in young people, usually before the age of two, but also in adults. In both cases, the clinical symptoms are more or less aspecific. The cause of the allergy is ascribed to the passage of macromolecules through the intestinal barrier. The estimated incidence of protein allergy is 3% of total cases of milk protein intolerance, but probably many of the unidentified disturbances are due to this factor.

In some Mediterranean countries, it is possible to fortify market (fluid) milk, yogurt milk, and cheese milk with proteins such as casein coprecipitates and milk powder; in others, for example Italy, the practice is prohibited by law (Navarro and Cezard 1983; Raiha 1983).

Mineral Salts.   Milks and other dairy products are rich in mineral salts; their contribution to the recommended daily intake (RDI) of calcium, magnesium, and some trace elements is particularly important, as can be seen in Tables 7-13 and 7-14. The role of dairy products in supplying calcium is obviously essential when we realize that without them, the daily intake rarely exceeds 300 mg out of an estimated 600–1000 mg requirement. Yogurt and rennetted cheeses maintain the salt content of the milk practically unchanged whereas acid-curdled cheese loses part of its salt in the whey, which, perhaps, explains the preference by Mediterranean people for yogurt and rennetted cheeses that better fulfill their calcium requirements (Gurr 1988b; Schaalsma 1983).

TABLE 7-13. Recommended Daily Intakes of Minerals and Amounts Supplied by One-Half Litre of Milk

	RDI (mg/day)	Supply in 1/2 l milk (percent)
Calcium	800	75
Phosphorus	800	60
Potassium	2000	38
Sodium	2000	24
Chlorine	3000	17
Magnesium	300	20

Source: Renner (1982).

TABLE 7-14. Recommended Daily Intakes of Trace Elements and Estimated Contribution to Diet from Dairy Products

	RDI (mg/day)	Contribution from Dairy Products (percent)
Chromium	0.05	20
Cobalt	0.003 (B12)	26
Copper	2.00	3
Iron	12–18	2
Fluorine	1.5–4.0	unknown
Iodine	0.15	20–36
Manganese	2.5–5.0	2–3
Molybdenum	0.15–0.5	unknown
Nickel	unknown	19
Selenium	0.05–0.20	unknown
Zinc	15	15.25

Source: Gurr (1988b).

Vitamins.   Milk is rich in vitamins (Table 7-15). The content of many vitamins, such as A, E, and D fluctuates widely with season and sun exposure. Processing may modify the content of some, even assuming relatively small losses except for C. According to investigations cited by Renner 1982, milk and milk products contribute to the following proportions of the total intake in diets of people in industrialized countries: vitamin A, 12–45%; thiamine, 6–20%; riboflavin, 35–70%; pyridoxine, 10–20%; nicotinic acid, 2–5%; pantothenic acids, 20–30%; ascorbic acid, 4–13%; vitamin D, 5–20%; vitamin E, about 10% (Alais 1984; Renner 1982).

Other Constituents.   In this list of ingredients in dairy products, by necessity incomplete, enzymes should also be mentioned: phosphatase, lactoperoxidase, catalase, lactase, lysozyme, lactoferrin, xanthinoxidase, plus hormones and organic acids (Reiter, 1985).

Dietary Aspects

Food Habits.   A comparison of amounts and kinds of dairy products consumed in several Mediterranean countries (see Table 7-16) can furnish a better understanding of the contribution of these foods to the RDI of some micronutrients (see Table 7-17). Familiar practices and organo-

TABLE 7-15. Average Vitamin Content of Milk

| | Content in Milk (mg/l) | |
	Mean Value	Range of Values
A	0.37	0.10 – 0.50
Carotene	0.21	0.05 – 0.40
B₁ (thiamine)	0.42	0.20 – 0.80
B₂ (riboflavin)	1.72	0.80 – 2.60
B₆ (pyridoxine)	0.0045	0.002 – 0.007
Nicotinic acid	0.92	0.30 – 0.20
Folic acid	0.053	0.01 – 0.10
Pantothenic acid	3.60	2.60 – 4.90
Inositol	160.0	30.00 – 400.00
C (ascorbic acid)	18.0	5.00 – 30.00
D (cholecalciferol)	0.0008	0.0001 – 0.002
E (tocopherol)	1.10	0.20 – 2.00
K	0.03	tr. – 0.17
Biotin	0.036	0.01 – 0.07
Choline	170.0	50.00 –450.00

Source: Renner (1982).

leptic preferences have certainly contributed to limiting daily milk consumption mainly to breakfast time. Actually, what is called the continental breakfast is practically the Mediterranean breakfast. This meal consists of bread or sometimes scones, a little butter, jam, honey, and a cup or bowl of milk, usually with coffee and sugar. Milk is used, though not to a large extent, in cooking.

Fermented milks are used in different ways according to national custom: as a dessert at lunchtime or as a snack during daily breaks. The use of yogurt is very popular in prepared dishes and sauces in Greece.

TABLE 7-16. Dairy Product Consumption in Some Mediterranean Countries (kg/capita/year)

	Milk	Fermented Milks	Butter	Cheese
France	70–100	>10	>5	>20
Italy	70–100	<5	1–5	15–20
Spain	>100	5–10	<1	<10
Greece	<70	5–10	<1	>20
Yugoslavia	>100	ND	<1	15–20
Malta	<70	ND	<1	<10
Israel	<70	>10	<1	15–20

Notes: Data elaborated from Table 7–3; ND = no data.

TABLE 7-17. Percentage of Daily Allowances of Microelements and Vitamins Provided by Dairy Products

	Ca	P	Fe	B_1	B_2	C	A
Yugoslavia	43.4	42.7	2.8	10.2	30.4	6.1	15.6
Malta	30.2	29.8	1.5	6.1	18.1	3.2	15.2
France	50.8	50.3	1.5	8.2	24.1	3.4	62.6
Greece	13.9	13.8	0.5	2.3	6.9	1.0	10.7
Italy	52.4	51.6	2.7	10.8	32.2	5.9	29.7
Spain	38.2	37.5	2.7	9.6	28.7	6.0	11.9
Israel	37.3	36.8	1.5	6.9	20.4	3.4	21.1

Notes: Daily dietary allowances are calculated for a 30- to 60-year-old male (L.A.R.N., or Livelli di Assunzione Raccomandati di Nutrienti [recommended dietary allowance]). Composition data are from tables by Instituto Nazionale della Nutrizione of Italy. Cheese composition is averaged for the four most representative items from consumption statistics: provolone, bel paese, crescenza, and grana.

Cheese, in ancient times considered a staple food and used alone as the principal source of protein, is now often included in meals as a second course or as a dessert.

Food Combinations. According to recent theories, combining dairy products with other foods is apparently nutritionally very significant (see Table 7–18). In this respect, it is important to emphasize the benefits of combining dairy products with nonanimal-derived foods such as cereals and vegetables. In the case of cereals, milk and other dairy products compensate for the shortage of lysine; in the case of vegetables and fruit, they add fiber in addition to mineral salts and vitamins.

The following paragraphs are keyed to Table 7–18.

A1. The association of nonamidaceous vegetables with dairy products is very popular. Noteworthy examples are Greek dishes such as salad made with lettuce, olives, tomatoes, cucumbers, and green pepper, plus feta cheese; salad with a dressing containing yogurt (sadziki); or the spinach and cheese pie spanakopita.

A2. Amidaceous vegetables and dairy products are combined to great advantage: Potatoes, eggplant, and pumpkin are used mashed or in pies with the addition of milk or cheese.

B. Pulses and cheese combine well, though the practice is not widespread. Broadbeans and pecorino is a well-known dish of central and southern Italy.

C1. Buttered bread is a staple of the Mediterranean breakfast. For centuries, cheese with bread has been a staple food for any meal.

C2. Cereal flour, rice, and pasta are universally used with dairy products and are excellent combinations from both organoleptic and nu-

TABLE 7-18. Combinations of Dairy Products with Nondairy Foods in the Mediterranean Diet

	Milk	Cream	Butter	Fermented Milks	Cheese fs[1]	mr[2]	lr[3]	Whey Cheese
A. Vegetables								
A1. Nonamidaceous (eg. salad)	■	■	−	+	+	+	+	+
A2. Amidaceous (eg. potato)	■	■	■	−	■	■	■	■
B. Pulses	■	■	■	−	■	+	+	■
C. Cereals								
C1. Bread	+	−	+	−	+	+	+	+
C2. Rice, Pasta	+	■	+	■	+	+	+	+
C3. Pizza	−	−	−	−	+	−	−	−
D. Fruits	+	+	−	+	+	−	−	+
E. Eggs	+	−	+	−	■	+	+	■
F. Fish	■	■	■	−	−	■	+	−
G. Meat	−	■	■	−	−	■	+	−
H. Spices	■	−	■	■	+	+	+	+
I. Alcoholic drinks	−	−	■	−	+	+	+	■

Note: ■ = rare, − = absent, + = frequent.
1. Fresh and soft
2. Medium ripened
3. Long ripened

tritional points of view. Polenta e latte (corn meal mush and milk), pasta and rice sprinkled with grated cheese, ravioli stuffed with spinach mixed with whey cheese: all are examples of Italian cooking, but similar dishes can found in other Mediterranean countries.

C3. The true pizza is made only with mozzarella, which is a buffalo or cow's milk pasta filata cheese.

D. Fruits match very well with dairy products; we can cite milk-shakes, ice cream, fruit yogurts, many fruit desserts, and, lastly, the proverbial cheese and pear.

E. Many recipes for omelettes and scrambled eggs call for milk or cheese.

F. Butter is rarely used for frying in Mediterranean countries, as the typical cook makes use mainly, if not exclusively, of olive oil. Cheese is sometimes used for stuffing clams or scallops.

G. Not everybody agrees that dairy products combine well with meat; for example, Jewish kosher laws prohibit the consumption of meat and dairy products at the same meal. In Mediterranean countries, dishes including both meat and cheese are rather common, such as

- Greek moussaka—grated hard cheese (kefalotyri) between layers of eggplant and meat
- Greek pastitsio—macaroni layered with meat sauce and kefalotyri cheese
- Italian cannelloni—rolls of pasta stuffed with meat, covered with bechamel (cream) sauce and sprinkled with Parmesan cheese
- Italian sartu—souffle made with rice, egg, chicken giblets, and mozzarella cheese

Combining meat with cheese is certainly more common today than in ancient times when a poor Mediterranean person's diet did not permit the luxury of two animal proteins at a single meal; such combinations, rather, occurred in the case of leftovers. It must also be emphasized that cheese often is only grated and sprinkled on top of the meat dish.

H.   Spices, such as black pepper and pimento, are sometimes embedded in cheeses. Some herbs, such as fennel, garlic, and parsley, are used today with dairy products, but ancient Roman recipes indicate that this practice was more common in that era.

I.   Light white wines team up very well with soft and short-ripened cheese, whereas red wines are more appropriate with medium and long-ripened cheese.

Beer, even if not a typically Mediterranean drink, is the most popular drink in pizza restaurants.

REFERENCES

Alais, C. 1984. *Science du lait. Principes des tecniques laitiers.* Paris: Société d'Edition et de Publicité Agricoles, Industrelles et Commerciales.

Associazione Italiana Lattiero-Casearia (ASSOLATTE). 1987. Relazione del Presidente. Supplemento della Rivista *Il Mondo del Latte.*

Battistotti, B., V. Bottazzi, A. Piccinardi, and G. Volpato. 1983. *Formaggi del mondo.* Milano: Arnoldo Mondadori.

Blanc, B. C. 1983. Caracterisation des souches microbienne intervenant dans la composition d'une culture fromagère. *Microb. Aliment, Nutr.* 1:321.

Bryan, F. L. 1982. *Diseases Transmitted by Foods (A Classification and Summary),* 2nd ed. Atlanta: Centers for Disease Control.

Burton, H. 1983. *Bacteriological, chemical, biochemical and physical changes that occur in milk at temperatures of 100–150°C.* In Part 1, Document 157, International Dairy Federation, ed. Brussels: IDF.

Cerutti, G. 1989. *Il rischio alimentare.* Milano: Techniche Nuove.

Cerutti, G., F. Semeraro, and R. Zappavigna. 1971. Tiramina ed altre ammine pressorie negli alimenti con particolare riguardo ai formaggi. Nota 2a. Esame di formaggi nazionali di varia origine ed eta. *Il Latte* **45**:15.

Costet, S. P., P. Rampal, M. Lonbiere, and J. Delmont. 1983. Do lipids play a role in milk intolerance? In *Milk Intolerances and Rejection,* J. Delmont, ed., p. 77. Basel: Merkur, Karger.

Dahlquist, A. 1983. Digestion of lactose. In *Milk Intolerances and Rejection,* J. Delmont, ed., p. 11. Basel: Merkur, Karger.

Davies, F. L., and B. A. Law. 1984. *Advances in the Microbiology and Biochemistry of Cheese and Fermented Milk.* London and New York: Elsevier.

Edwards, S. T., and W. E. Sandine. 1981. Public health significance of amines in cheese. *J. Dairy Sci.* **64**:2431.

Erkahof-Stork, N. 1976. *The World Atlas of Cheese.* United Kingdom: Paddington Press Ltd.

Gurr, M. I. 1983. Trans fatty acids from nutrition and metabolism. In *Nutrition and Metabolism,* International Dairy Federation, ed., p. 5. Document 166. Brussels: IDF.

Gurr, M. I. 1988a. Diet and cardiovascular disease: a strategy for IDF. In *Milk Products and Health,* International Dairy Federation, ed., p. 10. Document 222. Brussels: IDF.

Gurr, M. I. 1988b. Nutritional significance of essential trace elements in dairy foods. In *Milk Products and Health,* International Dairy Federation, ed., p. 18. Document 222. Brussels: IDF.

Hambreaeus, L. 1981. Comparative nutritive value of vegetable and milk proteins. In *Special Addresses at IDF Session,* International Dairy Federation, ed., p. 10. Document 136. Brussels: IDF.

Hentges, D. J. 1983. *Human Intestinal Microflora in Health and Disease.* New York: Academic Press.

International Dairy Federation. 1978. *Metal Contaminants in Milk and Milk Products.* Document 105. Brussels: IDF.

International Dairy Federation. 1979. *Residues in Milk.* Document 113. Brussels: IDF.

International Dairy Federation. 1980. *Behaviour of Pathogens in Cheese.* Document 122. Brussels: IDF.

International Dairy Federation. 1982. *Consumption Statistics for Milk and Milk Products Including Summary 1966–1980.* Document 144. Brussels: IDF.

International Dairy Federation. 1983. *Cultural Dairy Products in Human Nutrition.* Document 159. Brussels: IDF.

International Dairy Federation. 1988. *Fermented Milk Science and Technology.* Document 277. Brussels: IDF.

International Dairy Federation. 1989. *Consumption Statistics for Milk and Milk Products.* Document 237. Brussels: IDF.

Istituto Poligrafico e Zecca dello Stato. 1987. *A.A.:L'alimentazione nel mondo antico,* vols. 1–4, Rome.

Joosten, H. M. L. J., and M. D. Northolt. 1987. Conditions allowing the formation of biogenic amines in cheese: decarboxilative properties of some non-starter bacteria. *Neth. Milk Dairy J.* **41**:259.

Lawrence, R. C., T. D. Thomas, and B. E. Terzaghi. 1976. Reviews of the progress of dairy science: cheese starters. *J. Dairy Res.* **43**:141.

MacDonald, I., and C. A. Williams. 1983. Galactose tolerance in healthy subjects. In *Milk Intolerances and Rejection*, J. Delmont, ed., p. 77. Basel: Merkur, Karger.

Navarro, J., and J. R. Cezard. 1983. Intolerance to cow milk proteins before the age of two: diagnostic means, incidence and evolution. In *Milk Intolerance and Rejection*, J. Delmont, ed., p. 133. Basel: Merkur, Karger.

Ottogalli, G., and G. Caserio. 1989. Classical and recent methods for microbiological analysis of foods. In *Food Safety. New Methods for Research and Control*, E. De Poli, C. L. Galli, and P. Restani, eds., p. 37. Milan: Masson.

Ottogalli, G., A. Galli, and G. Rondinini. 1988. Cheese as a carrier of probiotic microflora in the diet. *Ann. Microbiol.* **38**:163.

Raiha, N. 1983. Milk proteins and the newborn. In *Nutrition and Metabolism*, International Dairy Federation, ed., p. 3. Document 166. Brussels: IDF.

Reiter, B. 1985. *Protective proteins in milk—biological significance and exploitation (lysozime, lactoferrin, lactoperoxidase, xanthineoxidase)*. International Dairy Federation, ed. Document 191. Brussels: IDF.

Renner, E. 1982. *Milk and Dairy Products in Human Nutrition*. Munich: Volkswirtschaftlicher Verlag.

Repelins, C. 1983. Technological production of lactase and lactose-hydrolysed milk. In *Milk Intolerances and Rejection*, J. Delmont, ed., p. 57. Basel: Merkur, Karger.

Robinson, R. K. 1986. *Dairy Microbiology*, vol. 1–2. London and New York: Elsevier.

Schaalsma, G. 1983. Milk and calcium. In *Nutrition and Metabolism*, International Dairy Federation, ed., p. 19. Document 166. Brussels: IDF.

Scott, R. 1986. *Cheesemaking Practice*. London and New York: Elsevier.

Thatcher, F. S., and D. S. Clark. 1986. *Microorganisms in Foods: Their Significance and Methods of Enumeration*. Toronto: University of Toronto Press.

Van der Merr, R. 1988. Species-dependent effects of dietary casein and calcium cholesterol metabolism from milk products and health. In *Milk Products and Health*, International Dairy Federation, ed., p. 24. Document 222. Brussels: IDF.

8

Grains, Legumes, Fruits, and Vegetables: Lente Carbohydrate Sources in the Mediterranean Diet

Thomas M. S. Wolever
Alexandra L. Jenkins
Peter J. Spadafora
David J. A. Jenkins

Foods of plant origin have always played a central role in the nutrition of Mediterranean peoples. The Roman conquest of Egypt was to secure a grain supply: Britain was valued by Rome as the granary of the North. Legumes also were highly prized in biblical times. Esau gave away his inheritance for a "mess of Pottage," a bowl of lentil soup. Cicero, the great republican Roman orator and statesman, derived his name from the chick-pea *(Cicer arietanum)* due to the pealike lesion on the nose of one of his ancestors. Cereals and legumes, therefore, represent foods that have been respected for their essential functions in the human diet since antiquity. We suggest that one of the reasons why many of these traditional foods have special health attributes, in addition to being low in saturated fat, is that they are also slowly absorbed.

At a time when many traditional eating patterns are changing radically, it is ironic that slowing carbohydrate absorption has now been designated a new therapeutic principle (Creutzfeldt and Folsh 1983). Already, a number of therapeutic approaches that rely on slowing the rate of carbohydrate absorption have been developed for the treatment of major chronic diseases. These treatment approaches include the use of (1) enzyme inhibitors (glucoxidase inhibitors), (2) soluble fiber, (3) diets of low glycemic index and, (4) increasing meal frequency (nibbling vs. gorging).

Enzyme inhibitors, for example, glucoxidase inhibitors, reduce small intestinal sucrase and maltase activity and pancreatic amylase activity. The enzyme inhibitors are being tested for their use on the treatment of diabetes (Hillebrand et al. 1979; Hillebrand and Boehma 1982) and hyperlipidemia (Maruhama et al. 1980). Over the last two decades, there has been much interest in the use of soluble fiber. In purified form, these have been shown to reduce the rate of diffusion of glucose (Jenkins et al. 1986a) and amino acids (Elsenhaus et al. 1980) in *in vitro* systems and to slow bulk diffusion in the small intestine (Blackburn et al. 1984). The effect appears to relate to increased luminal viscosity (Jenkins et al. 1986a; Blackburn et al. 1984). Soluble fibers in purified form (Bosello et al. 1984) and in foods (Gatti et al. 1984; Botha et al. 1981) have been associated with improved control of diabetes and reduced levels of serum cholesterol, specifically LDL cholesterol (Jenkins et al. 1979). Recent studies using low glycemic index diets have shown similar metabolic effects to fiber but with no increase in total fiber intake (Fontvieille et al. 1988; Brand et al. 1988); and increases in soluble fiber intake, where present, were small (Jenkins et al. 1985; Jenkins et al. 1987a).

In this context, the Mediterranean diet would be predicted to offer major nutritional advantages. Mediterranean foods are rich sources of fiber, especially soluble fiber. Many of the foods show slow rates of digestion *in vitro*, which make them valuable in reducing blood glucose rises and the need to secrete insulin. Foods in these categories may have special roles in maintaining low blood lipids and may favorably affect the progression and complications of non-insulin-dependent diabetes in the population as they age. In this respect, the Mediterranean diet has clear implications for the preservation of health through the prevention and the dietary treatment of hyperlipidemia, diabetes, and renal and hepatic diseases. A common denominator is that these diets are high in carbohydrate, low in saturated fats, and many of the carbohydrate foods are *slow release starch* or *lente carbohydrate* forms. The discussion will therefore focus on the effects of these foods with lente carbohydrate characteristics on (1) the physiology of carbohydrate, lipid, and nitrogen metabolism, (2) the implications in health and disease, and (3) the specific foods that may confer benefits.

PHYSIOLOGICAL EFFECTS OF SLOW RELEASE CARBOHYDRATE FOODS

Carbohydrate Metabolism—Slowing Absorption

Many factors in plant foods have been shown to reduce the rate of carbohydrate absorption. They include (1) food form (e.g., bread vs. pasta),

(2) particle size (flour vs. cracked wheat) (Heaton et al. 1988; Jenkins et al. 1988a), (3) amylose content (cereal vs. legumes), (4) protein content (starch protein interaction), (5) dietary fiber and, (6) various so-called antinutrients (Rea et al. 1985, Yoon et al. 1983), many of which may limit enzyme activity (lectins, phytates, tannins, saponins, amylose inhibitors).

It appears, for example, that the compact nature of pasta makes it less readily accessible to enzymatic digestion than bread. Similarly, the coarseness of a grain has a similar effect in reducing the rate of enzymatic attack. Amylose starch (Behall et al. 1988), as found in dried legumes and long-grain rice (Goddard et al. 1984), is less readily digested than amylopectin starch due to the linear structure of the former, which lacks the branch points. It therefore retains a more compact structure that tends to exclude water. Various enzyme inhibitors, such as phytate (Rea et al. 1985) and lectins (Yoon et al. 1983), are also found in high concentrations in dried beans. The activity of many of these compounds is reduced greatly on cooking, but normal cooking practises still preserve sufficient antinutrient to have an effect in reducing the rate of digestion. Protein-starch interactions in foods, especially wheat products (Anderson et al. 1981; Jenkins et al. 1987b), tend to reduce the rate of digestion, and plant protein sources appear to be less rapidly absorbed than many animal proteins and so cause less fluctuation in amino acid and insulin responses (Jenkins et al. 1989a). Finally, dietary fibers, especially soluble fibers, have well-documented effects in reducing the rate of glucose absorption and blunting the endocrine responses (Blackburn et al. 1984; Jenkins et al. 1978; Morgan et al. 1979).

Low Glycemic Indexes

One of the consequences of slow carbohydrate absorption is a flattened blood glucose response with its implication in the treatment of diabetes. In a food, any combination of the factors alluded to in the list on page 160 may be responsible for this effect. The flattening of glycemic response assessed by glycemic index is related to the rate at which the food is digested *in vitro* (Jenkins et al. 1982; Jenkins et al. 1984). The glycemic index (GI) itself is defined as (Jenkins et al. 1986a):

$$GI = \frac{\text{incremental blood glucose response to the food} \times 100}{\text{corresponding value for equi-carbohydrate portion of reference food}}$$

Initially, the reference food was glucose, but due to palatability and the possible osmotic effect of glucose in reducing gastric emptying, white bread was chosen as the reference food (Jenkins et al. 1986a). Although the glycemic index of a food relates well to its rate of digestion *in vitro*, the flattened blood glucose response cannot be explained by increased carbohydrate malabsorption since this, although a further feature of many low GI foods, is, nevertheless, relatively small (Jenkins et al. 1987c). Indeed, the effect of low GI foods can be mimicked in normal and diabetic volunteers by reducing the rate of nutrient delivery, by increasing meal frequency, and by reducing meal size proportionately (Gwinup et al. 1963a; Gwinup et al. 1963b; Jenkins et al. 1989b; Ellis 1934). Thus, when glucose is sipped at an even rate over 4 hours by healthy subjects, rather than being taken in 5 minutes as a bolus, the peak rise in blood glucose is markedly flattened as is the associated insulin response (Gwinup et al. 1963b). When normal foods are used and the number of meals per day are increased from three or less to eight or more, a similar picture is seen in the day-long glucose and insulin response. The insulin response is reduced after taking 17 meals compared to three (Gwinup et al. 1963a; Jenkins et al. 1989b). Perhaps even more dramatic is the fall in serum lipids including LDL cholesterol as meal frequency is increased (Gwinup et al. 1963a; Jenkins et al. 1989b).

In this respect, other approaches to reduce the glycemic response in foods including increased soluble fiber consumption, low glycemic index foods and the use of small intestinal enzyme inhibitors (alphaglycosidase inhibitors) have all been associated with favorable lipid profiles (Maruhama et al. 1982) and improved blood glucose control (Hillebrand et al. 1979; Hillebrand and Boehma 1982).

Reduced Insulin Requirements

As already mentioned, consumption of low glycemic index or lente carbohydrate foods is also associated with low postprandial insulin responses. In general, there is a highly significant relationship between the insulin and glucose responses to a wide range of starchy foods (Jenkins et al. 1982) and this, in turn, relates to the rates at which the foods are digested. Also, different protein sources evoke different insulin responses (Jenkins et al. 1989a). Thus, the insulin responses to proteins in plant foods appear to be less than that for proteins in milk and beef (Jenkins et al. 1989a). Since, in the Mediterranean diet, protein intakes are moderate and a substantial proportion is of vegetable origin, the rate of digestion is likely to have a major impact on the postprandial insulin response to a food.

Reduced insulin levels per se appear to have major health implications. Epidemiological studies in nondiabetic men have indicated that increased insulin levels are associated with increased risk of cardiovascular disease (Dulcimetiere et al. 1980). In support of these studies is the association of high circulating insulin levels with hypertension (Olefsky et al. 1982; De Fronzo 1982; Ferrannini et al. 1987), obesity (Olefsky et al. 1974) and the early stages of non-insulin-dependent diabetes (Stout 1968; Stout 1969; Stout et al. 1975). Furthermore, insulin has been shown *in vitro* to enhance proliferation of arterial smooth muscle cells and subintimal lipid accumulation (Stout 1968; Stout 1969; Stout et al. 1975). It is also a stimulant of HMG CoA reductase, a rate limiting step in cholesterol synthesis (Lakshmanan et al. 1973). High insulin levels may, therefore, have effects in enhancing atheroma formation in arterial walls and raising blood lipids. There also appears to be evidence for enhanced triglyceride synthesis associated with high postprandial insulin responses following low fiber carbohydrate foods (Albrink et al. 1979). It is therefore of interest that increased meal frequency as a model for slow release carbohydrate has not only been associated with reduced lipid levels (Gwinup et al. 1963a; Jagannathan et al. 1964; Young et al. 1971a; Young et al. 1971b) but also with a lower risk of cardiovascular disease (Gwinup et al. 1963a).

Lower Blood Lipids

As already mentioned, lower blood lipid levels have been shown to result from actions that reduce the rate of nutrient absorption. Studies where meal frequency has been increased at constant daily caloric intakes have shown decreases in LDL cholesterol and in some instances also of triglyceride (in women but not in men). The suggested mechanism involves reduced postmeal insulin peaks resulting in a lesser stimulus to hepatic lipogenesis, especially of HMG CoA reductase. This mechanism may be shared by other approaches such as the use of soluble fiber and low GI diets. However, in addition, it is suggested that soluble fiber may lower blood lipids by enhancing bile salt losses in the feces (Kritchevsky and Story 1974) and by increasing colonic fermentation with increased propionate generation (Chen et al. 1984). This so-called short-chain fatty acid is absorbed from the colon and, by a direct action on the liver, inhibits cholesterol synthesis.

Nitrogen Metabolism

Foods that are more rapidly digested raise blood amino acid levels more rapidly than more slowly digested food. In addition, they deliver less starch to the colon for fermentation. This typifies many processed carbohydrate foods in the North American and northern European diets and contrasts with many Mediterranean starchy staple foods. Thus, the amino acid responses following beans processed to increase their glycemic index demonstrated higher levels of branched chain and total amino acids postprandially by comparison with the normal nonprocessed low glycemic index form (Jenkins et al. 1987d). A similar finding has been made where high and low glycemic index diets have been compared in patients with cirrhosis (Jenkins et al. 1989a). This may have an effect in blunting the insulin response to a food and also the rate at which proteins are deaminated. Perhaps of greater significance was the finding in normal volunteers on fiber supplements that urea levels were reduced, suggesting increased colonic losses of nitrogen (Rampton et al. 1984). This ability of the colonic bacteria to trap urea nitrogen, which crosses the colonic epithelium from the blood, and assist in its elimination in the feces as bacterial cell proteins has been used in patients with chronic renal failure to lower serum urea levels. In these instances, soluble fiber has been added to the diets to enhance colonic bacterial cell activity and so achieve the reduction in serum urea levels (Rampton et al. 1984). The slow release carbohydrate diets may therefore have uses in renal disease. It may be that much of the pioneering work in renal diets was done in Italy and was made possible by the Mediterranean diet (Giordano 1985; Parillo et al. 1988a, 1988b).

Increased Colonic Fermentation

One of the results of delaying carbohydrate absorption is that a small increase can be predicted in the carbohydrate entering the colon. Many of the foods of the Mediterranean region share this attribute. The starch loss is in addition to the dietary fiber which, by definition, is not absorbed in the small intestine. This starch loss will increase colonic fermentation, possibly causing troublesome abdominal distension and flatulence in those unaccustomed to such diets.

Although there are obvious disadvantages to increasing colonic fermentation, a number of potential benefits have also been defined. These have been mentioned previously but will be explained in more detail.

All the dietary fiber in foods by definition reaches the colon where the so-called soluble fiber component, amounting to 30% or more of the total fiber in the diet and a proportion of the insoluble fiber is fermented (Cummings 1981). Starch in very significant amounts (10–20%) in the case of some foods, for example, legumes (Anderson et al. 1981; Jenkins et al. 1987c; Stephen et al. 1983; Wolever et al. 1986a), escapes digestion in the small intestine and enters the colon to contribute further substrate for fermentation. The amount of starch delivered to the colon appears to depend on the fiber content of the food. The higher the fiber content, the more starch it appears to carry with it to the colon (Jenkins et al. 1987c). In addition, mucins secreted in the gut contribute to the fermentable carbohydrate load.

The fermentation of carbohydrate produces short-chain fatty acids (SCFA) and reduces colonic luminal pH (Cummings 1981), a factor originally suggested to confer protection from colonic cancer, possibly through modification of gut flora. Changes in gut flora have been shown to occur on feeding fiber (Fuchs et al. 1976), together with changes in fecal bulk (Floch and Fuchs 1978). In this respect, an increase in fecal bulk and reduced synthesis of potential carcinogens are seen as advantageous. Furthermore, colonic fermentation of carbohydrate may liberate bound metal ions while their absorption may be enhanced in the presence of SCFA, a further potential advantage for absorption of such divalent cations as Ca^{++}, Mg^{++}, and Zn^{++} (James 1980). More recently, interest has shifted to the colon and nitrogen metabolism. It is recognized that fermentable carbohydrate that enters the colon may break the enterohepatic cycle of nitrogen in which urea from the blood compartment crosses the colonic mucosa, is hydrolyzed by bacterial urease to NH_3, and then diffuses out of the colon to be once more synthesized in the liver to urea. When carbohydrate is fermented, the lowering of pH converts NH_3 to NH_4^+ which crosses the colonic mucosa to the blood compartment less readily. Furthermore, the bacteria are provided with an energy source, through fermentation of carbohydrate, which enables them to fix the ammonia nitrogen for their own cell proteins. Nitrogen is thus eliminated from the body in the feces. Clinical use has been made of malabsorbed carbohydrate, as lactulose, in the treatment of hepatic encephalopathy. More recently, this approach has been used to eliminate urea nitrogen in chronic renal failure where the elevated urea levels in patients taking soluble fiber supplements has been shown to be significantly reduced (Rampton et al. 1984). These carbohydrate sources are the major substrates for short-chain fatty acid synthesis in the colon. The predominant SCFAs to which physiological functions have been ascribed are acetate, propionate, and butyrate, usually produced in the ratio 60:20:20 (Cummings 1981).

Butyrate appears to be a preferred substrate for energy utilization by the colonic mucosal cell and little enters the portal circulation (Cummings et al. 1987). One study (Kruk 1982) showed that butyrate reduces transformation in cells *in vitro*. *In vivo*, low butyrate concentrations have been found in fecal material from the colons of individuals subsequently found to have colonic neoplasms (Weaver et al. 1988). Early studies

(Roediger 1980) hypothesized that ulcerative colitis was an energy deficiency disorder. More recently, exclusion colitis has been successfully treated with butyrate enemata (Harig et al. 1989). The picture therefore emerges that luminal nutrition may be important for colonic health.

Propionate is largely taken up by the liver (Cummings et al. 1987). As an odd-chain fatty acid, it is also a gluconeogenic substrate and a major source of gluconeogenesis in ruminants (Judson et al. 1968; Ballard et al. 1969). Much of the current interest in propionate has related to its ability to inhibit cholesterol synthesis in hepatic tissue (Anderson and Bridges 1981; Bush and Milligan 1971) and in feeding studies of rats (Chen et al. 1984) and pigs (Thacker et al. 1981) to lower cholesterol. The suggestion has therefore been made that the hypocholesterolemic action of fiber is mediated by the propionate produced by fiber fermentation in the colon (Chen et al. 1984).

Of the three SCFA discussed, acetate is the only one that routinely appears in the peripheral circulation in significant amounts (Cummings et al. 1987). As with other short-chain acids (Balasse et al. 1967; Scheppach et al. 1988), it would be predicted to inhibit fatty acid mobilization from adipose tissue, and it has been suggested that this may result in improved carbohydrate tolerance. Recent studies with acetate have confirmed an effect of SCFA in suppressing FFA levels, although no improvement in carbohydrate tolerance (Scheppach et al. 1988). The effects of colonic fermentation and the synthesis of the SCFA produced may therefore influence the health attributes of the Mediterranean diet.

EFFECTS OF INDIVIDUAL FOODS

Cereals

To a very large extent cereal products take the place in terms of dietary calories that saturated fat occupies in the diets of northern European and North American communities. This fact in itself provides a reason for the positive health benefit of cereal foods as a replacement for saturated fat calories that will result in lower blood lipid, especially serum cholesterol levels.

However, there do not appear to be nutritional experiments where the carbohydrate elements of the Mediterranean diet have been isolated and compared with the effects of North American and northern European starchy foods while holding the fat and protein sources identical. It is therefore difficult to gauge the extent to which the different starchy foods and their amount in the Mediterranean diet are responsible for the observed good health by comparison with northern cultures and whether it is the presence of low glycemic index foods and fiber that are responsible. Nonetheless, likely benefits have been identified.

Of the cereal foods, pasta has been looked at in detail and studies have been carried out on cracked wheat, bulgur, oats, and barley. These results can possibly be extrapolated to some of the typical cereal dishes of the Mediterranean region, for example

Pasta
Bulgur (tabouli)
Malthouth
Oats and barley, whole or cracked
Coarse corn meal (polenta)

Pasta.   Pasta, which legend has it was brought from China by Marco Polo, has become the hallmark of the traditional Italian diet. Original concern over pasta as a fattening food is the result of accompanying sauces, especially those used in northern European and North American cultures in an attempt to enhance the popularity of pasta with the public in high saturated fat consuming areas. However, traditional pasta dishes may be useful in the dietary management of hyperlipidemia (Jenkins et al. 1987a), diabetes (Fontvieille et al. 1988; Parillo et al. 1988a; Jenkins et al. 1983; Wolever et al. 1986b) and possibly liver and renal diseases. Eaten with tomato and vegetable sauces, these foods allow displacement of saturated fats and cholesterol containing foods from the diet as has been shown for other carbohydrate food supplements. This intervention is likely to be of value in the management of hyperlipidemia and is probably one of the dietary reasons for the freedom from cardiovascular disease of those taking the Italian Mediterranean diet (Keys 1970). The popularity of pasta dishes may also allow displacement of the heavy meat dishes that increase protein intakes in many northern European and North American communities. This displacement may have advantages in liver disease and renal disease where in renal disease, early protein restriction is now advocated and in the later stages of both renal and liver diseases, diets may be unpalatable. It may be one of the reasons that Italian physicians Giovanetti and Giordano (Giordano 1985) first devised some of the most palatable low protein diets for the treatment of renal disease.

There are further reasons why pasta may have advantages related to the slower rates of digestion that they show. Earlier on, spaghetti and macaroni were shown to have low glycemic indexes in both normal and diabetic volunteers (Jenkins et al. 1983). The effect was independent of whether whole meal, whole wheat ("integrale") or white pasta was used. The effect has been demonstrated for a whole range of pastas. The degree to which the pasta must be *al dente* and retain its physical form is not established: It may loose its low glycemic effect when canned and where, as a result, the pasta has a much softer consistency. Addition of protein and, most especially, incorporation of soluble fiber, such as guar, into pasta has been shown to enhance the slow release prospective of pasta (Gatti et al. 1984). In longer term studies, guar pasta has been shown to have favorable effects on blood lipids (Gatti et al. 1984) and diabetes control (Bosello et al. 1984).

As part of low glycemic index diets where there was no increase in soluble fiber, consumption of pasta in exchange for breads was associated with improved glycemic control in type I and II diabetes (lower serum fructosamine and triglyceride levels) (Fontvieille et al. 1988; Brand et al. 1988). Low glycemic index diets where only a modest increase in soluble fiber was also present and which have also exchanged pasta for part of the bread in the diets have also shown reduced lipids in normals (Jenkins et al. 1987a), improved glycemic control in diabetes (Fontvielle et al. 1988; Parillo et al. 1988b; Jenkins et al. 1988b, 1988c), and lower LDL cholesterol and triglyceride levels in hyperlipidemic individuals, especially those with already increased triglyceride levels (type II and IV hyperlipidemias) (Bornet et al. 1987).

The mechanism by which pasta, or for that matter any other low glycemic index foods, may alter carbohydrate and lipid metabolism is still open to debate. The effects, however, are not confounded by fat and protein in mixed meals where comparisons have been made with bread, rice, or potatoes (Bornet et al. 1987), nor are they observed when used as part of a total diet. The effect may well relate to the slower rate of absorption of pasta as opposed to bread. The sequence of events may involve limited accessibility of amylolytic enzymes to the starch granules in protein as opposed to bread, for example, due to the more compact nature of pasta. Also, whole cylinders of spaghetti are likely to enter the duodenum and require a significant length of small intestinal digestion to break down all the starch to glucose, maltose, and maltotriose prior to small intestinal absorption by the brush border enzyme systems of the enterocytes. Certainly, pasta is digested less rapidly *in vitro* compared with bread (Jenkins et al. 1982). As a result, smaller GIP and insulin responses will be seen. The lower levels of these will result in a reduced stimulus to hepatic lipid synthesis, both of triglyceride and cholesterol, the latter being regulated by HMG-CoA reductase, which is an insulin sensitive enzyme (Lakshmanan et al. 1973).

The thesis developed for pasta in terms of mechanism and scope of effects is probably applicable to other low glycemic index foods with some modifications due to, for example, the presence of soluble fiber and antinutrients, which are notably low or absent in pasta.

Bulgur and Similar Cracked and Whole Grain Cereal Foods

Parboiled cracked wheat or bulgur is eaten around the Mediterranean basin and beyond throughout the Middle East. It may be eaten hot or cold as tabouli salad (mixed with parsley). These foods are eaten predominantly around the southern rim of the Mediterranean. In some countries (e.g., Tunisia), grains other than wheat are cracked (e.g., barley). The parboiling (boiling while unmilled in the seed coat and before the husk is removed) results in increased retention of vitamins and minerals. It also prevents expansion of the starch and so realigns the molecular structure such that subsequent hydration is limited. A slow release or lente carbohydrate form is therefore produced where, like pasta compared with bread, access of amylolytic enzymes is impeded.

In general, parboiled cereal foods have low glycemic indexes (Jenkins et al. 1986b) and in many ways are the dietary equivalent of the whole grain breads (rye, pumpernickel) of northern Europe. These breads are also slowly digested because of the particle size of the flour (Heaton et al. 1988; Jenkins et al. 1988a).

Barley is also used around the Mediterranean. It too is a low glycemic index food possibly in part due to its soluble beta-glucan fiber (Jenkins et al. 1988a). Farro was a similar popular cereal grain once used extensively in Italy. These foods also increase the carbohydrate entering the colon as starch as demonstrated in studies of human ileostomates (Jenkins et al. 1987c). In addition, when barley or oats are used, fermentable fiber as beta-glucan will also pass on to the colon. Starch and beta-glucan greatly increase the fermentable load entering the colon. These fermentable sources may confer benefit in terms of altered SCFA and nitrogen metabolism already discussed in relation to colonic fermentation.

Like pasta, bulgur is a very acceptable food to a wide range of tastes and has been used in low glycemic index diets to improve diabetic control. In the diets of hyperlipidemic patients its use, along with other low glycemic index foods, was associated with lower levels of serum LDL cholesterol and triglyceride (Jenkins et al. 1987a).

Couscous

Couscous is usually made from wheat flour but has a less dense texture than pasta. It is eaten in a similar geographic distribution to bulgur and can fill a similar niche in the diet.

It may have an advantage as a starchy food that would displace saturated fats and cholesterol from the diet when eaten as part of low fat dishes or meals. However, its glycemic index is not as low as bulgur and appears to be intermediate between pasta and bread. No formal studies of the longer-term dietary effects appear to have been carried out.

Polenta and Cereal Porridges

Ground cereals have been traditional Mediterranean foods for millennia. They may be made of flours from any of the cereals. Polenta from coarse ground corn would be expected to have a low glycemic index (Heaton et al. 1988) similar to coarse corn meal bread. Such foods may, therefore, have the spectrum of advantages similar to pasta and if they are derived from whole meal flours, they will also manifest the colonic effects relevant to an increase in insoluble dietary fiber.

Rice and Whole Grains

Rice is a less common food than wheat in Mediterranean cultures, but a number of Spanish rice dishes are well known. Long grain rices tend to be used. These are relatively high in amylose starch and thus are digested less rapidly than the lower amylose varieties of rice (Goddard et al. 1984). Rice has been classed as a lower glycemic index food than bread (Wolever et al. 1986b). This again probably depends on the type of rice used. When rice is parboiled first, its rate of digestion and glycemic effect are definitely reduced (Wolever et al. 1986b). Other cereals such as barley and oats may be eaten whole. These very definitely have a low rate of digestion and low glycemic index (Jenkins et al. 1988a).

Rice has been used as part of low glycemic index diets for type I diabetes and has been shown to lower serum fructosamine, triglyceride, and phospholipid levels. Effects have not been noted on serum cholesterol levels. Other whole grains have only been tested in acute studies. Longer term studies and studies of differing types of rice are required to define the spectrum of possible health advantages.

Legumes

Legumes are the archetypical slow release carbohydrate foods. Examples include

Chick-peas (dried) (ground as hummus)
Lentils (dried)
Large white beans (dried)
Kidney beans (dried)
Romano beans (dried)
Fava beans (dried)

Dried legumes have been eaten for millennia around the Mediterranean basin. Their use around the northern shores is likely to be diminishing together with the even more marked reduction experienced in the rest of Europe. Nevertheless, the large white bean and the pinto bean are still consumed as are lentils in the southeast and fava beans in the south. In Middle Eastern countries, a fava bean stew known as *foul* is popular and eaten in the same fashion as lentil *dahl* is in India.

Favism (associated with G-6-P dehydrogenase deficiency) was recognized in antiquity. It is said that Pythagoras suffered from favism and, despite being a vegetarian, advised his followers accordingly not to eat beans. Such was his sensitivity to beans that when his colony in southern Italy was attacked, rather than escape through a field of beans, he allowed himself to be caught and killed.

Nevertheless, dried legumes have much to recommend them nutritionally. They are rich sources of vegetable protein containing more than the required amounts of the essential amino acid lysine. They lack equivalent amounts of methionine but make very complete protein sources when combined with cereals that are complimentary in amino acid content having much methionine but a relative lack of lysine. Legumes are low in fat. Those that do contain fat, such as the soya bean and, to a lesser extent but more relevant to the Mediterranean diet, the chick-pea, the fat is unsaturated. Finally they contain fiber, including soluble fiber, antinutrients (lectins, phytates, tannins, etc.), and amylose starch, all of which result in the starch in legumes being digested slowly (Yoon et al. 1983; Jenkins et al. 1982; Thompson et al. 1984).

As a class, legumes have been shown to be digested more slowly than most other foods *in vitro* (Jenkins et al. 1982; Jenkins et al., 1984). *In vivo* they enhance colonic fermentation by virtue both of the soluble fiber and the legume starch, which escape digestion in the small intestine as has also been demonstrated in ileostomate volunteers (Jenkins et al. 1987c). Legumes fed in equi-carbohydrate portions, compared to other study foods, as a class, produce the flattest glycemic response (Jenkins et al. 1980). The flat glycemic response does not appear to be due to malabsorption but rather to slow absorption. The effect appears to be dependent on altered small intestinal events since gastric emptying rate is not related to the degree to which they reduce the peak postprandial glycemia (Torsdottir et al. 1984).

Legumes: Disease Treatment and Prevention

A number of studies have used legumes, often under the guise of dietary fiber, to demonstrate improved glycemic control in diabetes with favorable effects on blood lipids (Rivellese et al. 1980; Simpson et al. 1981; Anderson and Ward 1979). Notably, studies have used diets modeled on those eaten in southern Italy to increase soluble fiber intakes and produce reductions in LDL cholesterol (Rivellese et al. 1980). A number of studies have also shown the beneficial effects of legumes on LDL cholesterol and serum triglyceride in patients with hyperlipidemia (Jenkins et al. 1987a; Simpson et al. 1981; Anderson and Ward 1979). These diets have been aimed at raising fiber intake significantly from legumes or at lowering the glycemic index of the diet, in both instances, with increased legume intake as part of the strategy.

However, the fiber intakes have only been one of the alterations achieved in the diet. As shown in Behall et al. 1988, the role of amylose starch may be important. The antinutrients themselves may have effects on serum cholesterol. There is good evidence that vegetable proteins, especially of soya, as a model for legume proteins, has a fairly consistent effect in lowering serum cholesterol (Sirtori et al. 1977; Kritchevsky et al. 1978). The lack of effect of legumes in causing the expected increase in bile acid output (Anderson et al. 1984) may be a further indication that actions other than those related to fiber content are responsible for the lipid-lowering effect of fiber.

Furthermore, current studies suggest that vegetable proteins of legume origin may have specific benefits in the treatment of chronic post-systemic encephalopathy in liver disease (Shaw et al. 1983; De Bruijn et al. 1983) and possibly in maintaining low urea levels and sparing the progression of renal deterioration in kidney disease.

Finally, epidemiological studies appear to indicate a negative association between legume consumption and colonic cancer. At present, it is difficult to ascribe differences to different dried legumes. It can only be said that as a class of foods that are rapidly vanishing from the human diet, it would seem important by virtue of their health attributes to preserve their intake. In the Mediterranean diet it appears possible to achieve this aim.

Fruits and Vegetables

Fruits and vegetables feature strongly in the Mediterranean diet. Individually and even collectively little is known of their physiological effects. A number of them, for example, persimmons, okra, and eggplant, are rich sources of soluble fiber and would therefore be expected to slow absorption and possibly cause increased bile acid losses. As part of high fiber diets, fruits and vegetables have been associated with improved glycemic control in type II diabetes and lower LDL cholesterol levels (Rivellese et al. 1980). The exact role played by such foods is, however, unknown and requires considerable attention. Addition of vegetables such as zucchini and cabbage in normal meal portion sizes to carbohydrate meals made no difference to the postprandial glycemia (Wolever et al. 1988). The effects on lipids of supplements of individual vegetables has not been established. They may alter lipid metabolism by virtue of their content of such antinutrients as saponins or by displacement of foods containing saturated fat and cholesterol.

Epidemiological studies have suggested that green leafy vegetables of the brassica family may supply protection from cancer. Such vegetables are also potentially good sources of vitamin A. Despite relatively high tobacco consumption, lung cancer rates are lower than expected in the Mediterranean region. It is tempting to speculate that the negative association between lung cancer and vitamin A levels may relate to the lower rate seen in the Mediterranean region by virtue of the relatively high intakes of green vegetables.

CONCLUSION

The nature of many of the traditional carbohydrate and soluble fiber rich foods eaten in the Mediterranean region may be a reason for the apparent healthfulness of the Mediterranean diet. In many areas, starchy foods are eaten rather than saturated animal fats. As a result, foods that might otherwise raise serum lipids and increase the risk of cardiovascular disease are displaced from the diet.

In addition, many of the starchy foods have slow release, slow digestion profiles or lente carbohydrate characteristics. These attributes may allow the effect of high carbohydrate diets to be enhanced in maintaining flatter blood glucose profile, lower postprandial insulin responses, and, in the longer term, resulting in lower blood lipids.

Furthermore, these foods may allow more effective dietary treatment of other chronic diseases such as renal and liver diseases by virtue of their carbohydrate components (lente carbohydrate and fiber) and vegetable protein. The fiber and starch may enhance colonic fermentation and thus the bacterial trapping of NH_3, important in renal and liver diseases. The vegetable protein may contribute in ways as yet unspecified possibly related to the amino acid composition, including the presence or relative absence of specific amino acids or amines.

Finally, there is epidemiological evidence that the consumption of legumes and green vegetables as eaten in the Mediterranean diet may provide protection from neoplastic disease.

This field of nutrition is very promising. However, it now requires much more detailed research in specific clinical and food analytical areas combined with a thorough knowledge of food consumption patterns and chronic disease incidence.

REFERENCES

Albrink, M. J., T. Newman, and P. C. Davidson. 1979. Effect of high- and low-fiber diets on plasma lipids and insulin. *Am. J. Clin. Nutr.* **32**:1486–1491.

Anderson, I. H., A. S. Levine, and M. D. Levitt. 1981. Incomplete absorption of the carbohydrate in all-purpose wheat flour. *New Engl. J. Med.* **304**:891–892.

Anderson, J. W. and K. Ward. 1979. High carbohydrate, high fiber diets for insulin treated men with diabetes mellitus. *Am. J. Clin. Nutr.* **32**:2312–2321.

Anderson, J. W., and S. R. Bridges. 1981. Plant fiber metabolites alter hepatic glucose and lipid metabolism. *Diabetes* **30** (Suppl. 1):133A (Abstract).

Anderson, J. W., L. Story, B. Sieling, W. L. Chen, M. S. Petro, and J. A. Story. 1984. Hypercholesterolemic effects of oat-bran or bean intake for hypercholesterolemic men. *Am. J. Clin. Nutr.* **40**:1146–1155.

Balasse, E., E. Courturier, and J. R. M. Franckson. 1967. Influence of sodium beta-hydroxybutyrate on glucose and free fatty acid metabolism in normal dogs. *Diabetologia* **3**:488–493.

Ballard, F. J., R. W. Hanson, and D. S. Kronfell. 1969. Gluconeogenesis and lipogenesis in tissues from ruminant and non-ruminant animals. *Fed. Proc.* **28**:218–231.

Behall, K. M., D. J. Scholfield, and J. Canary. 1988. Effect of starch structure on glucose and insulin responses in adults. *Am J. Clin. Nutr.* **47**:428–432.

Blackburn, N. A., J. S. Redfern, H. Jarjis, A. M. Holgate, I. Hanning, J. H. B. Scarpello, I. T. Johnson, and N. W. Read. 1984. The mechanism of action of guar gum in improving glucose tolerance in man. *Clin. Sci.* **66**:329–336.

Bornet, F. R. J., D. Costagliola, A. Blayo, A. M. Fontvieille, M. J. Haardt, M. Letanoux, G. Tchobroutsky, and G. Slama. 1987. Insulinogenic and glycemic indices of six starch-rich foods taken alone and in a mixed meal by type 2 diabetics. *Am. J. Clin. Nutr.* **45**:588–595.

Bosello, O. L. Cominacini, I. Zocca, U. Garbin, F. Ferrari, and A. Davoli. 1984. Effect of guar gum on plasma lipoproteins and apolipoproteins C-II and C-III in patients affected by familial combined hyperlipoproteinemia. *Am. J. Clin. Nutr.* **40**:1165–1174.

Botha, A. P. J., A. F. Steyn, A. J. Esterhuysen, and M. Slabbdrt. 1981. Glycosylated hemoglobin, blood glucose and serum cholesterol levels in diabetics treated with guar gum. *S. Afr. Med. J.* **59**:333–334.

Brand, J. C., S. Colagiuri, S. Crossman, and A. S. Truswell. 1988. Comparison of low and high glycemic index diets in the management of diabetes. *Proc. Nutr. Soc.* **13**:150 (Abstract).

Bush, R. S., and L. P. Milligan. 1971. Study of the mechanism of inhibition of ketogenesis by propionate in bovine liver. *Can. J. Anim. Sci.* **51**:121–127.

Chen, W. J. L., J. W. Anderson, and D. Jennings. 1984. Propionate may mediate the hypocholesterolemic effects of certain soluble plant fibers in cholesterol fed rats. *Proc. Soc. Exper. Biol. Med.* **175**:215–218.

Creutzfeldt, W., and U. R. Folsh. 1983. *Delaying Absorption as a Therapeutic Principle in Metabolic Diseases.* New York: Thieme-Stratton.

Cummings, J. H. 1981. Short chain fatty acids in the human colon. *Gut* **22**:763–779.

Cummings, J. H., E. W. Pomare, W. J. Branch, C. P. E. Naylor, and G. T. Mcfarlane. 1987. Short chain fatty acids in human large intestine, portal, hepatic and venous blood. *Gut* **28**:1221–1227.

De Bruijn, K. M., L. M. Blendis, D. H. Zilm, P. L. Carlen, and G. H. Anderson. 1983. Effect of dietary protein manipulations in subclinical portal-systemic encephalopathy. *Gut* **24**:53–60.

DeFronzo, R. A. 1982. Insulin secretion, insulin resistance and obesity. *Internat. J. Obesity* **6**:73–79.

Ducimetiere, P., E. Eschwege, L. Papoz, J. L. Richard, J. R. Claude, and G. Rosselin. 1980. Relationship of plasma insulin levels to the incidence of myocardial infarction and coronary heart disease mortality in a middle-aged population. *Diabetologia* **19**:205–210.

Ellis, A. 1934. Increased carbohydrate tolerance in diabetes following hourly administration of glucose and insulin over long periods. *Quart. J. Med.* **27**:137–153.

Elsenhaus, B., U. Sufke, R. Blume, and W. F. Caspary. 1980. The influence of carbohydrate gelling agents on rat intestinal transport of monosaccharides and neutral amino acids in vitro. *Clin. Sci.* **59**:373–380.

Ferrannini, E., G. Buzzigoli, R. Bonadonna, M. A. Giorgio, M. Oleggini, L. Graziosi, R. Peorinelli, L. Brand, and S. Bevilaqua. 1987. Insulin resistance in essential hypertension. *New Engl. J. Med.* **317**:350–357.

Floch, M. H., and H. M. Fuchs. 1978. Modification of stool content by increased bran intake. *Am. J. Clin, Nutr.* **31**:S185–S189.

Fontvieille, A. M., M. Acosta, S. W. Rizkalla, F. Bornet, P. David, M. Letanoux, G. Tchobroutsky, and G. Slama. 1988. A moderate switch from high to low glycemic-index foods for 3 weeks improves the metabolic control of Type I (IDDM) diabetic subjects. *Diab. Nutr. Metabol.* **1**:139–143.

Fuchs, H. M., S. Dorfman, and M. H. Floch. 1976. The effect of dietary fiber supplementation in man. II. Alteration in fecal physiology and bacterial flora. *Am. J. Clin. Nutr.* **29**:1145–1147.

Gatti, E., G. Catenazzo, E. Camisasca, A. Torri, E. Denegri, and C. R. Sirtori. 1984. Effects of guar-enriched pasta in the treatment of diabetes and hyperlipidemia. *Ann. Nutr. Metab.* **28**:1–10.

Giordano, C. 1985. Early dietary protein restriction protects the failing kidney. *Kidney Int.* **28**(Suppl. 17):S66–S70.

Goddard, M. S., G. Young, and R. Marcus. 1984. The effect of amylose content on insulin and glucose responses to ingested rice. *Am. J. Clin. Nutr.* **39**:388–392.

Gwinup, G., R. C. Byron, W. H. Roush, F. A. Kruger, and G. J. Hamwi. 1963a. Effect of nibbling versus gorging on glucose tolerance. *Lancet* **2**:165–167.

Gwinup, G., R. C. Byron, W. H. Roush, F. A. Kruger, and G. J. Hamwi. 1963b. Effect on nibbling versus gorging on serum lipids in man. *Am. J. Clin. Nutr.* **13**:209–213.

Harig, J. M., K. H. Soergel, R. A. Komorowski, and C. M. Wood. 1989. Treatment of diversion colitis with short chain fatty acid irrigation. *New Engl. J. Med.* **320**:23–28.

Heaton, K. W., S. N. Marens, P. M. Emmett, and C. H. Bolton. 1988. Particle size of wheat, maize and oat test meals: effects of plasma glucose on insulin responses and on the rate of starch digestion. *Am. J. Clin. Nutr.* **47**:675–682.

Hillebrand, I., and K. Boehma. 1982. Clinical studies on acarbose during 5 years. In W. Creutzfeldt, ed., *Proceedings of First International Symposium on Acarbose*, Montreux, Oct. 1981. Amsterdam: Excerpta Medica, 445–450.

Hillebrand, I., K. Bochine, H. Kink, and P. Berchtold. 1979. The effects of the alpha-glucosidase inhibitor Bay g5421 (acarbose) on meal stimulated elevations of cirulating glucose, insulin and triglyceride levels in man. *Res. Exp. Med. (Berlin)* **175**:81–86.

Jagannathan, S. N., W. F. Connel, and J. M. R. Beveridge. 1964. Effect of gormandizing and semicontinuous eating of equicaloric amounts of formula type high fat diets on plasma cholesterol and triglyceride levels in human volunteer subjects. *Am. J. Clin. Nutr.* **15**:90–93.

James, W. P. T. 1980. Dietary fiber and mineral absorption. In *Medical Aspects of Dietary Fiber*, G. A. Spiller and R. McPherson-Kay, eds., pp. 237–259. New York: Plenum Press.

Jenkins, D. J. A. 1967. Ketone bodies and the inhibition of free fatty acid release. *Lancet* **2**:338–340.

Jenkins, D. J. A., T. M. S. Wolever, A. R. Leeds, M. A. Gassull, J. B. Dilawari, D. V. Goff, G. L. Metz, and K. G. M. M. Alberti. 1978. Dietary fibres, fibre analogues and glucose tolerance: importance of viscosity. *Br. Med. J.* **1**:1392–1394.

Jenkins, D. J. A., A. R. Leeds, B. Slavin, J. Mann, and E. M. Jepson. 1979. Dietary fiber and blood lipids: reduction of serum cholesterol in type II hyperlipidemia by guar gum. *Am. J. Clin. Nutr.* **32**:16–18.

Jenkins, D. J. A., T. M. S. Wolever, R. H. Taylor, H. M. Barker, and H. Fielden. 1980. Exceptionally low blood glucose response to dried beans: comparison with other carbohydrate foods. *Br. Med. J.* **281**:578–580.

Jenkins, D. J. A., H. Ghafari, T. M. S. Wolever, R. H. Taylor, A. L. Jenkins, H. M. Barker, H. Fielden, and A. C. Bowling. 1982. Relationship between rate of digestion of foods and post-prandial glycaemia. *Diabetologia* **22**:450–455.

Jenkins, D. J. A., T. M. S. Wolever, A. L. Jenkins, R. Lee, G. S. Wong, and R. G. Josse. 1983. Glycemic response to wheat products: Reduced response to pasta but no effect of fiber. *Diabetes Care* **6**:155–159.

Jenkins, D. J. A., T. M. S. Wolever, M. J. Thorne, A. L. Jenkins, G. S. Wong, R. G. Josse, and A. Csima. 1984. The relationship between glycemic response, digestibility, and factors influencing the dietary habits of diabetics. *Am. J. Clin. Nutr.* **40**:1175–1191.

Jenkins, D. J. A., T. M. S. Wolever, J. Kalmusky, S. Giudici, C. Giordano, G. S. Wong, J. Bird, R. L. Patten, M. Hall, G. Buckley, and J. A. Little. 1985. Low glycemic index carbohydrate foods in the management of hyperlipidemia. *Am. J. Clin. Nutr.* **42**:604–617.

Jenkins, D. J. A., M. J. A. Jenkins, T. M. S. Wolever, R. H. Taylor, and H. Ghafari. 1986a. Slow release carbohydrate: mechanism of action of viscous fibers. *J. Clin. Nutr. Gastroent.* **1**:237–241.

Jenkins, D. J. A., T. M. S. Wolever, A. L. Jenkins, C. Giordano, S. Giudici, L. U. Thompson, J. Kalmusky, R. G. Josse, and G. S. Wong. 1986b. Low glycemic response to traditionally processed wheat and rye products: bulgar and pumpernickel bread. *Am. J. Clin. Nutr.* **43**:516–520.

Jenkins, D. J. A., T. M. S. Wolever, J. Kalmusky, S. Giudici, C. Giordano, R. Patten, G. S. Wong, J. N. Bird, M. Hall, G. Buckley, A. Csima, and J. A. Little. 1987a. Low-glycemic index diet in hyperlipidemia: use of traditional starchy foods. *Am. J. Clin. Nutr.* **46**:66–71.

Jenkins, D. J. A., M. J. Thorne, T. M. S. Wolever, A. L. Jenkins, A. V. Rao, and L. U. Thompson. 1987b. The effect of starch-protein interaction in wheat on the glycemic responses and rate of in vitro digestion. *Am. J. Clin. Nutr.* **45**:946–951.

Jenkins, D. J. A., D. Cuff, T. M. S. Wolever, D. Knowland, L. U. Thompson, Z. Cohen, and E. J. Prokipchuk. 1987c. Digestibility of carbohydrate foods in an ileostomate: Relationship to dietary fiber, in vitro digestibility, and glycemic response. *Am. J. Gastroent.* **82**:709–717.

Jenkins, D. J. A., M. J. Thorne, R. H. Taylor, S. R. Bloom, D. L. Sarson, A. L. Jenkins, G. H. Anderson, and L. M. Blendis. 1987d. Effect of modifying the rate of digestion of a food on the blood glucose, amino acid, and endocrine responses in patients with cirrhosis. *Am. J. Gastroent.* **82**:223–230.

Jenkins, D. J. A., V. Wesson, T. M. S. Wolever, A. L. Jenkins, J. Kalmusky, S. Giudici, A. Csima, R. G. Josse, and G. S. Wong. 1988a. Wholemeal versus wholegrain breads: Proportion of whole or cracked grain and the glycemic response. *Br. Med. J.* **297**:958–959.

Jenkins, D. J. A., T. M. S. Wolever, and A. L. Jenkins. 1988b. Starchy foods and glycemic index. *Diabetes Care* **11**:149–159.

Jenkins, D. J. A., T. M. S. Wolever, G. Buckley, K. Y. Lam, S. Giudici, J. Kalmusky, A. L. Jenkins, R. L. Patten, J. Bird, G. S. Wong, and R. G. Josse. 1988c. Low glycemic index starchy foods in the diabetic diet. *Am. J. Clin. Nutr.* **48**:248–254.

Jenkins, D. J. A., N. Shapira, G. Greenberg, A. L. Jenkins, G. R. Collier, C. Poduch, T. M. S. Wolever, G. H. Anderson, and L. M. Blendis. 1989a. Low glycemic index foods and reduced glucose, amino acids, and endocrine responses in cirrhosis. *Am. J. Gastroent.* **84**:732–739.

Jenkins, D. J. A., T. M. S. Wolever, V. Vuksan, F. Brighenti, S. C. Cunnane, A. V. Rao, A. L. Jenkins, G. Buckley, R. Patten, W. Singer, P. Corey, and R. G.

Josse. 1989*b*. Nibbling versus gorging: Metabolic advantages of increased meal frequency. *New Eng. J. Med.* **321**:929–934.

Judson, G. J., E. Anderson, J. R. Luick, and R. A. Lang. 1968. The contribution of propionate to glucose synthesis in sheep given diets of different grain contents. *Br. J. Nutr.* **22**:69–75.

Keys, A. 1970. Coronary heart disease in seven countries. *Circulation* **41**:1–211.

Kritchevsky, D., and J. A. Story. 1974. Binding of bile salts in vitro by nonnutritive fiber. *J. Nutr.* **104**:458.

Kritchevsky, D., S. A. Tepper, and J. A. Story. 1978. Influence of soy protein and casein on atherosclerosis in rabbits. *Fed. Proc.* **37**:747.

Kruk, J. 1982. Effects of sodium butyrate, a new pharmacological agent, on cells in culture. *Mol. Cell. Biochem.* **42**:65–82.

Lakshmanan, M. R., C. M. Nepokroeff, G. C. Ness, R. E. Dugan, and J. W. Porter. 1973. Stimulation by insulin of rat liver Beta-hydroxy-Beta-methylglutaryl coenzyme A reductase and cholesterol-synthesizing activities. *Biochem. Biophys. Res. Commun.* **50**:704–710.

Maruhama, Y., A. Nagasake, Y. Kanazawa, H. Hirakawa, Y. Goto, H. Nishiyama, Y. Kishimoto, and T. Shimoyama. 1980. Effects of glucosidase-hydrolase inhibitor (Bay g5421) on serum lipids, lipoproteins and bile acids, fecal fat and bacterial flora and intestinal gas production in hyperlipidemic patients. *Tohoku J. Exp. Med.* **132**:453–562.

Morgan, L. M., T. J. Gondler, D. Tsiolakis, V. Marks, and K. G. M. M. Alberti. 1979. The effects of unabsorbable carbohydrate on gut hormones: modification of postprandial GIP secretion by guar. *Diabetologia* **17**:85–89.

Olefsky, J. M., G. M. Reaven, and J. W. Farquhar. 1974. Effects of weight reduction on obesity. Studies of lipid and carbohydrate metabolism in normal and hyperlipoproteinemic subjects. *J. Clin. Invest.* **53**:64–76.

Olefsky, J. M., O. G. Kolterman, and J. A. Scarlett. 1982. Insulin action and resistance in obesity and non-insulin dependent type II diabetes mellitus. *Am. J. Physiol.* **243**:E15–E30.

Parillo, M., R. Giacco, A. Rivellese, A. Giacco, C. Iovine, and G. Riccardi. 1988. Acute effects on pancreatic hormones and blood lipids of bread and spaghetti consumed within a meal. *Diab. Nutr. Metab.* **1**:133–137.

Parillo, M., G. Riccardi, D. Pacioni, C. Iovine, F. Contaldo, C. Isernia, F. De Marco, N. Perrotti, and A. Rivellese. 1988*b*. Metabolic consequences of feeding a high-carbohydrate, high-fiber diet to diabetic patients with chronic kidney failure. *Am. J. Clin. Nutr.* **48**:255–259.

Rampton, D. S., S. L. Cohen, V. deB. Crammond, J. Gibbons, M. F. Lilburn, J. Y. Rabet, A. J. Vince, J. D. Wagner, and O. M. Wrong. 1984. Treatment of chronic renal failure with dietary fiber. *Clin. Nephrol.* **21**:159–163.

Rea, R. L., L. U. Thompson, and D. J. A. Jenkins. 1985. Lectins in foods and their relation to starch digestibility. *Nutr. Res.* **5**:919–929.

Rivellese, A., G. Riccardi, A. Giacco, D. Pancioni, S. Genovese, P. L. Mattioli, and M. Mancini. 1980. Effect of dietary fiber on glucose control and serum lipoproteins in diabetic patients. *Lancet* **2**:447–450.

Roediger, W. E. W. 1980. The colonic epithelium in ulcerative colitis: An energy deficiency disease? *Lancet* **2**:712–715.

Scheppach, W., J. H. Cummings, W. J. Branch, and J. Schrezenmeir. 1988. Effect of gut derived acetate on oral glucose tolerance in man. *Clin. Sci.* **75**:355–361.

Shaw, S., T. M. Worner, and C. S. Lieber. 1983. Comparison of animal and vegetable protein sources in the dietary management of hepatic encephalopathy. *Am. J. Clin. Nutr.* **38**:59–63.

Simpson, H. R. C., R. W. Simpson, S. Lousley, R. D. Carter, M. Geekie, T. D. R. Hockaday, and J. I. Mann. 1981. A high carbohydrate leguminous fiber diet improves all aspects of diabetic control. *Lancet* **1**:1–5.

Sirtori, C. R., E. Agrandi, F. Conti, O. Mantero, and E. Gatti. 1977. Soybean-protein diet in the treatment of type II hyperlipoproteinemia. *Lancet* **1**:275–277.

Stephen, A. M., A. C. Haddad, and S. F. Phillips. 1983. Passage of carbohydrate into the colon. *Gastroenterology* **85**:589–595.

Stout, R. W. 1968. Insulin-stimulated lipogenesis in arterial tissue in relation to diabetes and atheroma. *Lancet* **2**:702–703.

Stout, R. W. 1969. Insulin stimulation of cholesterol synthesis by arterial tissue. *Lancet* **2**:467–468.

Stout, R. W., E. L. Bierman, and R. Ross. 1975. Effect of insulin on the proliferation of cultured primate arterial smooth muscle cells. *Circ. Res.* **36**:319–327.

Thacker, P. A., M. O. Salomons, F. X. Aherne, L. P. Milligan, and J. P. Bonland. 1981. Influence of propionic acid on the cholesterol metabolism of pigs fed hypercholesterolemic diets. *Can. J. Anim. Sci.* **61**:969–975.

Thompson, L. U., J. H. Yoon, D. J. A. Jenkins, T. M. S. Wolever, and A. L. Jenkins. 1984. Relationship between polyphenol intake and blood glucose response of normal and diabetic individuals. *Am. J. Clin. Nutr.* **39**:745–751.

Torsdottir, I., M. Alpsten, D. Andersson, R. J. M. Brammer, and H. Anderson. 1984. Effect of different starch foods in composite meals on gastric emptying rate and glucose metabolism: comparison between potatoes, rice and white beans. *Hum. Nutr. Clin. Nutr.* **38**:329–338.

Weaver, G. A., J. A. Krause, T. L. Miller, and M. J. Woolin. 1988. Short chain fatty acid distributions of enema samples from a sigmoidoscopy population: An association of high acetate and low butyrate ratios with adenomatous polyps and colon cancer. *Gut* **29**:1539–1543.

Wolever, T. M. S., and D. J. A. Jenkins. 1986. The use of the glycemic index in predicting the blood glucose response to mixed meals. *Am. J. Clin. Nutr.* **43**:167–172.

Wolever, T. M. S., Z. Cohen, L. U. Thompson, M. J. Thorne, M. J. A. Jenkins, E. J. Prokipchuk, and D. J. A. Jenkins. 1986a. Ileal loss of available carbohydrate in man: Comparison of a breath hydrogen method with direct measurement using a human ileostomy model. *Am. J. Gastroent.* **81**:115–122.

Wolever, T. M. S., D. J. A. Jenkins, J. Kalmusky, C. Giordano, S. Giudici, A. L. Jenkins, R. G. Josse, and G. S. Wong. 1986b. Glycemic response to pasta: effect of food form, cooking and protein enrichment. *Diabetes Care* **9**:401–404.

Wolever, T. M. S., D. J. A. Jenkins, J. Kalmusky, A. L. Jenkins, C. Giordano, S. Giudici, R. G. Josse, and G. S. Wong. 1986c. Comparison of regular and parboiled rices: explanation of discrepancies between reported glycemic responses to rice. *Nutr. Res* **6**:349–357.

Wolever, T. M. S., A. L. Jenkins, V. Vuksan, G. S. Wong., R. G. Josse, and D. J. A. Jenkins. 1988. Effect of "extra" vegetables added to a starchy meal on blood glucose responses in patients with type 2 diabetes. *J. Can. Diet. Assoc.* **49**:168–171.

Yoon, J. H., L. U. Thompson, and D. J. A. Jenkins. 1983. The effect of phytic acid on in vitro rate of starch digestibility and blood glucose response. *Am. J. Clin. Nutr.* **38**:835–842.

Young, C. M., S. S. Scanlan, C. M. Topping, V. Simko, and L. Lutwak. 1971*a*. Frequency of feeding, weight reduction and nutrient utilisation. *J. Am. Diet. Assoc.* **59**:473–480.

Young, C. M., S. S. Scanlan, C. M. Topping, V. Simko, and L. Lutwak. 1971*b*. Frequency of feeding, weight reduction and nutrient utilisation. *J. Am. Diet. Assoc.* **59**:466–472.

9

Physiological Effects
of Monounsaturated Oils

Gene A. Spiller

Early investigation into the effects of diet on serum cholesterol showed that vegetable oils were hypocholesterolemic when substituted for saturated fatty acids. Subsequent work by many investigators seemed to indicate that polyunsaturated fats (PFAs) were cholesterol-lowering, saturated fats (SFAs) were cholesterol-raising, and monounsaturated fats (MFAs) were neutral. Linoleic acid became the polyunsaturated fat of choice. The conclusions of these studies gained wide acceptance in the medical and scientific world. For nearly two decades following this early work, research on the connection between diet and coronary heart disease was focused almost exclusively on the ratio of polyunsaturated to saturated fats (expressed as the P/S ratio), with MFAs receiving little attention.

Extensive investigation that was gathered in the now classical book by Keys *Seven Countries. A Multivariate Analysis of Death and Coronary Heart Disease* published in 1980 showed that Mediterranean people who consumed their traditional high-MFA (olive oil) diet had comparatively low serum cholesterol levels and a low incidence of coronary heart disease (CHD).

At the same time, as more studies were carried out on the mechanism of action of *high intakes* of linoleic acid, some investigators found that along with lowering total serum cholesterol (TC) and low-density lipoprotein cholesterol (LDL-C) levels, these diets also reduced high density lipoprotein cholesterol (HDL-C) (Mattson and Grundy 1985, Grundy 1987).

Not all studies support this effect of linoleic acid intake on HDL-C (Mensink and Katan 1989; Dreon et al. 1990), and the different results may be linked to the level of total linoleic acid in the diet, the balance of other nutrients, or the specific fatty acid pattern of each oil used as in fact even different varieties of olive oil or different high polyunsaturated seed oil have often major differences in the amount of specific fatty acids.

No matter what the effect on HDL-C of high intakes of linoleic acid may be, there are important questions on how desirable a high polyunsaturated fat may be, questions based on results of many animal studies. These questions are not on the value of a reasonable intake of linoleic acid, undoubtedly an essential fatty acid that should be present in sufficient amounts in the diet but rather on the effect of making this fat the predominant fat present at fairly high levels in the diet for prolonged periods of time. Animal studies by Gammal (Gammal et al. 1967) and other studies that followed by various groups such as the American Health Foundation, raised the suspicion that such fat may favor tumor development in the presence of chemical carcinogens and that they may lead to immune suppression. Because of the unwillingness of many people to go on extremely low-fat diets, because of the desire of people to use some kind of *safe* fat in the diet, because of the need to have some fat to favor the absorption of oil soluble nutrients such as oil soluble vitamins, because of disagreement on the effect of high-carbohydrate diets, the need for a safe fat led to a renewed interest in monounsaturated fats.

Could monounsaturated fats be the answer in the search for a safe fat? In the 1980s the research on these fats blossomed and confirmed the value of Mediterranean diets in which the natural fat is usually mainly monounsaturated (olive oil) and the intake of meat fats is extremely low. The chapters in Part III of this book confirm the different disease pattern between populations eating different fats: An example is the difference between southern Italy where people consume little meat and use olive oil as the main free fat in the diet and northern Italy where some olive oil but mainly butter and a large amount of high-fat meat products are consumed.

Foods with a high ratio of monounsaturated to other fatty acids (Fig. 9–1) include olives, almonds, hazelnuts, and avocados. Whereas some animal foods such as chicken contain a reasonable amount of MFA, they also supply fairly large amounts of saturated fat. The aforementioned plant foods contain only a minimum level of saturated fatty acids.

Some key clinical studies have supported the epidemiological findings of the Seven Country Study (Keys 1980). Other chapters in this book cover other aspects of lipids and disease, and the facts presented here are intended to complement chapters 1, 10, and 12. It is also important to read chapter 6 on the chemistry and other aspects of oils used in Mediterranean diets.

Most studies used olive oil as the typical monounsaturated fat used since antiquity (see chapters 2 and 6).The majority of the studies support

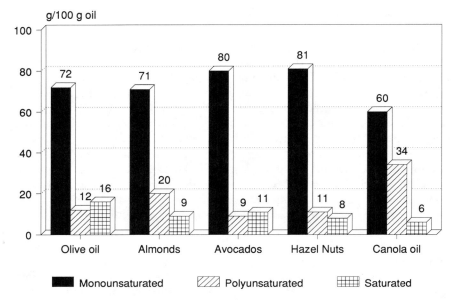

Figure 9-1.   Fatty acid pattern of some common foods high in monounsaturated fatty acids.

the effectiveness of olive oil, almonds (a high monounsaturated fat food), and canola oil, among others, as desirable replacements for saturated fat. The results of the effect of MFAs on HDL-C differ and these differences are probably caused by other factors in the diet, such as an oversimplistic approach to such complex oil as olive oil, the composition of which is affected by the state or ripeness of the olive, the methods of extraction, and even the climate where the olives are grown (Bailey 1951 and chapter 6).

OLIVE OIL STUDIES

It is interesting to review these studies in chronological order as it shows how the clinical research interest in this fat is a phenomenon of the 1980s.

In 1985, Mattson and Grundy (Mattson and Grundy 1985) conducted a study designed to examine the metabolic properties and lipid-lowering effects of MFAs fed as olive oil and to compare them with those of PFAs (linoleic acid). Briefly, the results of this study showed oleic acid to be as effective as linoleic acid in reducing TC and LDL-C levels. Furthermore, while linoleic acid caused a reduction in HDL-C, oleic acid did not.

In 1986, Grundy (Grundy 1986) compared a high-MFA diet with a low-fat diet in terms of effectiveness in lowering plasma cholesterol. When compared with a diet high in SFAs, both the high-MFA diet and the low-fat diet reduced TC and LDL-C levels, with the high-MFA diet proving somewhat more effective. The low-fat diet also caused a significant reduction of HDL-C and a rise in triglycerides. HDL-C was not affected by MFAs. Grundy suggested serious consideration be given to the use of MFA as a hypocholesterolemic agent. This liquid formula diet study needed support by studies with solid food as part of a normal diet.

In 1987, Mensink and Katan (Mensink and Katan 1987) conducted a study comparing the effects on TC and HDL-C of diets high in MFAs (in the form of olive oil) with those of diets high in carbohydrates. Results supported those of Grundy, with high-carbohydrate, high-fiber diets resulting in a reduction of TC and a concomitant reduction in HDL-C and high-MFA diets resulting in a comparable reduction in TC and an unchanged HDL-C level.

Many studies appeared in 1988. Grundy (Grundy et al. 1988) continued his investigations of the metabolic effects of MFAs with a study comparing a high-MFA diet with a high-SFA, high-cholesterol diet and with a low-fat, high-carbohydrate diet. In response to criticisms of his 1986 study, Grundy carried out this study using a solid food diet adhered to over a longer period of time. Results from this study confirmed earlier findings: high-MFA diets and low-fat diets both produced comparable reductions in TC and LDL-C. HDL-C levels, however, were significantly reduced by low-fat diets and remained essentially unchanged by diets high in MFAs or high in SFA and carbohydrate.

In the same year, Aravanis, Mensink, and colleagues (Aravanis et al. 1988) reported the results of a study on the long-term effects and serum lipid profiles of rural Cretan boys consuming a diet rich in olive oil. When compared with boys of other populations consuming a diet lower in MFAs, Cretan boys did not demonstrate lower levels of LDL-C, and their levels of TC were in fact higher than those of their counterparts in the United States. No explanation was offered for these findings.

Garg and co-workers (Garg et al. 1988) compared a high-carbohydrate diet with a high-MFA diet in patients with non-insulin-dependent diabetes mellitus in 10 patients receiving insulin therapy. The high-MFA diet contained 33% of the total energy in the form of monounsaturated fatty acids. Levels of TC and LDL-C cholesterol did not differ significantly in patients on the two diets. There appears to be better glycemic control in the patients on the high MFA diet.

The effect of olive-oil-enriched diet on serum lipoprotein levels and biliary cholesterol saturation was studied by Baggio (Baggio et al. 1988) in 11 young volunteers admitted to a metabolic ward. A significant decrease of mean total cholesterol (-9.5%), total apo-B (-7.4%), LDL-C (-12.2%), and total triglycerides (-25.5%) was observed after the olive-oil-enriched diet.

Total HDL-C and HDL-C subfractions cholesterol levels and serum apo A-I mean levels remained unchanged. The saturation index of the bile and fasting and after-meal gallbladder volumes were unaffected by the enriched diet. The authors concluded that olive oil may be a natural fat that can be used for the control of plasma and LDL cholesterol as a valid alternative to polyunsaturated fatty acids.

In 1989, Mensink and Katan (Mensink and Katan 1989) compared the effects of a high-MFA diet with a high-PFA diet on serum lipoprotein levels in healthy men and women. Both the high-MFA diet and the high-PFA diet produced significant reductions in TC, LDL-C, and serum apolipoprotein-B in both sexes, with the high-MFA diet producing a somewhat greater response. In contrast to the findings of Grundy and others, the high-PFA diet administered in this study did not result in a decrease in HDL-C or in apolipoprotein A-I. Men on both diets showed a very slight reduction of HDL-C that was statistically significant only in comparison with the women, none of whom showed any such decrease. The authors theorize that results obtained by Grundy and others that show high-PFA diets lowering HDL-C are caused by other factors in the composition of the experimental diets. The authors conclude that diets high in PFAs or MFAs are equally effective in reducing TC and LDL-C levels.

Mensink and co-workers (Mensink et al. 1989) studied the effects of monounsaturated fatty acids and complex carbohydrates on serum lipoproteins and apoproteins of 48 healthy men and women. The subjects were on a high-SFA diet for 17 days. For the next 36 days they consumed either a diet high in complex carbohydrates (24 subjects on MFA 9 kcal%, total fat 22 kcal%) or a high-fat, olive-oil-rich diet (24 subjects; MFA24 kcal%, total fat 41 kcal%). The amount of protein was 12% to 14%. PFA and cholesterol content were similar in all three diets. Serum cholesterol levels fell by 0.44 mmol/L (16 mg/dl) in subjects consuming the carbohydrate diet and by 0.52 mmol/L (20 mg/d) for those receiving the olive-oil-rich diet.

HDL$_2$ and LDL cholesterol levels fell to the same extent on both diets. There was no change in the composition of HDL$_3$, suggesting that the fall was caused by a decrease in the total number of circulating particles.

Ginsberg (Ginsberg et al. 1990) compared the effect on reduction of plasma cholesterol levels in normal men on an American Heart Association (AHA) Step 1 diet or a Step 1 diet with added MFA in 36 healthy young men. The Step 1 diet supplied 30% of the total calories as fat: 10% saturated, 10% monounsaturated, and 10% polyunsaturated fats, with 250 mg of cholesterol per day. The MFA-enriched Step 1 diet supplied 38% of the calories consumed as fat: 10% saturated, 18% monounsaturated, and 10% polyunsaturated fats, with 250 mg of cholesterol per day. The effects of these diets were then compared with those of an average American diet, in which 38% of the total calories were consumed as fat: 18% saturated, 10% monounsaturated, and 10% polyunsaturated fats, with 500 mg of cholesterol per day.

There were significant reductions ($P < 0.025$) in the plasma total cholesterol level in the group on the Step 1 diet (14 mg/dl) and in the group on the MFA-enriched Step 1 diet (-18 mg/dl). Neither the plasma triglyceride levels nor the HDL-C concentrations changed significantly with any diet. The authors concluded that enrichment of the AHA Step 1 diet with MFA does not alter the beneficial effects of the Step 1 diet on plasma lipid concentrations.

Trevisan (Trevisan et al. 1990), in a cross-sectional study on the consumption of olive oil and vegetable oils and coronary heart disease risk, found that in both men and women consumption of olive oil as well as other vegetable oils was inversely associated with serum cholesterol and glucose levels and systolic blood pressure.

OLIVE AND PEANUT OIL STUDIES

Dreon and co-workers (Dreon et al. 1990) compared two diets with 30% kcals from fat, one with MFA and the other with PFA as the major fat. The sources of MFAs were defined as *"olive oil and peanut oil products"* and the sources of PFA as *"primarily safflower and corn oil products."* Unfortunately the olive oil is not properly identified and it is not known how it was used, that is, as dressing for food in the raw state or for cooking. The same applies to the safflower and corn oil products. The PFA to SFA ratios were also quite different in the two diets. The study confirmed that both MFAs and PFAs are effective in lowering serum cholesterol but did not show any negative effect of PFAs on HDL-C. This result may be caused by the low-fat diet that actually limited the amount of PFA intake and thus the study was useful in relation to low-fat diet but did not test the hypothesis of whether larger amounts of PFAs lower HDL-C. In addition the subjects of this study were only mildly hypercholesterolemic. It is unfortunate that this study does not cast any light on the effect of larger doses of polyunsaturated fats.

ALMOND STUDIES

Spiller and co-workers (Spiller et al. 1989; Spiller et al. 1990) used whole high-MFA foods (almonds, see Fig. 9–1) in two different studies to confirm the effect on serum cholesterol of high-MFA diets.

In a long-term, nine-week study Spiller et al. (1989) studied the effect of a Mediterranean-type diet in which the predominant fat was supplied by raw almonds (100g/day; 636 kcal, MFA 34 g, PFA 11 g, and SFA 5 g) and almond oil was the only free fat allowed. All other fat sources were carefully controlled and the diet was high in plant foods and low-fat milk products. Twenty-six adults with mean TC of 238 mg/dl participated in the study. Serum cholesterol was measured at 3, 6, 8, and 9 weeks on the diet. There was a rapid initial and then a sustained reduction in serum cholesterol due to reduction in LDL-C, without significant changes in HDL-C, VLDL-C, or triglycerides. Serum cholesterol dropped at 6 weeks to 213 (− 25) mg/dl and remained at that level until the end of the study [at 9 weeks, 214 (− 24) mg/dl].

In another study (Spiller et al. 1990) a diet similar to the one just described was compared to a diet in which all the basic foods were the same except for the fat being supplied by cheese and butter at the same level as the fat supplied by the almonds. In this four-week study serum cholesterol dropped for the almond, high-MFA diet from an average of 257 to 220 mg/dl while there was no significant change for the SFA group. A separate control group on olive oil and on a similar diet also showed a significant drop in total serum cholesterol.

In both studies the almonds were fed raw to ensure a well-defined fatty acid pattern.

CANOLA OIL STUDY

Canola oil (see Fig. 9–1) has recently become popular in North America and has been studied by McDonald (McDonald et al. 1989). Canola oil was compared to highly polyunsaturated sunflower oil. The subjects of this study were normocholesterolemic young men with baseline total serum cholesterols that averaged approximately 190 mg/dl in one of the groups and 150 mg/dl in the other group. The number of subjects was very small (eight). Both canola oil and sunflower oil were equally effective in lowering total serum cholesterol as LDL cholesterol but did not lower HDL cholesterol or triglycerides. This study needs to be repeated with a hypercholesterolemic population.

CONCLUSION

Many studies on olive oil fail to define the olive oil properly. Olive oil (chapter 6 and Bailey 1951) varies in composition as the ripeness of the olive and the type of extraction have a major effect on the fatty acid pattern. This is not the case for many seed oils as commercially processed. Equating olive oil to MFA in a general way is bound to lead to confusion and conflicting results. In studies with free-living subjects often the way the oil was used is not stated (raw or in cooking).

It seems clear that: (1) Monounsaturated fats are a highly desirable replacement for excessive saturated fat in the diet and (2) They are probably one of the safest dietary fats.

Further study is needed to clarify the relative effect on HDL-C of various fatty acids. Some confusion is generated by the fact that many of the studies are difficult to compare as the hypocholesterolemia of the population at the beginning of the studies varies greatly.

The epidemiological evidence from Mediterranean regions is in overwhelming support of the benefits of MFA in the presence of a diet otherwise moderate in SFA and high in foods of plant origin.

One problem that arises in the study of MFAs as in many other studies in clinical nutrition is the tendency of many investigators to focus only on one part of the diet in a "reductionist" manner. This may also lead to problems in this case, as olive oil and other sources of MFAs contain various amounts of other PFAs and SFAs. Finally, not to be overlooked is the fact that olive oil and other typical Mediterranean foods such as almonds may need to be fed with a diet high in grain products and low in meats to be most effective in cholesterol-lowering diets.

The question of a safe level of fat when such MFAs are the main fats in the diet is a major challenge for cholesterol researchers and could lead to a revision of current thinking on low-fat diets. They are probably the only type of fat that could exceed the now popular recommendation of a 30% kcal of fat in diet and not lead to undesirable side effects even though some of these side effects have been tested only in animal models.

REFERENCES

Aravanis, C., R. P. Mensink, N. Karalias, B. Christodoulou, A. Kafatos, and M. B. Katan. 1988. Serum lipids, apoproteins and nutrient intake in rural Cretan boys consuming high olive oil diets. *J. Clin. Epidemiol.* **41**:1117–1123.
Baggio, G., A. Pagnan, M. Muraca, S. Martini, A. Opportuno, A. Bonanome,

G. B. Ambrosio, S. Ferrari, P. Guarini, and D. Piccolo. 1988. Olive-oil-enriched diet: effect on serum lipoprotein levels and biliary cholesterol saturation. *Am. J. Clin. Nutr.* **47**(6):960–964.

Bailey, A. E. 1951. *Industrial Oil and Fat Products.* New York: Interscience.

Dreon, G. A., K. M. Vranizan, R. M. Krauss, M. A. Austin, and P. Wood. 1990. The effects of polyunsaturated fat vs monounsaturated fat on plasma lipoproteins. *JAMA* **263**:2462–2466.

Gammal, E. B., K. K. Carroll, and E. R. Plunkett. 1967. Effect of dietary fat on mammary carcinogenesis by 7,12-dimethylbenz(alpha)anthracene in rats. *Cancer Res.* **27**:1737–1742.

Garg, A., A. Bonanome, S. M. Grundy, Z. J. Zhang, and R. H. Unger. 1988. Comparison of a high-carbohydrate diet with a high-monounsaturated-fat diet in patients with non-insulin-dependent diabetes mellitus. *New Engl. J. Med.* **319**:829–834.

Ginsberg, H. N., S. L. Barr, A. Gilbert, W. Karmally, R. Deckelbaum, K. Kaplan, R. Ramakrishnan, S. Holleran, and R. B. Dell. 1990. Reduction of plasma cholesterol levels in normal men on an American Heart Association Step 1 diet or a Step 1 diet with added monounsaturated fat. *New Engl. J. Med.* **322**(9):574–579.

Grundy, S. M. 1986. Comparison of monounsaturated fatty acids and carbohydrates for lowering plasma cholesterol. *New Engl. J. Med.* **314**(12):745–748.

Grundy, S. M. 1987. Monounsaturated fatty acids, plasma cholesterol, and coronary heart disease. *Am. J. Clin. Nutr.* **45**(suppl. 5):1168–1175.

Grundy, S. M., L. Florentin, D. Nix, and M. F. Whelan. 1988. Comparison of monounsaturated fatty acids and carbohydrates for reducing raised levels of plasma cholesterol in man. *Am. J. Clin. Nutr.* **47**(6):965–969.

Keys, A. 1980. *Seven Countries. A Multivariate Analysis of Death and Coronary Heart Disease.* Cambridge, Mass.: Harvard University Press.

McDonald, B. F., J. M. Gerrad, V. M. Bruce, and E. J. Corner. 1990. Comparison of the effects of canola oil and sunflower oil on plasma lipids and lipoproteins and on in vivo tromboxane A_2 and prostacyclin production in healthy young men. *Am. J. Clin. Nutr.* **50**:1382–1388.

Mattson, F. H., and S. M. Grundy. 1985. Comparison of effects of dietary saturated, monounsaturated, and polyunsaturated fatty acids on plasma lipids and lipoproteins in man. *J. Lipid Res.* **26**:194–202.

Mensink, R. P., and M. B. Katan. 1987. Effect of monounsaturated fatty acids versus complex carbohydrates on high-density lipoproteins in healthy men and women. *Lancet* **1**(8525):122–125.

Mensink, R. P., and M. B. Katan. 1989. Effect of a diet enriched with monounsaturated or polyunsaturated fatty acids on levels of low-density and high-density lipoprotein cholesterol in healthy women and men. *New Engl. J. Med.* **321**(7):436–441.

Mensink, R. P., M. J. de Groot, L. T. van den Broeke, A. P. Severijnen-Nobels, P. N. Demacker, and M. B. Katan. 1989. Effects of monounsaturated fatty acids v. complex carbohydrates on serum lipoproteins and apoproteins in healthy men and women. *Metabolism* **38**(2):172–178.

Spiller, G. A., J. E. Gates, D. J. A. Jenkins, O. Bosello, S. F. Nichols, and L. Cragen. 1990. Effect of two foods high in monounsaturated fat on plasma cholesterol and lipoproteins in adult humans. *Am. J. Clin. Nutr.* **51**(3):524.

Spiller, G. A., D. J. A. Jenkins, L. Cragen, O. Bosello, K. Berra, C. Rudd, and R. Superko. 1989. Sustained reductions of serum cholesterol over nine weeks on a diet with a high ratio of monounsaturated fats to other fats (Abstract). X Internat. Symp. Drugs Affecting Lipid Metabolism, Houston, Tex.

Trevisan, M., V. Krogh, J. Freudenheim, A. Blake, P. P. S. Muti, E. Farinaro, M. Mancini, A. Menotti, and G. Ricci. 1990. Consumption of olive oil, butter, and vegetable oils and coronary heart disease risk factors. *JAMA* **263**(5):688–692.

Part III

CLINICAL ASPECTS
AND EPIDEMIOLOGY

10

Lipids

Luciano Cominacini
Ulisse Garbin
Anna Davoli
Beatrice Cenci
Ottavio Bosello

EPIDEMIOLOGY

The Lipid Hypothesis

The relations between elevated cholesterol concentration and coronary heart disease is known to physicians as the lipid hypothesis. This theory breaks cholesterol into two components: low-density lipoprotein (LDL) or "bad" cholesterol and high-density lipoprotein (HDL) or "good" cholesterol. LDL usually deposits cholesterol on the inner walls of the arteries, whereas HDL works in the opposite manner. Therefore, a person who has a high total cholesterol and LDL level and a low level of HDL has an increased risk of developing coronary heart disease.

Many epidemiological studies have supported the lipid hypothesis. One of the first was the Framingham Heart Study in which the cardiac histories of the residents of Framingham, Massachusetts, were followed for 40 years (Kannel et al. 1979; Gordon et al. 1981). The Multiple Risk Factor Intervention Trial (MRFIT) started in the early 1970s and reported the health of more than 360,000 middle-aged men with no signs of coronary heart disease at the beginning of the study (Stamler et al. 1986). Both studies indicated that the risk of coronary heart disease increases steadily when the cholesterol concentration is over 160 mg/dl.

The seven-year Coronary Primary Prevention Trial (Lipid Research Clinics Program 1984) was probably the study that convinced most physicians of the close connection between cholesterol and coronary heart disease. About 3,800 middle-aged men with high cholesterol concentration but without clinical evidence of coronary heart disease were enrolled and randomly divided into a control group that received no drug treatment and a group treated with cholestyramine, the well-known cholesterol-lowering agent. The cholestyramine group had an average reduction of 9% in cholesterol and 19% in heart attacks. On the basis of these results, the "two-for-one" rule was established, which held that every 1% reduction in cholesterol produces a 2% reduction in heart disease risk. In the Oslo Study, a 13% decrease of cholesterol induced only by dietary changes was associated with a 40% reduction in coronary heart disease events after nine years of follow-up (Hjerman 1981).

With overwhelming evidence supporting the lipid hypothesis, the past few years have seen an extraordinary degree of interest in cholesterol and in coronary heart disease prevention. This interest has emanated from a variety of activities that have developed from programs in cholesterol education the world over. In the United States, the National Cholesterol Education Program (NCEP) was launched in 1985 by the National Heart, Lung, and Blood Institute of the National Institutes of Health. The NCEP was modeled on the National High Blood Pressure Education Program that had been in operation for well over a decade. The goal of the NCEP was to reduce the prevalence of elevated blood cholesterol in the United States and thereby reduce coronary heart disease morbidity and mortality. The NCEP has been developing its program through expert panels. The first of these, the adult treatment panel, was convened to develop recommendations for high-risk strategy and published its report (Consensus Development Conference 1985). It details criteria for the classification of patients according to their cholesterol levels and for the medical management of patients classified as being at high risk.

Treatment begins with dietary therapy. The minimal goals of therapy are to lower LDL cholesterol to levels below the cutoff points for initiating therapy, that is, to below 160 mg/dl, or to below 130 mg/dl if definite coronary heart disease or two other risk factors are present. The general aim of dietary therapy is to reduce elevated cholesterol levels while maintaining a nutritionally adequate and palatable eating pattern. Dietary therapy should occur in two steps designed to (1) progressively reduce intakes of saturated fatty acids and cholesterol and (2) promote weight loss in overweight patients by eliminating excess total calories.

Geographical Dietary Variations

Food patterns of a country are molded by its agricultural resources, technical progress, buying power, and cultural patterns. In trying to understand the food habits of a people, one needs to learn about their country or, in the case of immigrants or refugees, the country from which they came. The physical characteristics of a country have a strong influence on the eating habits of its people; for example, regions bordering on an ocean are likely to have a variety of fish in the diet, whereas in land-locked interior areas, fish constitute a minor part of the diet.

Confusion in interpreting the influence of diet on lipoproteins and lipids is caused by individual genetic response. Both genetic and environmental factors influence each person's lipid and lipoprotein levels, which can readily be seen by reviewing available study data. Individuals within a country or community often have widely divergent blood lipid and lipoprotein levels. When given the same diet in a maximally controlled environment, individuals within the group attain and maintain different average levels of lipids and lipoproteins. Such individual responses are affected by large, nondietary intrinsic factors that are probably genetic (McGandy et al. 1966). On the other hand, the effect of diet on lipid and lipoprotein levels has been clearly demonstrated. First, while holding constant other predisposing factors in the environment, it is possible to lower levels of lipids and lipoproteins in almost everyone by changing the diet (Stamler 1979; Keys 1975). Second, multifactorial population studies leave little doubt of the role of the diet in determining the average level of lipids and lipoproteins in different countries (Stamler 1979; Keys 1975). Such dietary influences are demonstrated by studies comparing ethnic Japanese populations in Japan, in Hawaii, and in California (Kato et al. 1973). The increased frequency of elevated cholesterol values among Japanese in Hawaii and California compared to those living in Japan suggests that hyperlipidemia is strongly affected by dietary factors.

In populations surveyed in the Seven Countries Study, most of the differences in average serum cholesterol levels among the populations were consonant with differences in the amount and kind of dietary fat consumed (Keys 1970). Populations manifesting high average cholesterol levels and higher levels of LDL have saturated fat intakes of 15% or more of calories. In contrast, populations with low average serum cholesterol levels have saturated fat intakes of 10% or less of calories. These dietary relationships are evident when we contrast the countries of Japan and Finland (Levy 1983). In Japan, where the studies were performed, the saturated fat intake was about 3% of calories and the average cholesterol was below 160 mg/dl with a coronary heart disease rate among the lowest of the industrial countries. In comparison, in eastern Finland (Levy 1983), where 22% of calories are from saturated fatty acids, the average cholesterol level is above 240 mg/dl, and the Finns have one of the highest atherosclerotic disease rates of any culture.

MEDITERRANEAN DIET CHARACTERISTICS
AND EURATOM STUDY RESULTS

The Seven Country Study demonstrated that people living in the area bordering the Mediterranean Sea had average cholesterol levels and risk of coronary heart disease much lower than those in other countries (Keys 1980). These findings were attributed to the specific characteristics of the food these populations were used to eating. But what are the peculiarities of the Mediterranean diet? When discussing this diet, the food habits of several different countries must be taken into consideration, that is, Spain, Portugal, Greece, Crete, Yugoslavia, Italy, and so forth. Unfortunately, sometimes statistics are lacking regarding the kind and quality of food the people bordering the Mediterranean Sea were and now are accustomed to eating. Therefore, very often data regarding the dietary practices in this area refer only to southern Italy.

At least two studies have described the food habits in this region: (1) the CNR study of 1930 (Galeotti 1936; Niceforo and Galeotti 1943) and (2) the European Atomic Energy Community (EURATOM) study begun in 1960 (Cresta et al. 1969).

The latter was particularly important, as it compared the food habits of different areas of Italy with north European populations presenting the highest incidence of coronary heart disease. In the study, the seven-day dietary recall of about 8,000 families was evaluated. First, it was demonstrated that the amount of calories derived from carbohydrates was higher (58%) among the people of southern Italy than among those of the other countries surveyed (between 43% and 52%). Not only was there a difference in the total amount of carbohydrates but also perhaps the most interesting difference was in the quality of carbohydrates. In the diet of southern Italy most sugar was derived from foods containing complex carbohydrates; the consumption of simplex carbohydrates was three times higher in the rest of Europe.

The EURATOM study also provided data demonstrating that the increased carbohydrate intake corresponded to a reduced consumption of food containing fat among the population of southern Italy (31%) compared with that of other areas (between 38% and 46%). Once again, however, the main difference was not in the quantity but in the quality of fat. The ratio between vegetable and animal fat was, in fact, about 3:1 in southern Italy and about 0.7:1 and 0.4:1, respectively, in northern Italy and the rest of Europe. The intake of animal fat, that is, saturated fatty acids, was therefore much lower in southern Italy than in any other European country. Interestingly, also, the consumption of polyunsaturates showed the same behavior; the ratio between saturated and poly-unsaturated fatty acid intake was even higher in southern Italy than in other European countries mostly as a consequence of the drastic reduction in animal fat intake. Conversely, according to the results of the EURATOM study (Cresta et al. 1969), in southern Italy, the majority of calories from fat were from monounsaturated fatty acids; so the ratio between monounsaturated and saturated fatty acids was particularly high in this area. An analysis of the sources of monounsaturates in southern Italy showed that the majority of these fatty acids derived from the consumption of olive oil and olives.

Consequently, the consumption of animal fat was very low and, given the monounsaturates derived from vegetables, the daily consumption of cholesterol was much lower in southern Italy than in northern Italy and the other countries involved in the EURATOM study. For example, the mean daily intake of cholesterol was about 200 mg in southern Italy, about 400 mg in northern Italy, and about 800 mg in Luxembourg.

The EURATOM study also provided data demonstrating that in absolute values there was not much difference between the daily protein intake in southern Italy and the other countries in the study. Once again, however, the great difference was in the kind of proteins. The consumption of animal proteins was much higher (90%) in northern Europe than in southern Italy, where the intake of vegetable protein, and in particular of leguminous protein, was prevalent.

Finally, the results of the EURATOM study showed that there was not much difference between the fiber content in the diet of southern Italy and that of diets in the other countries. However, in analyzing sources of fiber, the study revealed that the majority of the fiber was derived from potatoes in northern Europe and from other vegetables in southern Italy; the ratio of digestible carbohydrates to fiber, therefore, was very high in countries of northern Europe. Also, the ratios total fat to fiber and cholesterol to fiber were much higher in northern Europe than those in southern Italy. The results of the EURATOM study, therefore, seem to demonstrate that the Mediterranean diet is characterized by being (1) low in saturated fats and consequently in cholesterol, (2) low in animal protein, (3) rich in complex carbohydrates, and (4) rich in vegetable and leguminous fiber.

During the 1970s and 1980s, many studies tried to bring about an understanding of the relationship between dietary habit and hypercholesterolemia and lipoproteic pattern. Let us therefore consider the possible impacts of the characteristics of the Mediterranean diet on cholesterol levels and lipid pattern.

EFFECTS OF DIETARY CARBOHYDRATES
ON PLASMA LIPIDS

Effects of Refined Sugars and Starch
on Plasma Lipids

Several studies performed in the last few decades have shown that high carbohydrate feeding is associated with changes in levels, composition, and metabolism of serum lipoproteins. In particular, high carbohydrate feeding was found to be associated with fasting hypertriglyceridemia (Ahrens et al. 1967; Quarfordt et al. 1970; Ruderman et al. 1971; Reaven and Olefsky 1974; Schonfeld et al. 1976; Ginsberg et al. 1976; Nestel et al. 1979; Gonen et al. 1981; Lithell et al. 1982; Kashyap et al. 1982; Coulston et al. 1983; Liu et al. 1983; Hollenbeck et al. 1985) and with a decrease in HDL cholesterol levels (Schonfeld et al. 1976; Gonen et al. 1981; Lithell et al. 1982; Kashyap et al. 1982; Coulston et al. 1983). It should be pointed out, however, that the majority of these studies were carried out with formula diets (Ahrens et al. 1967; Ruderman et al. 1971; Reaven and Olefsky 1974; Schonfeld et al. 1976; Ginsberg et al. 1976; Gonen et al. 1981) and/or for a very short period of time (Ahrens et al. 1967; Quarfordt et al. 1970; Ruderman et al. 1971; Reaven and Olefsky 1974; Schonfeld et al. 1976; Ginsberg et al. 1976; Nestel et al. 1979; Gonen et al. 1981; Lithell et al. 1982; Coulston et al. 1983; Liu et al. 1983). Furthermore, another point must be stressed: The carbohydrate effects were often stated without specific consideration given to the kind of carbohydrate (Ahrens et al. 1967; Quarfordt et al. 1970; Ruderman et al. 1971; Reaven and Olefsky 1974; Schonfeld et al. 1976; Ginsberg et al. 1976; Gonen et al. 1981; Lithell et al. 1982; Kashyap et al. 1982; Coulston et al. 1983; Liu et al. 1983), and now there is considerable evidence showing that different carbohydrates produce different effects on serum lipids (MacDonald and Braithwaite 1964; Kuo and Basset 1965; Cohen et al. 1966; Kaufman et al. 1966; Nestel et al. 1970; Nikkila and Kekki 1972; Roberts 1973; Reiser et al. 1979; Srinivasan et al. 1983; Jenkins et al. 1985).

Actually, several studies demonstrated that, when solid diets containing large amounts of natural carbohydrates were used, an increase in plasma triglyceride levels was not observed (Ernest et al. 1962; Stone and Connor 1963; Ernest et al. 1965; Weinsier et al. 1974; Kiehm et al. 1976; Anderson et al. 1980; Rosenthal et al. 1985; Jenkins et al. 1985; Thuesen et al. 1986; Cominacini et al. 1988b).

The first point to be considered is that the Mediterranean diet is, in absolute values, rich in natural carbohydrates and that these carbohydrates are represented mostly by starch. Pasta and bread are indeed typical foods of southern Italy. The question is why complex carbohydrates do not cause hypertriglyceridemia and low HDL cholesterol levels. Indeed, several studies of diabetic and nondiabetic subjects have demonstrated that, when carbohydrates consumed were mainly starch in contrast to refined sugars, hypertriglyceridemia did not result (Ernst et al. 1962; Stone and Connor 1963; Ernst et al. 1965; Weinsier et al. 1974; Kiehm et al. 1976; Anderson et al. 1980; Rosenthal et al. 1985; Jenkins et al. 1985; Thuesen et al. 1986, Cominacini et al. 1988b). Conversely, those authors who specified the type of carbohydrates they used and found an increase in fasting triglyceride values generally gave small quantities of starch (Hollenbeck et al. 1985) and large amounts of refined sugars; in these tests, sucrose accounted for 22% to 25% of total carbohydrates (Coulston et al. 1983; Liu et al. 1983).

The Glycemic Index

Differences in amount and kind of ingested carbohydrates can affect glucose and insulin response in different ways (Crapo et al. 1976; Crapo et al. 1977; Reaven 1979). This information led to the introduction of the glycemic index to rank carbohydrate foods according to their postprandial blood glucose response (Jenkins et al. 1981; Jenkins et al. 1984). The glycemic index is determined by expressing individual results as a percentage of a reference food, thus allowing values obtained in different groups of subjects to be compared (Jenkins et al. 1981). The substantial differences that exist between the glycemic response to different starchy foods might be explained by the differences in digestibility of individual foods (Jenkins 1982; Jenkins et al. 1984). From such studies, the concept has arisen that the rate of carbohydrate digestion and absorption may be at least as important as the actual amount of carbohydrate eaten (Jenkins 1982).

For example, it is recognized that pasta produces one of the lowest glycemic indexes among starch foods (Jenkins 1983a). Because pasta forms a substantial part of the high-carbohydrate intake of the Mediterranean diet, one can anticipate that if such a diet gives the lowest postprandial glucose and insulin responses, the concentration of plasma triglycerides should not be affected. As a matter of fact, hyperinsulinemia can promote hypertriglyceridemia (Olefsky et al. 1974; Tobey et al. 1981), and therefore, as previously hypothesized (Cominacini et al. 1988b), the selection of foods that minimize the glucose and insulin response should reduce the stimulus to hepatic triglyceride synthesis. Cominacini et al (1988b) demonstrated that a low-fat, high-carbohydrate diet based on pasta and pumpernickel bread, that is, foods with the lowest glycemic index (Jenkins et al. 1983b; Jenkins et al. 1985), can reduce the triglyceride concentration even in patients affected by familial hypertriglyceridemia and that there was a close direct correlation between the variation in plasma triglyceride concentration and the variation of insulin secretion after oral glucose tolerance tests.

Can Low-Fat Diets Negatively Affect Plasma Lipids?

Another crucial point that may help to explain why a diet enriched in complex carbohydrates does not cause hypertriglyceridemia is the amount of fat administered during high-carbohydrate feeding. Because exogenous lipids are packaged in the intestine as chylomicrons, it is likely that a low-fat diet may reduce their production. Actually, previous reports have demonstrated lower postprandial triglyceride concentration after a low-fat diet (Ginsberg et al. 1976; Hayford et al. 1979; Anderson et al. 1979) and a decrease in VLDL secretion after reduction in absorptive lipoproteins (Cooper and Shewsbury 1979; Green et al. 1984).

High-Carbohydrate Feeding and HDL Cholesterol Levels

Finally, there is evidence that high-carbohydrate feeding is generally associated with low HDL cholesterol levels (Levy et al. 1966; Schonfeld et al. 1976; Blum et al. 1977; Shepherd et al. 1978; Gonen et al. 1981; Lithell et al. 1982). As already stated, however, the conclusions of these studies were generally drawn after a short-term feeding of a very-high-carbohydrate diet, and now there is evidence of augmented HDL cholesterol concentration after a long-term high-complex carbohydrate diet (Thuesen et al. 1986; Cominacini et al. 1988b; Cominacini et al. 1990). How this kind of diet may improve HDL cholesterol levels is not clear. However, since it was demonstrated that high-carbohydrate feeding mainly affects the less-dense HDL subfraction, that is, HDL^2 (Cominacini et al. 1988c), and the production of this lipoprotein is regulated also by the lipoprotein-lipase-induced catabolism of triglyceride-rich lipoproteins at adipose tissue level (Nikkila et al. 1978; Patsch and Gotto 1980), it is likely that the effect of complex, natural carbohydrates on HDL cholesterol levels may rely also on the accelerated removal of triglyceride-rich particles.

There is now evidence that hyperinsulinemia per se can negatively affect HDL cholesterol concentration (Cominacini et al. 1988a), so a diet giving the lowest postprandial glucose and insulin responses not only does not induce hypertriglyceridemia but also may prevent negative effects on HDL cholesterol levels. The results of the EURATOM study showed that the inhabitants of southern Italy consumed about 80% of the total carbohydrates as cereal carbohydrates (Cresta et al. 1969). The complex carbohydrates of the Mediterranean diet seem, once again, to contribute to the safest lipoprotein profile.

EFFECTS OF DIETARY FATS ON PLASMA LIPIDS

Excessive consumption of dietary fat has been indicated as a major risk factor in the development of atherosclerosis in general and coronary heart disease in particular. Several studies have provided evidence, possibly through an increase in plasma cholesterol levels, that high intakes of fat are associated with an increased prevalence of coronary heart disease (Keys et al. 1969; Hegsted et al. 1965; Keys 1970). The Mediterranean diet is, in absolute values, low in fat, and this characteristic per se could be favorable in preventing or retarding the progression of the atherosclerotic process. Indeed, populations that habitually consume low-fat diets have a low prevalence of coronary heart disease (Keys 1970).

The Impact of Different Kinds of Fatty Acids on Plasma Lipids

Although it has been generally believed that high dietary fat increases serum cholesterol concentration, one of the most important findings in recent years is that the components of dietary fat do not affect serum cholesterol and the different lipoproteins in the same manner. Indeed, the saturated fatty acids appear to be the most powerful LDL cholesterol-raising nutrients in the diet (Keys et al. 1957; Hegsted et al. 1965; Keys 1970). One of the important characteristics of the Mediterranean diet is that it is very low in saturated fatty acids. On the other hand, it is relatively rich in monounsaturated fatty acids, mainly derived from olive oil. Considerable data now demonstrate that these fatty acids have no effect on total cholesterol or LDL cholesterol (Keys et al. 1957; Hegsted et al. 1965; Mattson and Grundy 1985; Grundy 1986).

On the other hand, polyunsaturates have been shown to produce a reduction in plasma cholesterol levels (Keys et al. 1957; Ahrens et al. 1967; Hegsted et al. 1965; Grundy 1986). Ahrens et al. (1967) showed that linoleic acid, the major omega–6 polyunsaturated fatty acid in the diet, lowered the total cholesterol level when it was substituted for saturated fatty acids in the diet. The effect of linolenic acid, an omega–3 fatty acid found in several vegetable oils, has not been studied extensively regarding its effect on plasma cholesterol concentration, although it is probably similar to linoleic acid. Large quantities of omega–3 fatty acids are also contained in fish oils, and they are likely to have about the same effect as linoleic acid on plasma cholesterol (Grundy 1989). The effect of polyunsaturates in lowering total plasma cholesterol is mainly due to the decrease in LDL cholesterol (Grundy 1986). In addition to several other side effects (Gammal et al. 1967; Sturdevant et al. 1973; King and Spector 1978), polyunsaturated fatty acids have been found to greatly reduce HDL cholesterol levels (Shepherd et al. 1978; Vessby et al. 1980; Vega et al. 1982).

Dietary Fatty Acids and HDL Cholesterol

Since HDL may protect against coronary heart disease (Miller and Miller 1975), diets chosen for lowering total plasma cholesterol should not lower HDL cholesterol. Although the EURATOM study demonstrated that the ratio of polyunsaturated to saturated fatty acids in the diet was high in southern Italy, the contribution of polyunsaturates was, in absolute values, very low, mostly as a consequence of the generally lower fat intake apart from the olive oil (Cresta et al. 1969). So, while the Mediterranean diet does not seem to contain enough polyunsaturates to reduce HDL cholesterol levels, it must not be considered an extremely fat-poor diet. A series of observations of subjects consuming very-low-fat diets in short-term controlled studies showed a reduction of HDL cholesterol (Levy et al. 1966; Schonfeld et al. 1976; Blum et al. 1977; Shepherd et al. 1978; Gonen et al. 1981; Lithell et al. 1982). In these studies, however, the subjects consumed diets containing less than 2% of energy as fat, and the drastic reduction of the total amount of fat in the diet may also influence the HDL concentration by decreasing synthesis of lipoprotein that contains apoprotein A in the intestinal wall (Blum et al. 1977; Shepherd et al. 1978).

That, however, does not appear to be the case with the Mediterranean diet including an adequate intake of fat. Note also that the conclusions of the studies cited above were drawn after short-term feeding of a very-high-carbohydrate diet and that now there is evidence of increased HDL cholesterol levels after a long-term, low-fat diet in patients with coronary heart disease (Thuesen et al. 1986) and in subjects affected by type IV hyperlipoproteinemia (Cominacini et al. 1988b). Furthermore, in the Mediterranean diet, the fatty acids in the olive oil are a major source of fat and several studies demonstrate that the monounsaturates have no effect (Grundy 1986; Mensink and Katan 1987) or increasing effects (Ascaso et al. 1987; Grundy and Bonanome 1987) on HDL cholesterol levels.

These results were developed from data of the Seven Countries Study (Kannel et al. 1979) by evaluation of the effect of the Cretan diet on the incidence of coronary heart disease. The diet of the island population combined a low intake of saturated fatty acids with a high intake of total fat because of their liberal use of monounsaturated fatty acids in the form of olive oil. The incidence of coronary heart disease was lower than would be expected from their total fat consumption and plasma cholesterol levels, and this could not be explained by other concomitant risk factors.

Successively, on the basis of this evidence, Schlierf et al. (1979) found no effect of apoprotein A-I and A-II values of a diet rich in oleic acid in contrast to the same diet, except rich in corn oil, which greatly reduced the value of the apoproteins. Furthermore, Mattson and Grundy (1985) demonstrated that large amounts of olive oil had no effect on HDL cholesterol levels, whereas similar amounts of polyunsaturates significantly lowered the values of the lipoprotein. In another study, Grundy (1986) demonstrated that a formula diet rich in monounsaturates reduced total and LDL cholesterol to the same extent as a low-fat, high-carbohydrate diet and that plasma HDL cholesterol levels did not change significantly except during the high-monounsaturated fatty-acids period, while HDL was consistently reduced after the low-fat diet. These results were criticized because formula diets were employed; however, similar data were subsequently obtained by Mensink and Katan using natural diets (1987). It was also demonstrated that supplements of olive oil to a regular diet positively affected the lipid pattern. Jacotot et al. (1988) showed that a supplement of 40 g/day of olive oil produced not only an increase in LDL catabolism but also an increase in HDL cholesterol levels.

Similarly, long-term studies with natural diets containing olive oil or different seed oils were performed both with healthy subjects (Ascaso et al. 1987; Grundy and Bonanome 1987) and in familial hypertriglyceridemic patients (Cominacini et al. 1990). Significantly higher levels of HDL cholesterol were seen when the subjects enrolled in the study consumed olive oil. The Mediterranean diet, low in saturated and polyunsaturated fat and relatively rich in monounsaturates seems, therefore, to produce the best lipoprotein profile. In fact, the authors who studied the atherogenic index (total cholesterol/HDL cholesterol) found it significantly lower only when olive oil was used (Camena 1989).

EFFECTS OF DIETARY PROTEINS
ON PLASMA LIPIDS

Studies in experimental animals and in man have shown that the concentration of serum lipids, and in particular of cholesterol, can be affected by the kind and proportion of dietary protein (Kim et al. 1978; Kritchevsky 1979; Terpstra et al. 1983; Sirtori et al. 1977; Carrol et al. 1978; Holmes et al. 1980; Van Raaij et al. 1981; Verrillo et al. 1985; Bosello et al. 1988). It is now clear, for example, that feeding casein to rabbits in cholesterol-free, semipurified diets causes a hypercholesterolemia that increases with increasing amounts of casein (Huff et al. 1977; Terpstra et al. 1981). Similar diets containing soy protein have generally produced lower levels of serum cholesterol (Terpstra et al. 1983; Terpstra et al. 1984). The reduction in total serum and LDL cholesterol obtained in humans by substituting soy protein for animal protein seems to involve the same mechanisms as observed in rabbits. Although substitution of soy protein has not been demonstrated to increase fecal steroid in humans (Fumagalli et al. 1982) as it did in rabbits (Huff and Carrol 1980), there is evidence that dietary casein can down regulate LDL receptors (Lovati et al. 1987). So, the substitution of soybean protein for casein is likely to decrease plasma cholesterol, and in particular LDL cholesterol, by increasing the fractional catabolic rate of LDL, possibly by enhancing the number of LDL receptors.

Data on HDL cholesterol concentrations resulting from proteins from different sources can be extrapolated from the findings of Bosello et al. (1988), who studied the long-term effects of hypocaloric diets containing mainly casein or soy protein on the lipoproteins of obese subjects. While they confirmed that the soy protein diet had a greater effect than the casein diet in reducing LDL cholesterol levels, the results of this study seem to demonstrate that the well-known hypocaloric, diet-induced decrease in HDL cholesterol levels (Thompson et al. 1979; Brownell and Stunkard 1981; Tokunaga et al. 1982; Bosello et al. 1985) was more consistent in the group of obese subjects consuming casein. The reduction in HDL cholesterol occurred in both the HDL subfractions. However, the HDL^2 cholesterol fell more consistently in the group consuming casein, thus inducing a decrease in the HDL^2 to the HDL^3 cholesterol ratio. The fact that the apo A-I concentrations behaved the same as the HDL^2 cholesterol levels in the two groups supports the idea that the consumption of proteins from different sources may affect the HDL subfractions in a different manner. A factor that may have contributed to the lowering of plasma HDL cholesterol in both groups is the reduced intestinal synthesis of apo A-I and apo A-II, since oral nutrients and, in particular, fat are essential for their production (Blum et al. 1977; Shepherd et al.

1978). Furthermore, since HDL^2 is produced during catabolism of plasma-triglyceride-rich lipoproteins by lipoprotein lipase, especially at adipose tissue level (Nikkila et al. 1978; Patsch and Gotto 1980), and caloric restriction is said to decrease its activity (Taskinen and Nikkila 1981; Bosello et al. 1984a), it is likely that the more pronounced decrease in HDL^2 cholesterol found in the group consuming casein may indicate a prevalent decrease in triglyceride-rich lipoprotein catabolism. The demonstration that the turnover of VLDL apo B is augmented by the substitution of soybean protein for meat and daily protein (Huff et al. 1984; Cohn et al. 1984) agrees with that suggestion.

Finally, the study of Bosello et al. (1988) demonstrates that, in the group consuming mainly casein, there was a trend toward a decreased HDL to LDL cholesterol ratio while the ratio was unchanged with the soybean protein. Since current epidemiological data suggest that LDL cholesterol is a positive risk factor (Castelli et al. 1977), while HDL cholesterol, particularly HDL^2 is known to protect against cardiovascular disease (Miller and Miller 1975; Albers et al. 1978), the substitution of soy protein for casein can be beneficial in improving the lipoprotein pattern.

As demonstrated by the EURATOM study, the animal protein intake is about 90% lower in southern Italy than that in northern European countries (Cresta et al. 1969). Thus, the intake of vegetable protein provided by the typical Mediterranean diet could be a further contributing factor in reducing the risk of developing atherosclerosis.

EFFECTS OF DIETARY FIBERS ON PLASMA LIPIDS

The Fiber Hypothesis

It is now more than 35 years since Walker and Arvidsson (1954) first hypothesized that the low blood cholesterol levels of South African Bantu prisoners might be due, at least in part, to their high intakes of dietary fiber.

This premise was further developed by several other authors (Malhotra 1967; Trowell 1972; Burkitt 1973), and several studies demonstrate that dietary fiber can help considerably in improving the lipoprotein pattern. Basically, dietary fiber can be divided into two categories; water-soluble and water-insoluble fibers. Water-insoluble fibers, such as cellulose, lignin, and certain hemicelluloses, have great effect on fecal bulk and on gastrointestinal transit time but relatively little impact on intermediate metabolism (Munoz 1984; Crapo 1985). Thus cereal fiber, which is high in water-insoluble fibers, increases fecal bulk a great deal, approximately 3–9 g/g dietary fiber eaten, whereas it provides only meager amounts of energy for the growth of the colonic bacteria and is only slightly degraded by them (Kay 1982; Trowell and Burkitt 1986).

In contrast, water-soluble fibers, such as the pectins, hemicelluloses, and storage polysaccharides, have relatively little effect on fecal bulk, transit time, and mineral absorption but have great effects on intermediary metabolism (Kay 1982; Trowell and Burkitt 1986). Among the water-soluble fibers, the viscous polysaccharides such as pectin (Fisher et al. 1965; Palmer and Dickson 1968; Jenkins et al. 1975b; Jenkins et al. 1976; Durrington et al. 1976; Delbarre et al. 1977; Langley and Thye 1977; Miettinen and Tarpila 1977; Stasse-Wolthuis et al. 1980; Judd and Truswell 1982) and guar gum (Fahrenbach et al. 1965; Jenkins et al. 1976; Jenkins et al. 1979a; Miettinen 1983; Bosello et al. 1984b) seem to be the most potent hypocholesterolemic agents.

Dietary fibers exert their hypocholesterolemic effects mostly by decreasing LDL cholesterol (Kirby et al. 1981; Judd and Truswell 1982; Schwandt et al. 1982; Behall et al. 1984), while HDL cholesterol generally remains unchanged (Judd and Truswell 1985), indicating an increase in the DHL to LDL cholesterol ratio, a desirable effect, as higher HDL levels are associated with reduced risk of atherosclerotic heart disease (Castelli et al. 1977).

Plasma triglyceride levels have been unchanged in most reports of the hypolipidemic effects of dietary fiber (Judd and Truswell 1985), although there have been some reports of reductions in plasma triglyceride levels, usually in hyperlipidemic or diabetic patients (Rivellese et al. 1980; Jenkins et al. 1983b; Bosello et al. 1984b).

Mechanisms of the Lipid-Lowering Effects of Dietary Fiber

Several mechanisms have been suggested to explain the lipid-lowering effects of dietary fiber. Reduction in fat absorption, as demonstrated by augmented fecal fat excretion, has been reported mostly by using gel-forming fibers such as guar and pectin (Levine and Silvis 1980; Vahouney 1982; Sandberg et al. 1983; Judd and Truswell 1985). Furthermore, certain fibers can sequestrate bile acids like cholestyramine, inducing a decrease in LDL cholesterol levels via its accelerated excretion (Forman et al. 1968; Stanley et al. 1972; Jenkins 1977; Miettinen 1983). There is also evidence that dietary fiber and gel-forming products in particular can reduce postprandial hypertriglyceridemia, suggesting that these kinds of fiber may attenuate the postprandial rise in chilomicrons (Irie et al. 1982). Furthermore, if viscous polysaccharides alter the site of absorption in humans, and hence the composition of chilomicron particles, the subsequent utilization of the particles may be altered (Judd and Truswell 1985).

Finally, high-fiber diets and viscous polysaccharides in particular have been shown to reduce postprandial glucose and insulin response (Jenkins et al. 1976; Jenkins 1977; Peterson 1984). The reduction in insulin response has also been attributed to changes in gut hormones (Judd and Truswell 1985). Gastric inhibitory polypeptide and gut glucagonlike immunoreactivity are known to stimulate insulin secretion (Marks and Turner 1977), and they have appeared altered when high-fiber diets are fed (Morgan et al. 1979; Jenkins et al. 1980). As insulin can affect cholesterol (Bhathena et al. 1974) and triglyceride synthesis at liver level (Olefsky et al. 1974; Tobey et al. 1981), products that markedly alter insulin response appear to have the greatest effect on lipid pattern.

Dietary fiber seems to act almost synergistically with other characteristics of the Mediterranean diet in preventing and retarding the progression of atherosclerotic disease.

REFERENCES

Ahrens, E. H., J. Hirsh, K. Oette, J. W. Farquhar, and Y. Stein. 1967. Carbohydrate-induced and fat-induced lipemia. *Trans. Assoc. Am. Phys.* **74**:134–144.

Albers, J. J., M. C. Cheung, and W. R. Hazzard. 1978. High density lipoprotein in myocardial infarction survivors. *Metabolism* **27**:479–487.

Albrink, M. J., T. Newman, and P. C. Davidson. 1979. Effect of high- and low-fiber diets on plasma lipids and insulin. *Am. J. Clin. Nutr.* **32**:1486–1491.

Anderson, J. W., and W. L. Chen. 1979. Plant fiber. Carbohydrate and lipid metabolism. *Am. J. Clin. Nutr.* **32**:346–363.

Anderson, J. W., W. J. L. Chen, and B. Sieling. 1980. Hypolipidemic effects of high-carbohydrate, high-fiber diets. *Metabolism* **29**:551–558.

Ascaso, J. F., S. Serrano, and J. Martinez. 1987. Effecto del aceite de oliva de la dieta sobre las HDL. *Rev. Clin. Eso.* **180**:486–488.

Behall, K. M., K. H. Lee, and P. B. Mose. 1984. Blood lipids and lipoproteins in adult men fed four refined fibres. *Am. J. Clin. Nutr.* **39**:209–214.

Bhathena, S. J., J. Avigan, and M. E. Schreiner. 1974. Effect of insulin on sterol and fatty acids synthesis and hydroxymethylglutaryl coA reductase activity in mammalian cells grown in culture. *Proc. Natl. Acad. Sci.* **71**:2174–2178.

Blum, C. B., R. I. Levy, S. Eisemberg, M. Hall, R. H. Goebel, and M. Berman. 1977. High density lipoprotein metabolism in man. *J. Clin. Invest.* **60**:795–807.

Bosello, O., M. Cigolini, A. Battaglia, F. Ferrari, R. Micciolo, R. Olivetti, and M. Corsato. 1984a. Adipose tissue lipoprotein lipase in obesity. *Int. J. Obesity* **8**:213–220.

Bosello, O., L. Cominacini, I. Zocca, U. Garbin, F. Ferrari, and A. Davoli. 1984b. Effects of guar gum on plasma lipoproteins and apolipoproteins C-II and

C-III in patients affected by familial combined hyperlipoproteinemia. *Am. J. Clin. Nutr.* **40:**1165–1174.

Bosello, O., L. Cominacini, I. Zocca, U. Garbin, A. Davoli, and F. Ferrari. 1985. High density lipoprotein subfractions during semistarvation in obese women. *Ann. Nutr. Metab.* **29:**381–386.

Bosello, O., L. Cominacini, I. Zocca, U. Garbin, R. Compri, A. Davoli, and L. Brunetti. 1988. Short- and long-term effects of hypocaloric diet containing proteins of different sources on plasma lipids and apoproteins of obese subjects. *Ann. Nutr. Metab.* **32:**206–214.

Brownell, K. D., and A. J. Stunkard. 1981. Differential changes in plasma high-density lipoprotein-cholesterol levels in obese men and women during weight reduction. *Arch. Intern. Med.* **141:**1141–1146.

Burkitt, D. P. 1973. Some disease characteristics of modern Western civilisation. *Br. Med. J.* **1:**424–430.

Carmena, R. 1989. Monounsaturated fatty acids: a critical appraisal. In *Atherosclerosis VIII*, G. Crepaldi, A. M. Gotto, E. Manazato, and G. Baggio, eds., pp. 679–682. Amsterdam: Elsevier.

Carroll, K. K., P. M. Giovannetti, M. W. Huff, O. Moase, D. C. K. Roberts, and B. M. Wolfe. 1978. Hypocholesterolemic effect of substituting soybean protein for animal protein in the diet of healthy young women. *Am. J. Clin. Nutr.* **31:**1312–1321.

Castelli, W. P., J. T. Doyle, T. Gordon, C. G. Hames, M. C. Hjortland, S. B. Hulley, A. Kagan, W. J. Zukel. 1977. HDL-cholesterol and other lipids in coronary heart disease. The cooperative lipoprotein phenotyping study. *Circulation* **55:**767–772.

Cohen, A. M., N. A. Kaufmann, and R. Poznansky. 1966. Effect of starch and sucrose on carbohydrate-induced hyperlipaemia. *Br. Med. J.* **1:**339–340.

Cohn, J. S., W. G. Kimpton, and P. J. Nestel. 1984. The effect of dietary casein and soy protein on cholesterol and very low density lipoprotein metabolism in the rat. *Atherosclerosis* **52:**219–231.

Cominacini, L., I. Zocca, U. Garbin, A. Davoli, R. Micciolo, P. De Bastiani, and O. Bosello. 1988*a*. High density lipoprotein composition in obesity: interrelationships with plasma insulin levels and body weight. *Int. J. Obesity* **12:**343–352.

Cominacini, L., I. Zocca, U. Garbin, A. Davoli, R. Compri, L. Brunetti, and O. Bosello. 1988*b*. Long-term effect of a low-fat, high-carbohydrate diet on plasma lipids of patients affected by familial endogenous hypertriglyceridemia. *Am. J. Clin. Nutr.* **48:**57–65.

Cominacini, L., I. Zocca, U. Garbin, A. Davoli, L. Brunetti, M. Zamboni, C. Smacchia, R. Compri, and O. Bosello. 1988*c*. Effect of a low-fat, high-complex-carbohydrate diet on insulin response and plasma lipids in patients affected by endogenous hypertriglyceridemia. *Clin. Nutr.* **10:**54–59.

Cominacini, L., O. Bosello, U. Garbin, A. Davoli, L. Brunetti, and L. A. Scuro. 1990. Comparison of a low-fat, high-carbohydrate diet at two levels of polyunsaturates on plasma lipids of patients with familial endogenous hypertriglyceridemia. *J. Nutr. Med.* **1:**95–105.

Consensus Development Conference. 1985. Lowering blood cholesterol to prevent heart disease. *JAMA* **253:**2080–2086.

Cooper, A. D., and M. A. Shrewsbury. 1979. Effects of chilomicron remnants on hepatic lipoprotein metabolism. *Clin. Res.* **27:**363 (abstract).

Coulston, A. M., G. C. Liu, and G. M. Reaven. 1983. Plasma glucose, insulin and lipid response to high-carbohydrate, low-fat diets in normal humans. *Metabolism* **32**:52–56.

Crapo, P. A. 1985. Simple versus complex carbohydrate use in the diabetic diet. *Ann. Rev. Nutr.* **5**:95–114.

Crapo, P. A., G. Reaven, and J. Olefsky. 1976. Plasma glucose and insulin responses to orally administered simple and complex carbohydrates. *Diabetes* **25**:741–747.

Crapo, P. A., G. Reaven, and J. Olefsky. 1977. Postprandial plasma-glucose and insulin responses to different complex carbohydrates. *Diabetes* **26**:1178–1183.

Cresta, M., S. Lederman, A. Garnier, E. Lombardo, and G. Lacourly. 1969. *Etude des consommations alimentaires des populations de onze régions de la communauté européenne en vue de la détermination des niveaux de la contamination radioactive.* Rapport établi au centre d'Etude Nucléaire de Fontenay-aux-Roses, France: EURATOM, Commissariat à l'énergie atomique (C.E.A.)

Delbarre, F. J., J. Fondier, and A. De Gery. 1977. Lack of effect of two pectins on idiopathic or gout-associated hyperdyslipidemic hypercholesterolemia. *Am. J. Clin. Nutr.* **30**:463–464.

Durrington, P. N., J. P. Manning, C. H. Bolton, and M. Hartog. 1976. Effect of pectin on serum lipids and lipoproteins, whole gut transit time and stool weight. *Lancet* **2**:393–396.

Ernest, I., B. Hallgren, and A. Svanborg. 1962. Short term study of effect of different isocaloric diets in diabetes. *Metabolism* **11**:912–919.

Ernest, I., E. Linner, and A. Svanborg. 1965. Carbohydrate-rich, fat-poor diet in diabetes. *Am. J. Med.* **39**:594–602.

Fahrenbach, M. H., B. A. Riccardi, J. C. Saunders, N. Lourie, and J. C. Heider. 1965. Comparative effects of guar gum and pectin on human serum cholesterol levels. *Circulation* **31** (Suppl. II): 11–14.

Fisher, H., P. Griminger, E. R. Sostman, and M. K. Brush. 1965. Dietary pectin and plasma cholesterol. *J. Nutr.* **86**:113–118.

Forman, D. T., J. E. Garvin, J. E. Forestner, and C. B. Taylor. 1968. Increased excretion of faecal bile acids by an oral hydrophilic colloid. *Proc. Soc. Exp. Med.* **127**:1060–1063.

Fumagalli, R., R. Soleri, R. Farina, R. Musanti, O. Mantero, G. Noseda, E. Gatti, and C. R. Sirtori. 1982. Fecal cholesterol excretion studies in type II hypercholesterolemic patients treated with the soybean protein diet. *Atherosclerosis* **43**:341–350.

Galeotti, G. 1936. Primi risultati dell' inchiesta alimentare condotta in varie provincie d'Italia. *Quaderni della Nutrizione* **3**(1).

Gammal, E. B., K. K. Carroll, and E. R. Plunkett. 1967. Effects of dietary fat on mammary carcinogenesis by 7, 12-dimethylbenz(alpha)anthracene in rats. *Cancer Res.* **27**:1737–1742.

Ginsberg, H., J. M. Olefsky, G. Kimmerling, P. Crapo, and G. M. Reaven. 1976. Induction of hypertriglyceridemia by a low-fat diet. *J. Clin. Endocr. Metab.* **42**:729–735.

Gonen, B., W. Patsch, I. Kuisk, and G. Schonfeld. 1981. The effect of short-term feeding of high carbohydrate diet on HDL subclasses in normal subjects. *Metabolism* **30**:1125–1129.

Gordon, T., W. Kannel, W. P. Castelli, and T. R. Dawber. 1981. Lipoproteins, cardiovascular disease and death. The Framingham Study. *Arch. Intern. Med.* **141**:1128–1131.

Green, M. H., E. R. Massaro, and J. B. Green. 1984. Multicompartmental analy-

sis of the effects of dietary fat saturation and cholesterol on absorptive lipoprotein metabolism in the rat. *Am. J. Clin. Nutr.* **40**:82–94.

Grundy, S. M. 1986. Comparison of monounsaturated fatty acids and carbohydrates for lowering plasma cholesterol. *N. Engl. J. Med.* **314**:745–748.

Grundy, S. M. 1989. What is the desirable fat intake? In *Atherosclerosis VIII*,
G. Crepaldi, A. M. Gotto, E. Manzato, and G. Baggio, eds., pp. 665–672.
Amsterdam: Elsevier.

Grundy, S. M., and A. Bonanome. 1987. Summary of the Second Colloquium
on Monounsaturates, Bethesda, 1987. *Arteriosclerosis* **7**:644–648.

Hayford, J. T., M. M. Danney, D. Wiebe, S. Roberts, and R. G. Thompson.
1979. Triglyceride integrated concentrations: effect of variation of source and
amount of dietary carbohydrate. *Am. J. Clin. Nutr.* **32**:1670–1678.

Hegsted, D. M., R. B. Mc Gandy, M. L. Myers, and F. J. Stare. 1965. Quantitative effects of dietery fat on serum cholesterol in man. *Am. J. Clin. Nutr.*
17:281–295.

Hjerman, I. 1981. Effect of diet and smoking intervention on the incidence of
coronary heart disease. Report from the Oslo Study Group of a randomized
trial in healthy men. *Lancet* **2**(8259):1303–1310.

Hollenbeck, C. B., M. C. Riddle, W. E. Connor, and J. E. Leklem. 1985. The
effects of subject-selected high carbohydrate, low fat diets on glycemic control in insulin dependent diabetes mellitus. *Am. J. Clin. Nutr.* **41**:293–298.

Holmes, H. L., G. B. Rubel, and S. S. Hood. 1980. Comparison of the effect of
dietary meat versus dietary soybean protein on plasma lipids of hyperlipidemic individuals. *Atherosclerosis* **36**:379–387.

Huff, M. W., and K. K. Carrol. 1980. Effects of dietary protein turnover, oxidation and absorption of cholesterol on steroid excretion in rabbits. *J. Lipid Res.*
21:546–558.

Huff, M. W., R. M. G. Hamilton, and K. K. Carrol. 1977. Plasma cholesterol
levels in rabbits fed low-fat, cholesterol-free, semipurified diets: effects of
dietary protein hydrolysate and amino acid mixtures. *Atherosclerosis* **28**:187–
195.

Huff, M. W., P. M. Giovannetti, and B. M. Wolfe. 1984. Turnover of very low-
density lipoprotein-apoprotein B is increased by substitution of soybean protein for meat and dairy protein in the diets of hypercholesterolemic men. *Am.
J. Clin. Nutr.* **39**:888–897.

Irie, N., T. Hara, and Y. Goto. 1982. The effects of guar gum on post-prandial
chylomicronemia. *Nutr. Rep. Int.* **26**:207–214.

Jacotot, B., M. F. Baudet, and M. Lasserre. 1988. Olive oil and the lipoprotein
metabolism. *Rev. Fran. Corps Gras.* **35**:51–56.

Jenkins, D. J. A. 1977. Action of dietary fibre in lowering fasting serum cholesterol and reducing post-prandial glycemia. In *International Conference on Atherosclerosis*, L. A. Carlson, R. Paoletti, and G. Weber, eds., pp. 173–178. New
York: Raven Press.

Jenkins, D. J. A., 1982. Lente carbohydrate: a new approach to the dietary management of diabetes. *Diabetes Care* **5**:634–641.

Jenkins, D. J. A., M. S. Hill, and J. K. Cummings. 1975a. Effect of wheat fiber
on blood lipids, fecal steroid excretion and serum iron. *Am. J. Clin. Nutr.*
28:1408–1411.

Jenkins, D. J. A., A. R. Leeds, C. Newton, and J. H. Cumming. 1975b. Effect of
pectin, guar gum and wheat fibre on serum cholesterol. *Lancet* **1**:1116–1117.

Jenkins, D. J. A., A. R. Leeds, M. A. Gassul, H. Houston, D. V. Goff, and M. J. Hill. 1976. The cholesterol lowering effect of guar and pectin. *Clin. Sci. Mol. Med.* **51**:8–12.

Jenkins, D. J. A., A. R. Leeds, B. Slavin, J. Man, and E. M. Jepson.1979*a*. Dietary fibre and blood lipids: reduction of serum cholesterol in Type II hyperlipidemia by guar gum. *Am. J. Clin. Nutr.* **32**:16–18.

Jenkins, D. J. A., D. Reynolds, A. R. Leeds, A. L. Waller, and J. H. Cummings. 1979*b*. Hypocholesterolemic action of dietary fibre unrelated to fecal bulking effect. *Am. J. Clin. Nutr.* **32**:2430–2435.

Jenkins, D. J. A., S. R. Bloom, R. H. Albuquerque, A. R. Leeds, D. L. Sarson, G. L. Metz, and K. G. M. M. Alberti. 1980. Pectin and complications of gastric surgery: normalisation of post-prandial glucose and endocrine responses. *Gut* **21**:574–579.

Jenkins, D. J. A., T. M. S. Wolever, and R. H. Taylor. 1981. Glycemic index of foods: a physiological basis for carbohydrate exchange. *Am. J. Clin. Nutr.* **34**:362–366.

Jenkins, D. J. A., T. M. S. Wolever, A. L. Jenkins, R. Lee, G. S. Wong, and R. Josse. 1983*a*. Glycemic response to wheat products: reduced response to pasta but no effect of fiber. *Diabetes Care* **1**:155–159.

Jenkins, D. J. A., G. S. Wong, R. Pattern, J. Bird, M. Hall, G. C. Buckley, V. McGuire, R. Reichart, and J. A. Little. 1983*b*. Leguminous seeds in the dietary management of hyperlipidemia. *Am. J. Clin. Nutr.* **38**:567–573.

Jenkins, D. J. A., T. M. S. Wolever, A. L. Jenkins, R. G. Josse, and G. S. Wong. 1984. The glycemic response to carbohydrate foods. *Lancet* **2**:388–391.

Jenkins, D. J. A., T. M. S. Wolever, and J. Kalmusky. 1985. Low glycemic index foods in the management of hyperlipidemia. *Am. J. Clin. Nutr.* **42**:604–617.

Judd, P. A., and A. S. Truswell. 1982. Comparison of the effects of high- and low-methoxyl pectins on blood and fecal lipids in man. *Br. J. Nutr.* **48**:451–458.

Judd, P. A. and A. S. Truswell. 1985. Dietary fibre and blood lipids in man. In *Dietary Fibre Perspectives*. A. R. Leeds, ed., pp. 23–39. London: John Libbey.

Kannel, W. B., W. P. Castelli, and T. Gordon. 1979. Cholesterol in the prediction of atherosclerotic disease. New perspectives based on the Framingham Study. *Ann. Intern. Med.* **90**:85–91.

Kashyap, M. L., R. L. Barnhart, and S. Srivastava. 1982. Effects of dietary carbohydrate and fat on plasma lipoproteins and apolipoproteins C-II and C-III in healthy men. *J. Lip. Res.* **23**:877–886.

Kato, H., J. Tillotson, M. Nichman, G. Rhoades, and H. Hamilton. 1973. Epidemiologic studies of coronary heart disease and stroke in Japanese men living in Japan, Hawaii and California: Serum lipids and diet. *Amer. J. Epidemiol.* **97**:372–380.

Kaufmann, N. A., S. R. Poznansky, S. H. Blondheim, and Y. Stein. 1966. Changes in serum lipid levels of hyperlipemic patients following the feeding of starch, sucrose and glucose. *Am. J. Clin. Nutr.* **18**:261–269.

Kay, R. M. 1982. Dietary fiber. *J. Lipid Res.* **23**:221–242.

Keys, A., J. T. Anderson, and F. Grande. 1957. Prediction of serum-cholesterol responses of man to changes in fats in the diet. *Lancet* **2**:959–969.

Keys, A., J. T. Anderson, and F. Grande. 1969. Serum-cholesterol response to changes in the diet. II. The effect of cholesterol in the diet. *Metabolism* **14**:759–765.

Keys, A. 1970. Coronary heart disease in seven countries. *Circulation* **41** (supplement):1–10.

Keys, A. 1975. Coronary heart disease. The global picture. *Atherosclerosis* **22**:149–156.

Keys, A. 1980. *Seven Countries. A multivariate analysis of death and coronary heart disease*. Cambridge, Mass.: Harvard University Press.

Kiehm, T. G., J. W. Anderson, and K. Ward. 1976. Beneficial effects of a high carbohydrate, high fiber diet on hyperglycemic diabetic men. *Am. J. Clin. Nutr.* **29**:895–899.

Kim, D. N., K. T. Lee, and W. A. Thomas. 1978. Effect of soy protein on serum cholesterol in swine fed fat and cholesterol. *Exp. Mol. Pathol.* **29**:385–389.

King, M. E. and A. A. Spector. 1978. Effect of specific fatty acyl enrichments on membrane physical properties detected with a spin label probe. *J. Biol. Chem.* **253**:6493–6501.

Kirby, R. W., J. W. Anderson, B. Sieling, E. D. Rees, W. J. L. Chen, R. E. Miller, and R. M. Kay. 1981. Oat bran selectivity lowers serum low-density lipoprotein concentration: studies of hypercholesterolemic men. *Am. J. Clin. Nutr.* **34**:824–829.

Kritchevsky, D. 1979. Vegetable protein and atherosclerosis. *J. Amer. Oil Chem. Soc.* **56**:135–139.

Kuo, P. T., and D. R. Basset. 1965. Dietary sugar in the production of hypertriglyceridemia. *Ann. Intern. Med.* **62**:1199–1212.

Langley, N. J., and F. W. Thye. 1977. The effect of wheat bran and/or citrus pectin on serum cholesterol and triglycerides in middle aged men. *Fed. Proc.* **36**:1118 (abstract).

Levine, A. S., and S. E. Silvis. 1980. Absorption of whole peanuts, peanut oil and peanut butter. *N. Engl. J. Med.* **303**:1729–1733.

Levy, R. I. 1983. Intervention on single risk factors. hyperlipoproteinemia. In *Atherosclerosis VI*, G. Schettler, A. M. Gotto, G. Middelhoff, A. J. R. Habenicht, and K. R. Jurutka, eds., pp. 759–766. Berlin:Springer-Verlag.

Levy, R. J., R. S. Lees, and D. S. Frederickson. 1966. The nature of pre-beta (very low-density) lipoproteins. *J. Clin. Invest.* **45**:63–77.

Lipid Research Clinics Program. 1984. The Lipid Research Clinics Coronary Prevention Trial results: II. The relationship of reduction in incidence of coronary heart disease to cholesterol lowering. *JAMA* **251**:365–374.

Lithell, H., I. Jacobs, B. Vessby, K. Hellsing, and J. Karlsson. 1982. Decrease of lipoprotein lipase activity in skeletal muscle during a short-term carbohydrate-rich dietary regime. With special reference to HDL-cholesterol, apolipoprotein and insulin concentration. *Metabolism* **31**:994–998.

Liu, G. C., A. M. Coulston, and G. M. Reaven. 1983. Effect of high carbohydrate-low fat diets on plasma glucose, insulin and lipid responses in hypertriglyceridemic humans. *Metabolism* **32**:750–753.

Lovati, M. R., C. Manzoni, A. Canavesi, M. Sirtori, V. Vaccarino, M. Marchi, G. Gaddi, and C. R. Sirtori. 1987. Soybean protein diet increases low density lipoprotein receptor activity in mononuclear cells from hypercholesterolemic patients. *J. Clin. Invest.* **80**:1498–1502.

MacDonald, I., and D. M. Braithwaite. 1964. The influence of dietary carbohydrate on the lipid pattern in serum and in adipose tissue. *Clin. Sci.* **27**:23–30.

Malhotra, S. L. 1967. Serum lipids, dietary factors and ischemic heart disease. *Am. J. Clin. Nutr.* **20**:462–474.

Marks, V., and D. S. Turner. 1977. The gastrointestinal hormones with particular reference to their role in the regulation of insulin secretion. *Essay Biochem.* **3**:109–152.

Mattson, F. H., and S. M. Grundy. 1985. Comparison of effects of dietary saturated, monounsaturated and polyunsaturated fatty acids on plasma lipids and lipoproteins in man. *J. Lipid Res.* **26**:194–202.

McGandy, R. B., D. M. Hegsted, M. L. Myers, and F. J. Stare. 1966. Dietary carbohydrate and serum cholesterol levels in man. *Am. J. Clin. Nutr.* **18**: 237–242.

Mensink, R. P., and M. B. Katan. 1987. Effect of monounsaturated fatty acids versus complex carbohydrates on high-density lipoproteins in healthy men and women. *Lancet* **1**:122–125.

Miettinen, R. A., and S. Tarpila. 1977. Effect of pectin on serum cholesterol, fecal bile acids and biliary lipids in normolipidemic and hyperlipidemic individuals. *Clin. Chim. Acta* **79**:471–477.

Miettinen, R. A. 1983. Effects of dietary fiber on cholesterol metabolism in man. In *Fibre in Human and Animal Nutrition*, G. Wallace and L. Bell, eds., pp. 173–177. *Roy. Soc. N.Z. Bull.* 20.

Miller, G. J., and N. E. Miller. 1975. Plasma high density lipoprotein concentration and development of ischaemic heart disease. *Lancet* **1**:16–19.

Morgan, L. M., I. J. Goulder, D. Tsiolakis, V. Marks, and K. G. M. M. Alberti. 1979. The effect of unabsorbable carbohydrates on gut hormones. *Diabetologia* **17**:85–89.

Muñoz, J. 1984. Fiber and diabetes. *Diabetes Care* **7**:297–298.

Nestel, P. J., K. F. Carrol, and N. Havenstein. 1970. Plasma triglyceride response to carbohydrates, fats and caloric intake. *Metabolism* **19**:1–18.

Nestel, P. J., M. Rearden, and N. H. Fidge. 1979. Sucrose-induced changes in VLDL- and LDL-B apoprotein removal rates. *Metabolism* **28**:531–535.

Niceforo, A., and G. Galeotti. 1943. Primi risultati dell' inchiesta alimentare condotta in varie provincie d'Italia. *Quaderni della Nutrizione* **1**(1).

Nikkila, E. A., and M. Kekki. 1972. Effects of dietary fructose and sucrose in plasma triglyceride metabolism in patients with endogenous hyper-triglyceridemia. *Acta Med. Scand.* **542** (suppl):221–229.

Nikkila, E. A., M. R. Taskinen, and M. Kekki. 1978. Relation of plasma high density lipoprotein cholesterol to lipoprotein-lipase activity in adipose tissue and skeletal muscle of man. *Atherosclerosis* **29**:497–501.

Olefsky, J. M., J. W. Farquhar, and G. M. Reaven. 1974. Reappraisal of the role of insulin in hypertriglyceridemia. *Am. J. Med.* **57**:551–560.

Palmer, G. H., and D. G. Dixon. 1968. Effect of pectin dose on serum cholesterol levels. *Am. J. Clin. Nutr.* **18**:437–442.

Patsch, J. R., and A. M. Gotto, Jr. 1980. Role of high density lipoprotein (HDL) in the catabolism of triglyceride-rich lipoproteins. In *Lipoprotein and Coronary Heart Disease*. M. Greten, P. D. Land, and G. Schettler, eds., pp. 16–24. Baden-Baden, Cologne: G. Witzstock.

Peterson, D. B., P. R. Ellis, J. M. Baylis, P. G. Frost, A. R. Leeds, and A. M. Jepson. 1984. Effects of guar on diabetes and lipids. Food and pharmacology compared. *Diabetologia* **27**:319A.

Quarfordt, S. H., A. Frank, D. M. Shames, M. Berman, and D. Steinberg. 1970. Very low density lipoprotein triglyceride transport in type IV hyperlipoproteinemia and the effects of carbohydrate-rich diets. *J. Clin. Invest.* **49**:2281–2297.

Reaven, G. M. 1979. Effects of differences in amount and kind of dietary carbohydrate on plasma glucose and insulin responses in man. *Am. J. Clin. Nutr.* **32**:2568–2578.

Reaven, G. M., and J. M. Olefsky. 1974. Increased plasma glucose and insulin response to high carbohydrate feeding in normal subjects. *J. Clin. Endocr. Metab.* **38**:151–154.

Reiser, S., J. Hallfrisch, O. E. Michaelis, F. L. Lazar, R. E. Martin, and E. S. Prather. 1979. Isocaloric exchange of dietary starch and sucrose in humans. Effects on levels of fasting blood lipids. *Am. J. Clin. Nutr.* **32**:1659–1669.

Rivellese, A., G. Riccardi, A. Giaco, D. Pacioni, S. Gebivesem, P. L. Mattioli, and M. Mancini. 1980. Effect of dietary fibre on glucose control and serum lipoproteins in diabetic patients. *Lancet* **2**:447–450.

Roberts, A. M. 1973. Effects of a sucrose-free diet on the serum lipid levels of men of Antarctica. *Lancet* **1**:1201–1204.

Rosenthal, M. B., R. J. Barnard, D. P. Rose, S. Inkeles, J. Hall, and N. Pritikin. 1985. Effects of a high-complex-carbohydrate, low-fat, low-cholesterol diet on levels of serum lipids and estradiol. *Amer. J. Med.* **78**:23–27.

Ruderman, N. B., A. L. Jones, R. M. Krauss, and E. Shafrir. 1971. A biochemical and morphologic study of very low density lipoproteins in carbohydrate-induced hypertriglyceridemia. *J. Clin. Invest.* **50**:1355–1368.

Sandberg, A. T. S., R. Ahderinne, H. Anderson, B. Hallgren, and L. Hutten. 1983. The effect of citrus pectin on the absorption of nutrients in the small intestine. *Hum. Nutr. Clin. Nutr.* **37**:171–184.

Schlierf, G., T. Nikolaus, and A. Stiehel. 1979. The effect of a lipid-lowering diet on biliary and plasma lipids in healthy subjects. *Proc. Third Int. Congr. on Biology Value of Olive Oil, I.O.O.C., Crete*, pp. 212–220.

Schonfeld, G., S. W. Weidman, J. L. Witztum, and R. M. Bowen. 1976. Alterations in levels and interrelations of plasma apolipoproteins induced by diet. *Metabolism* **25**:261–265.

Schwandt, P., W. O. Richter, P. Weiweiler, and G. Neureuther. 1982. Cholestyramine plus pectin in treatment of patients with familial hypercholesterolemia. *Atherosclerosis* **39**:379–383.

Shepherd, B., C. J. Packard, J. P. Patsch, A. M. Gotto, Jr., and O. D. Taunton. 1978. Effects of polyunsaturated fat on the properties of high density lipoproteins and the metabolism of apoprotein A-I. *J. Clin. Invest.* **61**:1582–1592.

Sirtori, C. R., E. Agradi, F. Conti, O. Mantero, and E. Gatti. 1977. Soybean-protein diet in the treatment of type-II hyperlipoproteinemia. *Lancet* **1**:275–277.

Srinivasan, S. R., B. Radhakrishnamurthy, T. A. Foster, and G. S. Berenson. 1983. Divergent responses of serum lipoproteins to changes in dietary carbohydrate and cholesterol in cynomolgus monkeys. *Metabolism* **32**:377–386.

Stamler, J. 1979. Population studies. In *Nutrition, Lipids and Coronary Heart Disease—A Global View.* R. I. Levy, B. M. Rifkind, B. H. Denis, and N. Ernst, eds., pp. 25–31. New York: Raven Press.

Stamler, J., D. Wentworth, and J. Neaton. 1986. Is the relationship between serum cholesterol and risk of death from coronary heart disease continuous and graded? *JAMA* **256**:2823–2828.

Stanley, M. M., D. Paul, D. Gacke, and J. Murphy. 1972. Effect of cholestyramine, metamucil and cellulose on fecal bile acid excretion in man. *Gastroenterology* **65**:889–894.

Stasse-Wolthuis, M., H. F. F. Abers, J. G. C. van Jeveren, J. Wil de Jong, J. G.

A. J. Hautvast, R. J. J. Hermus, M. B. Katan, W. C. Brydon, and M. A. East-wood. 1980. Influence of dietary fiber from vegetables and fruits, bran or citrus pectin on serum lipids, fecal lipids and colonic functions. *Am. J. Clin. Nutr.* **33**:1745–1756.

Stone, D. B., and W. E. Connor. 1963. The prolonged effects of a low cholesterol, high carbohydrate diet upon the serum lipids in diabetic patients. *Diabetes* **12**:127–132.

Sturdevant, R. A., M. L. Pearce, and S. Dayton. 1973. Increased prevalence of cholelithiasis in men ingesting a serum-cholesterol-lowering diet. *N. Engl. J. Med.* **288**:24–27.

Taskinen, M. R., and E. A. Nikkila. 1981. Lipoprotein lipase of adipose tissue and skeletal muscle in human obesity: response to glucose and to semistarvation. *Metabolism* **30**:810–817.

Terpstra, A. H. M., L. Harkes, and F. H. van der Veen. 1981. The effect of different proportions of casein in semipurified diets on the concentration of serum cholesterol and the lipoprotein composition in rabbits. *Lipids* **16**:114–119.

Terpstra, A. H. M., R. J. J. Hermus, and C. E. West. 1983. Dietary protein and cholesterol metabolism in rabbits and rats. In *Animals and Vegetable Proteins in Lipid Metabolism and Atherosclerosis*, pp. 19–49. New York: Alan R. Liss, Inc.

Terpstra, A. H. M., C. E. West, J. T. C. M. Fenis, J. A. Schouten, and E. A. van de Veen. 1984. Hypocholesterolemic effects of dietary soy protein versus casein in rhesus monkey. *Am. J. Clin. Nutr.* **39**:1–7.

Thompson, P. D., R. W. Jeffery, R. R. Wing, and P. D. Wood. 1979. Unexpected decrease in plasma high density lipoprotein cholesterol with weight loss. *Am. J. Clin. Nutr.* **32**:2016–2021.

Thuesen, L., L. B. Henriksen, and B. Engby. 1986. One-year experience with a low-fat, low-cholesterol diet in patients with coronary heart disease. *Am. J. Clin. Nutr.* **44**:212–219.

Tobey, T. A., M. Greenfield, F. Kraemer, and G. M. Reaven. 1981. Relationship between insulin resistance, insulin secretion, very low density lipoprotein kinetics and plasma triglyceride levels in normotriglyceridemic man. *Metabolism* **30**:165–171.

Tokunaga, K., K. Ishikawa, and Y. Matsurawa. 1982. Lipids and lipoproteins during a very low caloric diet. *Int. J. Obesity* **6**:416.

Trowell, H. C. 1972. Ischaemic heart disease and dietary fiber. *Amer. J. Clin. Nutr.* **25**:926–932.

Trowell H., and D. Burkitt. 1986. Physiological role of dietary fiber: a ten year review. *Contemp. Nutr.* **11**:1–2.

Trowell, H. C., N. Painter, and D. P. Burkitt. 1974. Aspects of epidemiology of diverticular disease and ischaemic heart disease. *Am. J. Dig. Disease* **19**:864–873.

Vahouney, G. V. 1982. Dietary fibers and intestinal absorption of lipids. In *Dietary Fiber in Health and Disease*, G. V. Vahouney and D. Kritchevsky, eds., pp. 203–227. New York and London: Plenum Press.

Van Raaij, J. M. A., M. B. Katan, J. G. A. Hautvast, and R. J. J. Hermus. 1981. Effects of casein versus soy protein diets on serum cholesterol and lipoproteins in young healthy volunteers. *Am. J. Clin. Nutr.* **34**:1261–1271.

Vega, G. L., E. Grozsek, R. Wolf, and S. M. Grundy. 1982. Influence of polyunsaturated fats on composition of plasma lipoproteins and apolipoproteins. *J. Lipid Res.* **23**:811–822.

Verrillo, A., A. De Teresa, P. Giarrusso, and S. La Rocca. 1985. Soybean protein diets in the management of type II hyperlipoproteinemia. *Atherosclerosis* **54**:321–333.

Vessby, B., I. B. Gustaffson, J. Boberg, B. Karlstrom, H. Lithell, and I. Werner. 1980. Substituting polyunsaturated for saturated fat as a single change in a Swedish diet: effects on serum lipoprotein metabolism and glucose tolerance in patients with hyperlipoproteinemia. *Eur. J. Clin. Invest.* **10**:193–202.

Walker, A. R. P., and U. B. Arvidsson. 1954. Fat intake, serum cholesterol concentration and atherosclerosis in the South African Bantu. *J. Clin. Invest.* **33**:1358–1365.

Weinsier, R. L., A. Seeman, G. Herrera, J. P. Assal, J. S. Soeldner, and R. E. Gleason. 1974. High and low-carbohydrate diets in diabetes mellitus. Study of effects on diabetic control, insulin secretion, and blood lipids. *Ann. Internal. Med.* **80**:332–341.

11

Hypertension

Pasquale Strazzullo
Alfonso Siani

The expression *Mediterranean diet,* found more and more often in the medical literature in recent years, is unfortunately vague and its definition largely incomplete, as pointed out by Ferro-Luzzi and Sette (1989). There are, in fact, several dietary patterns in the Mediterranean area that differ in many respects. For practical reasons in this paper in speaking of the Mediterranean diet, we shall refer to the most prevalent dietary pattern in southern Italy in the early 1960s (Cresta et al. 1969), according to Ferro-Luzzi and Sette (1989).

The first historical description of the traditional dietary habits of southern Italy was found in the archives of the Kingdom of Naples (Verrastro et al. 1989). It was part of a detailed investigation of socioeconomic conditions in the kingdom, carried out by the local authority in 1811. By means of this document, it has been possible to construct a complete picture of the dietary model adopted by a Mediterranean population in the nineteenth century. The diet was based on a large consumption of cereals, particularly bread and pasta, plus vegetables and fruit. The only source of visible fat was olive oil, while the consumption of meat and fish was generally very low. Almost the only source of animal protein was a limited quantity of dairy products. Wine production and consumption was widespread in all social classes.

Historically, therefore, what is now defined as the Mediterranean diet arises from an inability to procure much food of animal origin and from poor socioeconomic conditions. It may not be surprising that the legacy of an era of extreme poverty may be useful today in fighting the so-called civilization diseases of affluent societies.

Whether the characteristics of the Mediterranean diet have a relevant impact on blood pressure is still an open question. During the 1970s and 1980s, clinical researchers have become increasingly interested in the possible role of a number of nutritional factors in the prevention and treatment of high blood pressure (Joint National Committee 1988). In addition to the widely recognized deleterious effect of excess sodium intake (MacGregor 1985; Intersalt 1988), recent works investigated the role of such factors as potassium (Intersalt 1988; Treasure and Ploth 1983), calcium (McCarron 1985; Cappuccio et al. 1989), various kinds of fat (Pietinen and Huttunen 1987), and fiber (Margetts et al. 1987) intake. These studies have provided a fairly large body of evidence to support the concept that some of these nutrients may be individually relevant to the control of blood pressure. Nevertheless, very few studies tested the effects on blood pressure of a complex dietary pattern as a whole.

Examples of such studies are the intervention trials carried out with vegetarians (Rouse and Beilin 1984). In general, the interpretation of this type of study is made difficult by a number of methodological problems, the most important being the covariability of changes in the intake of multiple nutrients. In addition, some studies demonstrating significant changes in blood pressure cannot, in fact, be interpreted because of the failure to control for changes in potentially confounding factors, namely physical activity, smoking habits, alcohol consumption, psychosocial behavior, and others.

With these limits in mind, we will review the epidemiological, experimental, and clinical evidence relating the so-called Mediterranean diet to the control of blood pressure.

EPIDEMIOLOGICAL ASPECTS

Several population studies support the hypothesis that lifestyle and dietary habits may significantly influence blood pressure; in particular, a number of studies suggested that vegetarians have lower blood pressure than omnivorous people (Rouse and Beilin 1984). A few studies also deal with the hypothesis that the Mediterranean diet might exert a beneficial influence on blood pressure.

A pilot epidemiological study (Iacono et al. 1982), involving relatively small Finnish, Italian, and U.S. population samples, showed that the Finnish sample had higher blood pressure levels than the Italians and Americans. At the same time, large differences in the average diet of the three populations were documented. Of these, the most striking differences were the high intake of saturated fatty acid by the Finns and the low intake by the Italians; the very low dietary polyunsaturated/saturated fat (P/S) ratio of the Finns; and the high alcohol intake (primarily wine) of the Italian sample.

In their report on the 15-year follow-up of the Seven Countries Study, Keys and coworkers (1986) emphasized the beneficial effects of monounsaturated fatty acids (i.e., from olive oil) on total and coronary heart disease mortality.

In another study of coronary heart disease and fatty acid composition of the adipose tissue carried out with middle-aged men in northern Karelia and southwest Finland, Scotland, and southern Italy, significantly lower blood pressures were once again observed in the Italian as compared to the Finnish and Scottish men (Riemersma et al. 1986). Interestingly they reported significant differences in mortality rates for coronary heart disease for the populations of these geographical areas: 140/100,000 in Scotland, 212/100,000 in northern Karelia, 146/100,000 in southwest Finland, and 43/100,000 in southern Italy. Likewise, significant differences in the composition of the adipose tissue were observed; in particular, higher proportions of oleic and linoleic acid were found in the Italian sample, a fact that probably reflects the differences in diet.

A cross-sectional comparison of risk factors for atherosclerosis in nine representative samples of healthy people from eight Italian regions showed decreasing mean levels of serum cholesterol and blood pressure when proceeding from northern Italy, where lifestyles and dietary patterns are more similar to those of highly industrialized Western countries, to southern and insular Italy, where the modification of the traditional diet toward models typical of affluent societies still lags behind (Italian National Research Council 1981).

The interpretation of these findings in terms of a possible relationship between the Mediterranean diet and blood pressure is attractive but still open to question, as the results are often based on small samples and poorly standardized measurement techniques. However, while this chapter was in preparation, the results of a cross-sectional study on a large Italian population sample again strongly suggested that olive oil consumption may be associated with a lower coronary risk profile. In particular, significantly lower blood pressure and serum cholesterol levels were found to be associated with higher levels of olive oil intake; in contrast, butter consumption was associated with a higher cardiovascular risk (Trevisan et al. 1990).

In addition to the widespread use of olive oil, the Mediterranean dietary pattern is characterized by a large consumption of vegetables (legumes, cereals, fruit) (Ferro-Luzzi and Sette 1989). A corollary of this inclination toward vegetables is the relatively high potassium and fiber intake.

There is now growing evidence that high-potassium diets may be beneficial in both human and rat genetic hypertension (Treasure and Ploth 1983; Tobian 1988). Epidemiological data on dietary potassium intake and blood pressure come mainly from American and Japanese studies (Langford 1982; Sasaki 1962; Yamori et al. 1981). In particular, the hypothesis that a high potassium intake may be associated with lower blood pressure levels has received further support from the results of the INTERSALT study (1988).

Added to the evidence of a cross-cultural association between high dietary potassium intake and lower blood pressure levels is a 12-year prospective population study (Khaw and Barrett-Connor 1987) on a co-hort of 859 men and women in southern California that suggested that a high potassium intake protects against stroke-associated mortality. In this study, a 10-mmol increase in daily potassium intake was associated with a 40% reduction in the risk of stroke. The principle sources of dietary potassium in this population sample were fruit and vegetables.

There is, at present, no convincing epidemiological evidence of the influence of dietary fiber intake on blood pressure; clinical studies on this issue will be discussed in the section Blood Pressure: Fiber.

INTERVENTION STUDIES

Blood Pressure: Lipids

Experimental evidence of a relationship between the Mediterranean diet and blood pressure has been provided by a set of intervention trials carried out as part of an international collaborative project involving Finland and Italy. The principal objective of the project was to investigate the influence of the type and amount of dietary fat on serum lipids and blood pressure in populations with largely different dietary patterns (northern Karelia, Finland, and Cilento, southern Italy).

One study was carried out in northern Karelia, a region with a particularly high rate of cardiovascular disease (Iacono et al. 1983). The customary diet of this community is characterized by a high animal fat intake and a low P/S ratio. Fifty-four middle-aged normotensive volunteers participated in this trial, which consisted of a 2-week baseline period, a 6-week dietary intervention, and a 6-week switchback period. During the intervention period, the composition of the habitual diet was modified to resemble that of Mediterranean countries. Animal fat was reduced and replaced mainly by polyunsaturated fatty acid, resulting in a very high P/S ratio.

As a result of the intervention, the proportion of energy derived from fat decreased from 39% during baseline to 24% during the intervention period, with a compensatory 10% increase in energy from carbohydrates. Dietary P/S increased from 0.15 to 1.18 during the intervention; all the dietary changes were reversed during the switchback period. At the end of the intervention, a significant decrease was observed in both systolic and diastolic blood pressure ($-7.5/-2.8$ mmHg) compared to the baseline period. When the subjects resumed their habitual diet, their blood pressure increased progressively, reaching the initial values again. In the course of this study, the intake of both sodium and potassium was kept constant. The change in blood pressure was associated with a significant change in the serum lipid profile: a significant decrease was observed in total cholesterol, LDL cholesterol, HDL cholesterol, and apoprotein-B.

This study was followed by another intervention trial also in northern Karelia, and it aimed at reproducing the results of the first study under better-controlled conditions and at comparing the effects on blood pressure of changes in dietary fats and salt intake (Puska et al. 1983). In this trial, 57 married couples (normotensive or untreated mildly hypertensive subjects) were randomly allocated to one of three groups: (I) low-fat diet, (II) low-sodium diet, and (III) control diet. While the control diet derived 38% of total energy from fat, the low-fat diet derived only 25% of energy from fat, with a P/S of 1.0. The low-salt diet was similar to the control diet but contained approximately 80 mmol sodium/day instead of 190 mmol/day. As with the previous study, this study also consisted of three periods: baseline, 2 weeks; intervention, 6 weeks; and switchback, 4 weeks.

The results of this controlled trial confirmed those of the former study. In group I (low-fat diet), a significant blood pressure decrease was observed (8.9/7.6 mmHg) during the intervention period, with a subsequent rise to baseline values after switchback. The blood pressure changes in group II (low-salt) and III (control diet) were small and not significantly different from each other.

As part of the same international collaborative project, an intervention trial was implemented in a rural area of southern Italy (Strazzullo et al. 1986; Ferro-Luzzi et al. 1984). The study was designed to investigate in a free-living situation the changes induced in the blood pressure and serum lipid levels of a group of middle-aged men and women by manipulation of their customary Mediterranean-style diet.

Current trends in Italy are indeed marked by a gradual evolution from the Mediterranean type of diet toward dietary models similar to those established in most Western industrialized countries. The Cilento area was selected for this study because the local population still maintains to a great extent traditional models of life and diet, in particular the use of olive oil as the only visible fat employed in cooking.

The design of the study was similar to that of the two Finnish trials, with a 2-week baseline period and two consecutive 6-week intervention and switchback periods; the participants, 29 men and 28 women, were normotensive volunteers. The goal of dietary intervention was, in this case, to raise to 40% the fat contribution to total energy intake and to lower the P/S ratio to about 0.2. This dietary modification was obtained by substituting foods rich in saturated fatty acids such as butter, dairy cream, cheese, and meat for specific items of the habitual diet: olive oil, cereals, and vegetables.

As a result of the intervention, during which consumption of saturated fatty acids was increased by 70%, P/S changed significantly (baseline was 0.44, intervention 0.22 and switchback 0.40). Systolic blood pressure had increased significantly at the end of the intervention period. Diastolic pressure increased to a lesser extent but was significantly higher compared with that observed at the end of the switchback period (Strazzullo et al. 1986) (Table 11-1). Figure 11-1 depicts the time trend of blood pressure during the intervention and switchback periods. The increase in systolic and diastolic pressure was continuous during the intervention period; a rapid decrease in blood pressure levels to pre-intervention values was observed after return to the customary diet. The increase in the saturated-fat content of the diet was associated with a remarkable increase in total cholesterol of 15% and LDL cholesterol of 19% (Ferro-Luzzi et al. 1986).

The joint results of the studies conducted in Finland and Italy support the concept that modifications of the diet may influence blood pressure. In particular, the current trend toward replacing the traditional diet with patterns typical of Western industrialized societies may have a deleterious impact on cardiovascular risk in Mediterranean populations.

TABLE 11-1. Blood Pressure at the End of Each Study Period

	Baseline (mmltg)	Intervention (mmHg)	Switchback (mmHg)
Males (n = 29)			
Systolic	$115.7 \pm 9.8^*$	118.3 ± 10.0	$115.6 \pm 9.1^*$
Diastolic	77.4 ± 8.2	78.8 ± 8.1	$75.2 \pm 8.3^{**}$
Females (n = 28)			
Systolic	$103.7 \pm 10.7^*$	108.5 ± 9.9	$105.2 \pm 9.6^{**}$
Diastolic	68.6 ± 7.6	70.6 ± 8.6	$66.6 \pm 7.8^{***}$

Source: Strazzullo et al. (1986).
Notes: Values are mean ± SD.
   $^*p < 0.05$.
  $^{**}p < 0.01$.
$^{***}p < 0.001$.

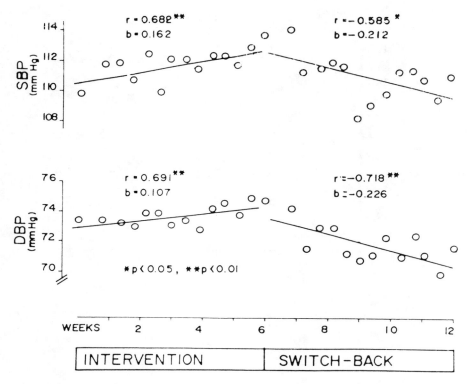

Figure 11-1. From Mediterranean diet to Western: means of the individual blood pressure values every third day in each period were regressed against time. Data for men and women were combined. (SBP and DBP = systolic and diastolic blood pressure; r = correlation coefficient; b = regression coefficient.)

Blood Pressure: Potassium

The effects of high potassium intake on blood pressure are still under investigation. The majority of controlled clinical trials suggest that oral potassium supplementation lowers blood pressure in a significant proportion of hypertensive patients, although often to a small degree (MacGregor et al. 1982; Kaplan et al. 1985; Siani et al. 1987). However, no data are yet available on the effectiveness of an increased potassium intake from natural foods.

To test the hypothesis of an antihypertensive effect of high potassium intake, we carried out a long-term controlled trial of moderate oral potassium supplements in patients with mild hypertension (Siani et al. 1987). The study was conducted with 37 patients randomly allocated to

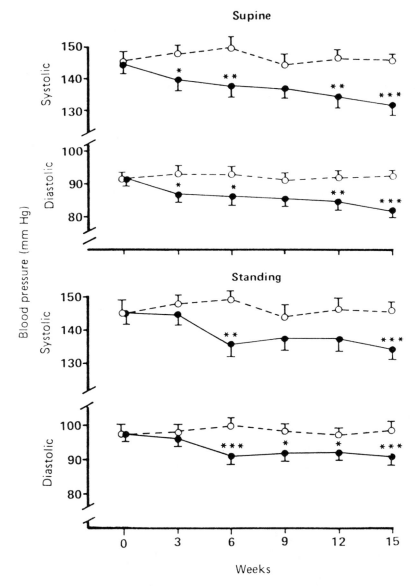

Figure 11–2. Average supine (*top*) and standing (*bottom*) blood pressures of 18 hypertensive patients receiving oral potassium supplement of 48 mmol/day (closed circles) and of 19 patients receiving placebo (open circles) over 15 weeks. *p < 0.05; ** < 0.01; ***p < 0.001.

receive a 48-mmol/day oral potassium supplement (n = 18) or an identical placebo (n = 19) for 15 weeks. A significant blood pressure decrease was observed in patients who received potassium treatment (Fig. 11–2) compared to the placebo group. Normalization of blood pressure values was attained by 14 of 18 patients. No changes were observed in the plasma potassium concentration, while 24-hour urinary potassium excretion increased significantly in patients taking potassium, from 57 ± 4 to 87 ± 4 mmol/24 hours. All patients completed the trial without any adverse effects. The decrease in blood pressure associated with oral potassium supplement was biologically and clinically significant, suggesting that moderate potassium supplements might be a valuable non-pharmacological intervention in controlling blood pressure. These results warrant further studies to explore the possibility of achieving an increase in potassium intake by means of simple dietary modifications.

Blood Pressure: Fiber

Data on the effects of an isolated increase in dietary fiber on blood pressure have thus far been inconclusive due to the lack of controlled studies in hypertensive patients. Wright et al. (1979) suggested that a high-fiber diet lowered the blood pressure of normotensive volunteers accustomed to a low-fiber diet, but in the same study, a subset of 12 hypertensive patients showed no blood pressure decrease after 6 weeks of high fiber intake. In another trial, 12 patients with type I diabetes mellitus were given a high-fiber diet (65 g/day); after 2 weeks of treatment, there was roughly a 10% decrease in blood pressure values (Anderson 1983). In both studies, the fall in blood pressure could not be distinguished from the effects of familiarization or other confounding dietary factors.

Brussard et al. (1981) found that a diet containing about 40 g/day of fiber had no effect in normotensive individuals. The controlled, randomized trial of Margetts et al. (1987) showed no effect on blood pressure in healthy, normotensive men after a 6-week period of high fiber intake (57 g/day). Finally, a controlled trial conducted by Swain et al. (1990) confirmed that in normotensive volunteers, blood pressure was unaffected by high-fiber diet (39 g/day). The relationship between dietary fiber intake and blood pressure needs to be investigated further, using controlled trials with hypertensive patients.

EXPERIMENTAL STUDIES

Few biochemical data address the possible role of nutritional changes on blood pressure regulation in humans. Because a large number of plasma membrane abnormalities have been reported in hypertensive patients, however, two studies examined whether changes in dietary fat composition might alter the structure and function of plasma membranes so as to affect the ion transport systems.

The first study was a randomized double-blind trial with normotensive healthy volunteers to investigate the effects of an increase in dietary linoleic acid on leucocyte membrane sodium transport and on blood pressure. The study showed that this dietary intervention caused a significant activation of the sodium pump in leucocytes, accompanied by an increased incorporation of linoleic acid into the erythrocyte membranes; a small blood pressure decrease was also observed (Heagerty et al. 1986).

A more recent study tested the possibility that a diet rich in olive oil might influence the membrane lipid composition and cation transport in erythrocytes; the study was carried out with 11 normotensive, healthy volunteers. The dietary modification was obtained by adding 100 g/day of olive oil (36% of total calories) for 3 weeks; the resulting diet was isocaloric to the subjects' customary diet. At the end of the study, a 15.7% increase in the oleic acid content of the plasma membrane was observed. It was reported that the maximal rates of Na-K pump and Na-K cotransport were significantly increased (Pagnan et al. 1989).

These results suggest a relationship between dietary modifications and changes in cation transport systems, probably mediated by changes in membrane composition. The therapeutic implications of these findings remain to be investigated in further studies.

CONCLUSIONS

Evidence is increasing from both epidemiological and clinical studies, that a dietary model similar to that prevalent in many countries of the Mediterranean area may be beneficial to the control of high blood pressure. The studies reviewed here lead to the conclusion that the Mediterranean diet may have a favorable effect on the cardiovascular risk profile. In particular, the unfavorable changes in plasma cholesterol and blood pressure observed when a sample of Mediterranean population was temporarily switched to a Western-style diet strongly support this view.

The component or components of the Mediterranean diet that are associated with the effects on blood pressure are still uncertain: an independent role for any one nutrient—for example, fat, potassium, or fiber—has not yet been conclusively demonstrated.

Further studies should be encouraged to ensure firm scientific evidence for the hypothesis that is being investigated; it is hoped that the results of such studies will offer expanded options in the area of non-pharmacological treatment of high blood pressure.

Acknowledgments

The authors thank Ms. Rosanna Scala for her assistance in the preparation of the manuscript.

REFERENCES

Anderson, J. W. 1983. Plant fiber and blood pressure. *Ann. Intern. Med.* **98**:842.

Brussard, J. H., J. M. A. van Raaiji, M. Stasse-Wolthius, M. B. Katan, and J. G. A. J. Hautvast. 1981. Blood pressure and diet in normotensive volunteers: absence of an effect of dietary fiber, protein or fat. *Am. J. Clin. Nutr.* **34**:2023.

Cappuccio, F. P., A. Siani, and P. Strazzullo. 1989. Oral calcium supplementation and blood pressure: an overview of randomized controlled trials. *J. Hypertension* **7**:941.

Cresta, M., S. Ledermann, A. Garnier, E. Lombardo, and G. Lacourly. 1969. *Etude des consommations alimentaires des populations de onze régions de la communaute européenne en vue de la détermination des niveaux de contamination radioactive.* Rapport etabli au Centre d'Etude Nucléaire de Fontenay-Aux-Roses, France: EURATOM, Commissariat à l'énergie atomique (CEA).

Ferro-Luzzi, A., and S. Sette. 1989. The Mediterranean Diet: An attempt to define its present and past composition. *Eur. J. Clin. Nutr.* **43**(92):13.

Ferro-Luzzi, A., P. Strazzullo, C. Scaccini, A. Siani, S. Sette, M. A. Mariani, P. Mastranzo, R. M. Doughtery, J. M. Iacono, and M. Mancini. 1984. Changing the Mediterranean diet: effects on blood lipids. *Am. J. Clin. Nutr.* **40**:1027.

Heagerty, A. M., J. D. Ollerenshaw, D. I. Robertson, R. F. Bing, and J. D. Swales. 1986. Influence of dietary linoleic acid on leucocyte sodium transport and blood pressure. *BMJ* **293**:295.

Iacono, J. M., R. M. Doughtery, and P. Puska. 1982. Reduction of blood pressure associated with dietary polyunsaturated fat. *Hypertension* **4**(S III):III–34.

Iacono, J. M., P. Puska, R. M. Doughtery, P. Pietinen, E. Vartiainen, U. Leino, M. Mutanen, and M. Moisio. 1983. Effect of dietary fat on blood pressure in a rural Finnish population. *Am. J. Clin. Nutr.* **38**:860.

Intersalt Cooperative Research Group. 1988. INTERSALT: an international study of electrolyte excretion and blood pressure. Results for 24-hour urinary sodium and potassium excretion. *BMJ* **297**:319.

Joint National Committee. 1988. The 1988 report of the Joint National Committee on detection, evaluation and treatment of high blood pressure. *Arch. Intern. Med.* **148**:1023.

Kaplan, N. M., A. Carnegie, F. Raskin, J. A. Heller, and M. Simmons. 1985. Potassium supplementation in hypertensive patients with diuretic-induced hypokalemia. *New Engl. J. Med.* **290**:110.

Keys, A., A. Menotti, M. J. Karvonen, et al. 1986. The diet and 15-year death rate in the Seven Countries Study. *Am. J. Epidemiol.* **124**:903.

Khaw, K. T., and E. Barrett-Connor. 1987. Dietary potassium and stroke-associated mortality. A 12-year prospective population study. *New Engl. J. Med.* **316**:235.

Langford, H. G. 1982. Dietary potassium and hypertension: epidemiologic data. *Ann. Intern. Med.* **96**:770.

McCarron, D. A. 1985. Is calcium more important than sodium in the pathogenesis of essential hypertension? *Hypertension* **7**:607.

MacGregor, G. A. 1985. Sodium is more important than calcium in essential hypertension. *Hypertension* **7**:607.

MacGregor, G. A., S. J. Smith, N. D. Markandu, R. A. Banks, and G. A. Sagnella. 1982. Moderate potassium supplementation in essential hypertension. *Lancet* **2**:567.

Margetts, B. M., L. J. Beilin, R. Vandongen, and B. K. Armstrong. 1987. A randomized controlled trial of the effect of dietary fiber on blood pressure. *Cli. Sci.* **72**:343.

Pagnan, A., R. Corrocher, G. B. Ambrosio, S. Ferrari, P. Guarini, D. Piccolo, A. Opportuno, A. Bassi, O. Olivieri, and G. Baggio. 1989. Effects of an olive-oil rich diet on erythrocite membrane lipid composition and cation transport systems. *Cli. Sci.* **76**:87.

Pietinen, P., and J. K. Huttunen. 1987. Dietary fat and blood pressure—a review. *Eur. Heart J.* **8(S B)**:8.

Puska, P., J. M. Iacono, A. Nissinen, H. J. Korhonen, E. Vartiainen, P. Pietinen, R. Doughtery, U. Leino, M. Mutanen, S. Moisio, and J. Huttunen. 1983. Controlled, randomized trial of the effect of dietary fat on blood pressure. *Lancet* **i**:1.

Research Group, The, ATS-RF2 of the Italian National Research Council. 1981. Distribution of some risk factors for atherosclerosis in nine Italian population samples. *Am. J. Epidemiol.* **113**:338.

Riemersma, R. A., D. A. Wood, S. Butler, R. A. Elton, M. Oliver, M. Salo, T. Nikkari, E. Vartiainen, P. Puska, F. Gey, P. Rubba, M. Mancini, and F. Fidanza. 1986. Linoleic acid content in adipose tissue and coronary heart disease. *BMJ* **292**:1423.

Rouse, I. L., and L. J. Beilin. 1984. Editorial Review: vegetarian diet and blood pressure. *J. Hypertension* **2**:231.

Sasaki, N. 1962. High blood pressure and the salt intake of the Japanese. *Japan Heart J.* **3**:313.

Siani, A., P. Strazzullo, L. Russo, S. Guglielmi, L. Iacoviello, L. A. Ferara, and M. Mancini. 1987. Controlled trial of long term oral potassium supplements in patients with mild hypertension. *BMJ* **294**:1453.

Strazzullo, P., A. Ferro-Luzzi, A. Siani, et al. 1986. Changing the Mediterranean diet: effects on blood pressure. *J. Hypertension* **4**:407.

Swain, J. F., I. L. Rouse, C. B. Curley, and F. M. Sacks. 1990. Comparison of the effects of oat bran and low-fiber wheat on serum lipoprotein levels and blood pressure. *New Engl. J. Med.* **322**:147.

Tobian, L. 1988. The Volhard lecture: potassium and sodium in hypertension. *J. Hypertension* **6**(suppl. 4):S12.

Treasure, J., and D. Ploth. 1983. Role of dietary potassium in the treatment of hypertension. *Hypertension* **5**:864.

Trevisan, M., V. Krogh, J. Freudenheim, A. Blake, P. Muti, S. Panico, E. Farinaro, M. Mancini, A. Menotti, G. Ricci, and Research Group ATS-RF2 of the Italian National Research Council. 1990. Consumption of olive oil, butter and vegetable oils and coronary heart disease risk factors. *JAMA* **263**:688.

Verrastro, V., A. M. Giambersio, and A. M. Verrastro. 1989. Il cibo dei meschini. *Il Polso*, 15 November.

Wright, A., P. G. Burstyn, and M. J. Gibney. 1979. Dietary fiber and blood pressure. *BMJ* **2**:1541.

Yamori, Y., M. Kihara, Y. Nara, et al. 1981. Hypertension and diet: multiple regression analysis in a Japanese farming community. *Lancet* **i**:1204–1205.

12

Cardiovascular Diseases

Alessandro Menotti

The concept of a Mediterranean diet was first developed by Professor Ancel Keys in his book *How to Eat Well and Stay Well, The Mediterranean Way* (Keys and Keys 1975). The book is basically a cookbook, full of recipes from different areas of the Mediterranean coast; but each recipe is complemented, on a scientific basis, by a quantitative description of its principal nutrients. Moreover, some long introductory chapters clearly describe the scientific background that led to the concept of a Mediterranean diet. In addition, the entire work focuses on cardiovascular diseases and mainly on atherosclerotic coronary heart disease (CHD).

All this is to say that the Mediterranean diet has been known, described, and appreciated chiefly in connection with its possible influence in limiting the incidence of cardiovascular diseases and mortality and especially of CHD.

The first speculations in the 1950s about a possible relationship between the typical diets of common people and a low incidence of coronary heart disease, including the intermediate role of low serum cholesterol levels, were founded on exploratory surveys conducted by Prof. Keys, Dr. Paul White, and a number of their colleagues and friends in southern Italy, in Spain, and in Greece. In fact, the reported rarity of cases of hospitalized myocardial infarction, as observed by the local clinicians, was paralleled by demonstrated low mean levels of serum cholesterol as measured in small population samples (Keys et al. 1954a; Keys et al. 1955; Keys et al. 1954b). These observations were particularly impressive when compared with similar data reported from the United States and Finland, where higher levels of serum cholesterol corresponded to everyday observation of many cases of myocardial infarction and similar conditions encountered in medical practices (Keys et al. 1958; Keys et al. 1963; Keys 1952, 1957; Keys and White 1956). The Mediterranean populations did show, again in simple, exploratory surveys, a dietary pattern different from that of the North American and northern

European populations, where fat consumption was particularly elevated.

These observations, based on nonsystematic approaches (mainly for the measurement of morbidity and for sampling procedures) became the basis for methodologically more valid approaches, which led to the organization of the Seven Countries Study. This enterprise produced a major demonstration of the role of the Mediterranean diet as a protective factor against coronary heart disease.

EARLY HOSPITAL OBSERVATIONS

Several of the early clinical observations on the problems of coronary heart disease in the countries of the Mediterranean basin came from areas that did not contribute, later on, to the scientific demonstration of the role of the diet in coronary heart disease.

In 1959, a complete issue of *Acta Cardiologica* reviewed the epidemiology of heart diseases, and mainly of coronary heart disease, that had been elicited from clinical data. Hospital studies conducted in Spain showed that, of all the organic heart diseases, only 7% were diagnosed as coronary heart disease (Gilbert-Queralto and Balaguer-Vintro 1959). A report from Syria showed that less than 40% of all heart disease could be attributed to atherosclerosis, whereas the majority were diagnosed as being due to rheumatic fever or other conditions (Latham 1959). In France only 12–13% of all patients requiring medical attention for heart disease were diagnosed as ''coronary'' (Froment 1959).

In hospital statistics from Morocco, fewer than 5% of cardiac patients were diagnosed with myocardial infarction or angina pectoris, whereas rheumatic heart disease was much more common and represented the dominant heart condition (Delanoe 1959). Somewhat similar statistics were reported from Italy and Yugoslavia (Puddu 1989; Plavsic et al. 1959). In 1963, two reports from the Tripolitania region in Libya disclosed that typical coronary heart disease, manifested as myocardial infarction or angina pectoris, represented only 2% of all hospital cardiac patients (Menotti et al. 1963), while the ratio of stroke to myocardial infarction was over 10:1 (Menotti 1963). A report from the Food and Agriculture Organization of the United Nations (FAO 1958) indicated that the average diet measured in a population sample in Libya provided 1880 kcal, with a contribution of 12.9% from fat. Such a diet included only 54 g proteins (9 from animal origin), whereas 95% of all calories were from vegetable foods.

Many limitations are built into these data since they do not provide a population denominator. Conversely, a common feature was the dominating role of rheumatic heart disease, which could also be influenced by malnutrition caused by protein and vitamin deficiencies and by poor hygienic conditions. The situation in Libya may represent an extreme in terms of a diet low in calories, total fats, and animal products and relatively rich in vegetable foods. In the same years, a population sample studied in southern Italy showed a total caloric intake of 2467 kcal with 31% from fats, 58% from carbohydrates and 6.5%, 16.8%, and 2.8% respectively from saturated, monounsaturated, and polyunsaturated fatty acids, and a 2:1 ratio of vegetable to animal proteins (Cresta et al. 1969). The possibility that the study was being conducted in areas and in a historic period characterized by a special dietary pattern and by a limited incidence of coronary heart disease was legitimate but could not be demonstrated by such simple approaches.

MORTALITY DATA

A relationship between food consumption and official mortality data would provide more information on the possible role of the Mediterranean diet in protecting against coronary heart disease. This approach must, however, be limited to historic periods of several decades ago, before those important changes in eating habits that have altered part of the picture. In the 1950s and early 1960s, the FAO produced data derived from National Food Balance Sheets (FAO 1966) showing a clearly inverse relationship between the proportion of calories from animal sources and those from grains and potatoes. All the Mediterranean countries included in that analysis showed low animal-food consumption and high grain and potato consumption: Italy, Greece, Egypt, Turkey, and Israel, with France as the exception, where consumption was roughly evenly divided. The same countries were known to have had few cases of coronary heart disease during those years.

A similar study published in 1970 by the World Health Organization (WHO) analyzed 37 countries including some of the Mediterranean area, such as Yugoslavia, Greece, France, Spain, Israel, and Italy (Masironi 1970). Correlations were studied between dietary factors estimated from national food balance sheets in 1960 to 1962 and death rates from atherosclerotic heart disease in 1965. Strong correlations were found between total caloric intake ($r = 0.77$), fat consumption ($r = 0.84$), saturated fats ($r = 0.81$), sucrose ($r = 0.56$), simple sugars ($r = 0.24$), complex carbohydrates ($r = -0.72$) and atherosclerotic heart disease. Fat consumption and saturated fat consumption in the Mediterranean countries were among the lowest of the entire set (except in France), and the mortality rates were also among the lowest (except in Israel). Conversely, carbohydrate consumption was among the highest of the 37 countries. Similar relationships were found comparing the estimated food consumption of the 1940s and 1950s with 1955 death rates in a subset of 25 out of the 37 countries.

Armstrong et al. (1975) analyzed both nutrients and food groups from 1963 to 1965 and age-standardized mortality rates for men and women aged 35 to 64 for 1968 or 1969. The 30 countries involved were Canada, Chile, the United States, Israel, Japan, Austria, Belgium, Bulgaria, Czechoslovakia, Denmark, Finland, France, German Democratic Republic, German Federal Republic, Greece, Hungary, Ireland, Italy, Malta, the Netherlands, Norway, Poland, Romania, Spain, Sweden, Switzerland, United Kingdom, Australia, and New Zealand, plus Hong Kong. Some dietary variables such as saturated fats, total fat, animal protein, total protein, total calories, meat, eggs, milk, sugar, tea, and coffee were significantly correlated with CHD mortality, whereas significant negative correlations were recorded for cereals and vegetables. Among the Mediterranean countries that exhibited both low consumption of foods positively correlated with CHD and low mortality from CHD, were Israel, Italy, Malta, Spain, and Greece.

A review of the influence of fats on health was published by the Commission of the European Communities (1977). Eight countries were included in the analysis but only Italy was strictly Mediterranean. Again, Italy showed the lowest consumption of total fat and saturated fat but the highest consumption of monounsaturated fats and the lowest death rates from coronary heart disease.

This kind of analysis clearly has several limitations. The national food balance sheets on one side and the official mortality data on the other are not among the most accurate estimates of the two phenomena. Moreover, the relationships between individual values might be biased by several factors that have not always been taken into consideration in the analysis. Among these are a number of socioeconomic indicators that frequently have the same direct correlation with both dietary pattern and mortality from CHD. Coronary heart disease, moreover, was likely to be underdiagnosed at that time in relatively underindustrialized countries.

THE SEVEN COUNTRIES STUDY

The Seven Countries Study probably represents the major investigation contributing to knowledge about the relationship between the Mediterranean diet and CHD. The study was designed in the late 1950s with the purpose of answering three major questions: (1) whether real differences existed in terms of mortality, prevalence, and incidence from CHDs among different population samples who contrasted in life style and mainly in dietary habits; (2) whether such differences, if any, could be at least partly explained by the general characteristics of the populations involved; and (3) whether, within single populations, some individual characteristics would be identified that could be correlated with the development of the disease.

The methodology and principal results of the study have been published in some monographs and major papers (Keys et al. 1967; Den Hartog et al. 1968; Keys 1970; Keys et al. 1980; Keys et al. 1981; Keys et al. 1984; Keys et al. 1986). It is worthwhile, however, to recall some details. The study was conducted on almost 13,000 men aged 40 to 59 at entry examination, enrolled in 16 population samples located in seven different countries: United States (1 sample), Finland (2), the Netherlands (1), Italy (3), Yugoslavia (5), Greece (2), and Japan (2). Of the 16 cohorts, 11 were of rural nature; two were made up of railroad workers in the United States and Italy; one was a probabilistic sample drawn from the small town of Zutphen, the Netherlands; one was made up of men working in an agroindustrial cooperative at Zrenjanin, Yugoslavia; and one was comprised of university professors in Belgrade, Yugoslavia.

After a period dedicated to conducting pilot studies and validating methodologies, the real study started in 1957. The enrollment of the various samples, including the entry examination, proceeded until 1964, and the follow-up included two direct examinations carried out after 5 and 10 years. The collection of data on mortality and causes of death was continuous from the beginning in 1957, and almost complete data on 25-year mortality are now available for all the cohorts.

The methodology concerning the measurement of individual characteristics supposed to be coronary risk factors has been described several times elsewhere, together with the diagnostic procedures for the classification of incidence and for the allocation of causes of death (Keys et al. 1967; Keys 1970; Keys et al. 1980). Dietary data were collected at different time points, using several methodologies (Den Hartog 1968; Keys 1970; Keys et al. 1981; Keys et al. 1986). For the purpose of this presentation, reference is made to data from measurements in subsamples of each cohort, following procedures validated by or including chemical measurements of nutrients in food portions taken at home in different seasons. All the dietary data will be expressed as percent of total caloric intake.

Most of the data presented here refer to the relationship between levels of nutrients at entry into the study and incidence or mortality in 10 or 15 years. Such a period of follow-up permits analysis of a sufficient number of events for proper intercohort comparisons. At the same time, the relationships should not be much biased by changes of eating habits that occurred over time in many areas. Complete mortality data in 15 years are available for all cohorts with the only exception being Belgrade.

Some variations in the analysis and results are affected by the inclusion or exclusion in the denominator of men already carriers of major cardiovascular disease at entry examination or of men who died from violent causes, and by the inclusion or exclusion of alcohol in the computation of total calories.

For some purposes, the cohorts were analyzed in pools of Mediterranean areas (Dalmatia, in Yugoslavia; Montegiorgio and Rome railroad in Italy; Crete and Corfu in Greece, all located within 100 km of the shores of the Mediterranean Sea); southern European cohorts which, in addition to the Mediterranean, include also the Crevalcore region in Italy, Slavonia, Velika Krsna, and Zrenjanin in Yugoslavia; northern Europe cohorts, which include the two Finnish areas (east and west), plus Zutphen in the Netherlands; and North America, represented by the U.S. sample.

Table 12-1 reports consumption of some nutrients expressed as percent of total calories, together with the coronary death rates in 15 years. The linear correlation coefficients of Table 12-2 suggest positive and significant relationships between total fats, saturated fat, and CHD death rates and negative and significant correlations between the polyunsaturated/saturated ratio (P/S) and the monounsaturated/saturated (M/S) ratio on one side and the CHD death rates on the other.

A graphic example of the saturated-fat/CHD-mortality relationship is given in Fig. 12-1. The coefficients of monounsaturated fat and of carbohydrates are negative but not significant. When the same analysis was done excluding alcohol from the total calorie computation, the picture was similar, although total fat was no longer significant ($r = 0.41$), and carbohydrates yielded a larger but still not significant negative correlation coefficient ($r = -0.42$). Similar results were obtained when computing partial correlation coefficients (i.e., everything else being equal) of death rates related to single nutrients. When the major nutrients were fed into a multiple linear regression, protein consumption was discarded because it was not significant, and carbohydrates were excluded because of their high dependence on fats. The three fat types produced significant coefficients (positive for saturated fat, negative for mono- and polyunsaturated fats).

An analytical inspection of Table 12-1 indicates that the people of the Mediterranean areas, and also the majority of those defined as southern European, are among those characterized by low saturated-fat consumption, high monounsaturated-fat consumption and relatively high

TABLE 12-1. Average Estimated Consumption of Some Nutrients and Death Rates from Coronary Heart Disease

Cohort	T-Fat	S-Fat	M-Fat	P-Fat	CH	P/S	M/S	CHD
			Percent of Total Calories					*(per 10,000 in 15 years)*
US	38.0	16.2	16.2	4.8	43.7	0.30	1.00	773
EF	38.5	23.7	11.9	2.9	53.9	0.12	0.50	1202
WF	34.3	19.4	11.3	3.0	50.8	0.85	0.58	741
ZU	38.0	20.2	12.5	5.4	45.3	0.27	0.62	636
CR	27.0	8.9	11.4	3.2	50.2	0.36	1.28	424
MO	24.5	9.6	11.6	3.3	54.3	0.34	1.21	447
RR	27.4	7.6	17.1	2.7	51.2	0.36	2.25	515
DA	25.6	9.1	13.4	6.9	43.2	0.75	1.47	216
SL	31.9	13.6	13.3	3.4	49.8	0.25	0.98	389
VK	21.9	5.7	14.6	1.9	60.1	0.33	2.56	67
ZR	32.6	9.7	20.1	3.1	50.0	0.32	2.07	297
CT	36.1	7.7	25.8	2.5	49.4	0.33	3.35	38
CO	33.0	6.4	18.3	3.5	47.6	0.54	2.86	202
TA	9.0	2.9	2.9	2.9	73.3	1.00	1.00	144
UH	9.0	2.9	2.9	2.9	73.6	1.00	1.00	127

Source: Keys et al. (1986).

Notes: Men with major cardiovascular disease at entry are excluded, as well as those who died from accidents. Proportion of calories on total calories incuding alcohol.

US = U.S. Railroad; EF = Eastern Finland; WF = Western Finland; ZU = Zupthen, The Netherlands; CR = Crevalcore, Italy; MO = Montegiorgio, Italy; RR = Rome Railroad, Italy; DA = Dalmatia, Yugoslavia; SL = Slavonia, Yugoslavia; VK = Velika Krsna, Yugoslavia; ZR = Zrenjanin, Yugoslavia; CT = Crete, Greece; CO = Corfu, Greece; TA = Tanushimaru, Japan; UH = Ushibuka, Japan.

T-FAT = total fats; S-FAT = saturated fats; M-FAT = monounsaturated fats; P-FAT = polyunsaturated fats; CH = carbohydrates; P/S = ratio of polyunsaturated fats to saturated fats; M/S = ratio of monounsaturated fats to saturated fats; CHD = death rates per 10,000 in 15 years.

consumption of carbohydrates. These seem to be the major characteristics of these samples, together with low death rates from CHD.

The overall picture was clearly influenced by the coexistence in the analysis of other cohorts that largely differed from the Mediterranean. However, when similar computations were repeated after excluding the Japanese cohorts or the Japanese and U.S. cohorts, the overall results did not differ substantially from the previous ones.

The early analyses performed on data from 5 and 10-year follow-up periods yielded, for saturated fats, correlation coefficients of the same

TABLE 12-2. Simple Linear Regression and Correlation of 15-year Death Rates from CHD on Some Nutrients in 15 Cohorts of the Seven Countries Study

	Intercept (a)	Slope (b)	Linear Correlation Coefficient (r)	r	t Value of b and r
Total Fats	−140	19.5	0.57	0.33	2.51*
Saturated Fats	−107	49.2	0.91	0.83	7.96***
Monosaturated Fats	498	−6.7	−0.14	0.02	0.51
Polyunsaturated Fats	291	35.4	0.14	0.02	0.51
P/S Ratio (×100)	714	−7.0	−0.60	0.36	2.70**
M/S Ratio (×100)	759	−2.3	−0.63	0.40	2.93**
Carbohydrates	468	−0.7	−0.20	0.04	0.74

Source: Computed from data of Keys et al. (1986).

Notes: the symbols a, b, and r pertain to the regression-correlation equations and t refers to the t test applied to the linear correlation coefficient.

*$p < 0.05$
**$p < 0.02$
***$p < 0.001$

size (5 years: $r = 0.84$ for CHD incidence; 10 years: $r = 0.84$ for CHD death: $r = 0.73$ for CHD incidence) (Keys 1970; Keys et al. 1980).

Three important issues are worthy of comment:

- The major differences in food consumption between the Mediterranean areas and northern Europe and the United States were in the proportions of saturated fat and not necessarily in overall fat consumption.
- The polyunsaturated fat consumption has relatively minor relevance since the intercohort differences are limited.
- The monounsaturated fat consumption is important since it influences the M/S ratio, which is another possible protective characteristic; but more than that, the M/S ratio was shown to be negatively and significantly correlated not only with CHD death rates but also with cancer death rates and death rates from all causes. It was the only dietary characteristic so related to all such major fatal events in a systematic analysis based on 15-year follow-up data (Keys et al. 1986).

Other types of comparisons permit a more intensive view of the problem. Table 12–3 shows the differences in the consumption of certain nutrients between the pool of the Mediterranean areas, the pool of the southern European areas, and the pool of the northern European plus-the-U.S. cohorts. Once more a striking difference appears in the con-

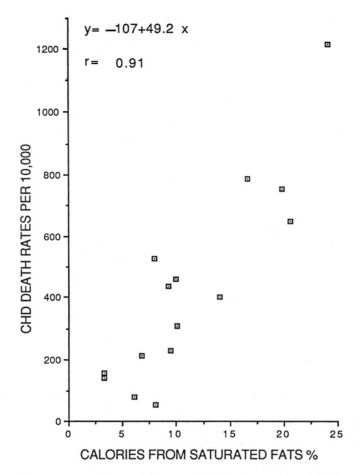

Figure 12-1.   Seven Countries Study. Relationship of CHD death rates per 10,000 in 15 years on entry levels of saturated fat consumption in 15 cohorts (after Keys et al. 1986).

sumption of saturated fats and monounsaturated fats and consequently in the M/S ratio. Also, the combined death rates from CHD and all causes of death are largely different (Menotti and Seccareccia 1986).

Kromhout et al. (1989) published a systematic review and recoding of food consumption in the Seven Countries cohorts. Table 12-4, based on that paper, compares the pool of the three northern European cohorts to the pool of the five strictly Mediterranean cohorts for food consumption, as defined by large food groups. The three northern European cohorts are a little higher in the consumption of cereals, bread, and po-

TABLE 12-3. Consumption of Some Nutrients, CHD and All Causes of Mortality in Subsets of Cohorts of the Seven Countries Study

	Saturated Fats (% cal)	Monoun-saturated Fats (% cal)	M/S Ratio	Carbohy-drates (% cal)	CHD Mortality (15 yr/10K)	All Causes of Mortality (15 yr/10K)
Mediterranean[a]	8.4	19.6	2.33	49.3	284	1550
Southern Euro-pean[b]	9.4	19.2	2.04	50.5	288	1756
Northern European plus U.S.[c]	19.5	15.0	0.76	46.8	838	2070

Source: Menotti and Seccareccia (1986).
[a]Damatia, Yugoslavia; Montegiorgio and Rome railroad, Italy; Corfu and Crete, Greece.
[b]The Mediterranean plus Crevalcore, Italy; Slavonia, Velika Krsna, and Zrenjanin, Yugoslavia.
[c]Eastern Finland and Western Finland; Zupthen, the Netherlands; U.S. railroad.

TABLE 12-4. Average Consumption of Some Foods in Five Mediterranean Cohorts and Three Northern European Cohorts of the Seven Countries Study

	Mediterranean[a] (g/day)	Northern European[b] (g/day)
Bread, Cereals, Potatoes	567	665
Vegetables, Pulses	226	150
Fruit	222	51
Meat, Eggs, Cheese	139	179
Milk	114	927
Fish	48	26
Fat	74	82
Pastries, Other Sugar Products	28	119
Alcoholic Beverages	489	24

Source: Kromhout et al. (1989); © Am. J. Clin. Nutr. (American Society of Clinical Nutrition).
[a]Dalmatia, Yugoslavia; Montegiorgio and Rome railroad, Italy; Corfu and Crete, Greece.
[b]Eastern Finland; Western Finland; Zutphen, the Netherlands.

tatoes (mainly due to the potato component), of meat, eggs, and cheese, of milk and fats (mainly of animal origin), and of pastries and other sugar products. The five Mediterranean cohorts consume more vegetables, pulses, fruit, fish, and much greater quantities of alcoholic beverages. The two patterns are extremely different and largely reflect the tendency toward high consumption of animal products in the north and of vegetable products in the Mediterranean area. A large proportion of fat in the Mediterranean cohorts consisted of olive oil.

When comparing the different cohorts, the strict relationship between eating habits and CHD incidence or mortality has an immediate biological explanation that is worth mentioning, although the problem has been dealt with in other chapters of this book. Positive and highly significant correlations were found between saturated-fat consumption in the different cohorts and mean levels of serum cholesterol on the one hand and between serum cholesterol and incidence of mortality from CHD on the other. Table 12-5 and Fig. 12-2 summarize some of these relationships.

Within the European cohorts of the Seven Countries, an attempt was made to identify the precise amount of difference in CHD incidence that could be explained by the main coronary risk factors during a follow-up period of 10 years. The net result was that only serum cholesterol explained the differences in incidence between northern and southern European countries; this difference was about 50% (Mariotti et al. 1982). Significantly, mean levels of serum cholesterol of 235 mg/dl in the Netherlands and 255 mg/dl and 265 mg/dl in the two Finnish cohorts contrasted with mean levels around or less than 200 mg/dl in all the southern European cohorts.

It would be unwise to conclude that cardiovascular illness in Mediterranean areas is a minor problem, because conditions other than CHD compete as causes of death. In particular, the epidemic of stroke does not spare those populations. Stroke death rates in the Mediterranean cohorts of the Seven Countries are among the highest in the study. Still,

TABLE 12-5. Relationship Between Mean Levels of Serum Cholesterol and Saturated-fat Consumption and CHD Incidence or Mortality in the Seven Countries Study

Relationship			Cohorts (n)	Linear Correlation Coefficient
Mean saturated fat consumption	vs.	Mean serum cholesterol	16	0.89
Mean serum cholesterol	vs.	CHD incidence hard criteria 5 years	13	0.76
Mean serum cholesterol	vs.	CHD mortality 10 years	16	0.80
Mean serum cholesterol	vs.	CHD mortality 15 years	15	0.87

Sources: Keys (1970); Keys et al. (1980); Keys et al. (1984).

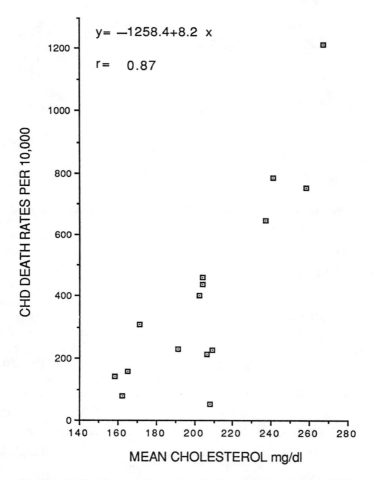

Figure 12-2.   Seven Countries Study. Relationship of CHD death rates per 10,000 in 15 years on entry mean levels of serum cholesterol in 15 cohorts (after Keys et al. 1984; Keys et al. 1986).

the sum of CHD plus stroke death rates is again lower in the Mediterranean countries compared with those of the northern European or North American areas. This fact is clearly shown by the data of Table 12-6. In addition, it appears that the mean age of stroke deaths is higher than that of CHD deaths, which provides an additional advantage in terms of life expectancy to those populations who have low CHD death rates, although the stroke death rates are relatively high. For example, in the

TABLE 12-6. Fifteen-year Death Rates per 10,000 from CHD, from Stroke and Total in the Seven Countries Study

	CHD	Stroke	CHD + Stroke
Five Mediterranean cohorts[a]	331	253	584
Three Northern European cohorts[b]	1134	170	1304

[a] Dalmatia, Yugoslavia; Montegiorgio and Rome railroad, Italy; Corfu and Crete, Greece.
[b] Eastern Finland and Western Finland; Zutphen, the Netherlands.

20-year follow-up period, the mean age of death was almost two years higher for stroke deaths than it was for CHD deaths.

RECENT TRENDS

Data reported thus far are from observations of dietary habits in some countries of the Mediterranean basin as they were in the 1950s and 1960s together with the consequences to health and disease as measured in the following few years. It is well known that changes in eating habits have occurred in the Mediterranean world since those years and that some changes moved far away from the old model. As shown in Table 12-7, for example, in a three-decade period in Italy, increases in the con-

TABLE 12-7. Changes in Dietary Habits in Italy Between 1952-54 and 1982-84

Nutrients	1952–54	1962–64	1972–74	1982–84
Proteins				
Vegetable (g)	58	59	60	59
Animal (g)	22	33	46	58
Total (g)	30	92	106	117
Fats				
Vegetable (g)	31	49	72	70
Animal (g)	23	28	37	50
Total (g)	54	77	109	120
Carbohydrates (g)	412	434	473	475
Calories	2350	2690	3180	3330
Calories From Alcohol	190	240	270	260
Total Calories	2540	2930	3450	3590

Source: Mariani Costantini (1986).

sumption of animal proteins, total proteins, vegetable and animal fats, total carbohydrates, alcohol, and total calories have completely distorted the 1952–1954 diet (Mariani Costantini 1986).

Trends in CHD morbidity could not be followed, but CHD mortality is known to have dramatically increased at least until the late seventies (Capocaccia et al. 1984; Menotti 1976). The relationship between the two phenomena cannot be demonstrated as causal but it is highly suggestive. Incidentally, mean serum cholesterol levels also increased in Italy during those years. Within single areas, differences of 20 mg/dl, representing levels measured in different generations reaching the same age 10 years apart, were followed by a CHD incidence rate 19% higher in the generation with higher levels of serum cholesterol (Menotti et al. 1985). The most recent mortality trends, again in Italy, which tend toward a slight decline, are much more difficult to explain. Beyond diet and cholesterol, they are probably associated with better control of hypertension, a reduction in the prevalence of smoking (at least among men), a decrease of body mass index in women, and improvement in medical and surgical treatment (Menotti et al. 1985; Menotti 1989; Italian National Research Council 1987).

Similar changes are likely to have occurred in other Mediterranean countries. In terms of mortality, the age-standardized rates for CHD in people aged 30 to 65 during the period 1970 to 1985 increased in Greece, Spain, and Yugoslavia and decreased slightly in Italy and Malta (more in females than in males). When heart diseases were considered (to avoid the bias due to different diagnostic practices), the increase in Greece and Yugoslavia was less evident and practically absent in Spain, and the decrease was less marked in Italy and Malta. In all these countries, there was a decrease of stroke mortality except in Yugoslavia, where there was still an increase (Uemura and Pisa 1988) (Table 12-8).

The interpretation of these trends is complex and cannot be resolved in this paper. Trends in other factors—mainly in smoking habits and control of hypertension—have probably contributed to modulating the amount and rate of disease and mortality beyond dietary habits. The Mediterranean countries still enjoyed a relatively low mortality from cardiovascular disease even in the 1980s compared to other countries whose mortality statistics are available (Uemura and Pisa 1988).

INTERVENTION

The Mediterranean diet has probably influenced to some extent those who, from the 1950s to the 1980s, have conducted intervention trials targeted at reducing CHD incidence and mortality. A systematic review

TABLE 12-8. Changes in Death Rates from Heart Diseases in Men and Women aged 30-69 in Some Mediterranean Countries Between 1970 and 1985

	IHD		HD		CVD		ACVD	
	M	F	M	F	M	F	M	F
Greece	+ +	+	+ +	0	0	−	+	−
Israel	− −	− − −	− −	− − −	− − −	− − −	− −	− − −
Italy	−	− −	−	− −	− −	− −	−	− −
Malta	0	− −	−	− −	− −	− − −	−	− −
Spain	+ +	+	0	− −	− −	− −	−	− −
Yugoslavia	+ + +	+ +	+ +	+	+	0	+ +	+

Source: Uemura and Pisa (1988).

Notes: IHD = ischaemic heart disease; HD = heart disease; CVD = cerebrovascular disease; ACVD = all cardiovascular diseases.

    0 = no change or less than + 10%
    + = rise 10% or more
  + + = rise 30% or more
+ + + = rise 50% or more
    − = fall 10% or more
  − − = fall 30% or more
− − − = fall 50% or more

of such trials is not appropriate, but some comments might be worthwhile, mainly because some differences between the Mediterranean diet and the experimental ones are clear.

Sometimes, changing a current diet has been used as a single tool for the preventive experiment; sometimes it has been used in combination with other adjustments. In the second instance, it has not been easy to discriminate the role of the diet (and of the subsequent cholesterol changes) from that of the other adjustments. There were a number of pure dietary trials, which were known as the Anti-Coronary Club (Christakis et al. 1966), the Veterans Administration Study (Dayton et al. 1969), the Finnish Mental Hospital Study (Miettinen et al. 1972). Multifactor trials including dietary changes were the Coronary Prevention Evaluation Program of Chicago (Inter-Society Commission for Heart Disease Resources 1970), the Multiple Risk Factor Intervention Trial (MR-FIT Research Group 1982), the North Karelia Project (Puska et al. 1985), the WHO European Multifactor Preventive Trial of CHD (WHO Collaborative Group 1986), the Oslo Preventive Trial (Hjermann et al. 1981), and the Gotenburg Trial (Wilhelmsen 1986).

The suggested or imposed changes in dietary habits were frequently oriented toward a net increase of polyunsaturated fat, possibly accompanied by a reduction of saturated fats; none of the original Mediterranean diets were particularly rich in polyunsaturated fats. Also, none of the experimental diets were particularly high in monounsaturated fat, the use of which is typically Mediterranean because of the high consumption of olive oil.

The satisfactory or positive results of saturated-fat reduction obtained in the majority of the mentioned above trials demonstrate, at least, the need to reduce the amount of saturated fats in the diet. On the other hand, not a single trial including hard end-points has been organized with the purpose of testing typical Mediterranean dietary habits.

Still, other intervention studies with soft end-points (such as changes in blood lipids) support, at least indirectly, the usefulness of a diet that resembles that used in the 1950s or 1960s in some Mediterranean areas (Enholm et al. 1982; Grundy 1986). Several statements have been made by different bodies and organizations that suggest preventive diets rather similar to the Mediterranean ideal diet (American Heart Association 1982; WHO 1982; Consensus Conference 1985; European Atherosclerosis Society Study Group 1987; Consensus Conference Italiana 1986). As an example, in the final document of the Italian Consensus Conference on Cholesterol and in a recent Italian book on the Mediterranean diet (Consensus Conference Italiana 1986; Agradi 1988), it is stated that in a healthful diet, total fat should not exceed 30% of total calories, of which saturated fats should be less than 10%, polyunsaturated fats should be around 5% to 6% and, as a consequence, monounsaturated fats should range from 15% to 17% or more, with the specific indication for a large use of olive oil as basic fat. In addition to stipulations regarding fat, it is recommended that abundant use be made of grains (bread, pasta), legumes, and fresh vegetables and fruits, and that use of dairy and other animal products be limited.

The final experimental proof of the specific role of such a diet has not been given, but much circumstantial evidence is pointing to its efficacy; more research on the problem is needed and will be enthusiastically received.

SUMMARY

The Mediterranean diet has been identified and studied mainly in connection with cardiovascular disease and with CHD in particular. Clinical observations from hospitals were already suggesting, in the 1950s, the existence of low rates of CHD in the area.

Correlation studies between food balance sheets and official mortality data indicated the association between low-fat, low-saturated-fat, high-monounsaturated-fat and high-carbohydrate consumption and low rates from CHD.

The Seven Countries Study involving, among others, three Mediterranean Countries (Italy, Yugoslavia, and Greece) gave the best scientific proof of the association between a diet low in animal products and saturated fat and low mean population levels of serum cholesterol and with low incidence and mortality from CHD.

These correlations have probably become distorted during the 1970s and 1980s by the changes that have occurred both in terms of eating habits (departing from the traditional diet) and of CHD mortality, which is increasing, at least in some countries.

Mediterranean dietary habits have been used as a model, although never exactly replicated, for primary prevention trials of CHD and as guidelines for primary prevention recommended by several bodies and organizations.

REFERENCES

Agradi, E. 1988. *Le basi scientifiche della dieta mediterranea.* Rome: Verduci Editore.

American Heart Association. 1982. Committee report: Rationale of the Diet Heart Statement. Report of Nutrition Committee. *Circulation* **65**:839A.

Armstrong, B. K., J. I. Mann, A. M. Adelstein, and F. Eskin. 1975. Commodity consumption and ischaemic heart disease mortality with special reference to dietary practices. *J. Chron. Dis.* **28**:455.

Capocaccia, R., G. Farchi, S. Mariotti, A. Verdecchia, A. Angeli, P. Morganti, and M. L. Panichelli-Fucci. 1984. *La mortalita' in Italia nel periodo 1970–79.* Rapporti ISTISAN, ISSN–0391–1675. Istituto Superiore di Sanita', Roma.

Christakis, G., G. Winslow, S. Jampel, J. Stephenson, G. Friedman, H. Fein, A. Krans, and G. Hames. 1966. The Anti-Coronary Club: A dietary approach in the prevention of coronary heart disease. A seven year report. *Am. J. Pub. Health* **56**:299.

Commission of the European Communities, Directorate General for Agriculture. 1977. *Influence on health of different fats in food,* Information on Agriculture No. 40. Brussels and Luxembourg: EEC.

Consensus Conference. 1985. Lowering blood cholesterol to prevent heart disease. *JAMA* **253**:2080.

Consensus Conference Italiana. 1986. *Abbassare la colesterolemia per ridurre la cardiopatia coronarica.* CNR, Italian National Research Council, Rome.

Cresta, M., S. Ledermann, A. Garnier, E. Lombardo, and G. Lacourly. 1969. *Etude des consommations alimentaires des onze régions de la communaute Européene en vue de la détermination des niveaux de contamination radioactive.* Rapport établi au Centre d'Etude Nucléaire de Fontenay-Aux-Roses, France: EURATOM, Commissariat à l'énergie atomique (CEA).

Dayton, S., M. L. Pearce, S. Hashimoto, W. J. Dixon, and U. Tomiyasu. 1969. A controlled clinical trial of a diet high in poly-unsaturated fat. *Circulation* 40, suppl 2.

Delanoe, G. 1959. Consideration sur une statistique des 500 malades hospitalises dans un service de cardiologie. *Arch. Mal Coeur* **52**:361.

Den Hartog, C., K. Buzina, F. Fidanza, A. Keys, and P. Roine, eds. 1968. *Dietary Studies and Epidemiology of Heart Disease*. The Hague: Stichting tot wetenschappelijke Voorlichting op Voedingsgebied.

Enholm, C., J. K. Huttunen, P. Pietinen, U. Leino, M. Mutanen, E. Kostiainen, J. Pikkarainen, R. Dougherthy, J. Jacono, and P. Puska. 1982. Effect of diet on serum lipoproteins in a population with a high risk of coronary heart disease. *N. Engl. J. Med.* **307**:850.

European Atherosclerosis Society Study Group. 1987. Strategies for the prevention of coronary heart disease. A policy statement of the European Atherosclerosis Society. *Eur. Heart J.* **8**:77.

FAO. 1958. *Report to the Government of Libya on Nutrition*. FAO Report 920, Rome.

FAO. 1966. Food Balance Sheets: 1954–56, FAO Rome, 1958; 1957–59, FAO Rome, 1963; 1960–1962, FAO Rome.

Froment, R. 1959. La maladie coronarienne en France. *Acta Cardiol.* **14**(suppl. 8):39.

Gibert-Queralto, J., and I. Balaguer-Vintro. 1959. La frequence de la maladie coronarienne en Espagne. *Acta Cardiol.* **14**(suppl. 8):70.

Grundy, S. M. 1986. Comparison of monounsaturated fatty acids and carbohydrates for lowering plasma cholesterol. *N. Engl. J. Med.* **314**:745.

Hjermann, I., K. Velve Byre, I. Holme, and P. Leren. 1981. Effect of diet and smoking intervention on the incidence of coronary heart disease. Report from the Oslo Study Group of a randomized trial in healthy men. *Lancet* **2**:1303.

Inter-Society Commission for Heart Disease Resources. 1970. Report: Primary prevention of atherosclerotic diseases. *Circulation* **42**:A55.

Italian National Research Council. 1987. Research Group ATS-RF2-OB43. Time trends of some cardiovascular risk factors in Italy. *Am. J. Epidem.* **126**:95.

Keys, A. 1952. Human atherosclerosis and the diet. *Circulation* **5**:115.

Keys, A. 1957. Diet and epidemiology of coronary heart disease. *JAMA* **164**:1912.

Keys, A., ed. 1970. Coronary heart disease in Seven Countries. *Circulation* **41**(suppl 1):1.

Keys, A., and M. Keys. 1975. *How To Eat Well and Stay Well, The Mediterranean Way*. Garden City, N.Y.: Doubleday and Co.

Keys, A., and P. D. White. 1956. *World Trends in Cardiology. I. Cardiovascular epidemiology*. New York: Hoeber-Harper.

Keys, A., F. Vivanco, J. L. Rodriguez-Minon, M. H. Keys, and H. C. Mendoza. 1954*a*. Studies on the diet, body fatness and serum cholesterol in Madrid, Spain. *Metabolism* **3**:195.

Keys, A., M. J. Karvonen, and F. Fidanza. 1958. Serum cholesterol studies in Finland. *Lancet* **2**:175.

Keys, A., F. Fidanza, U. Scardi, G. Bergami, M. H. Keys, and F. Di Lorenzo. 1954*b*. Studies on serum cholesterol and other characteristics on clinically healthy men in Italy. *Arch. Int. Med.* **93**:328.

Keys, A., F. Fidanza, and M. H. Keys. 1955. Further studies on serum cholesterol of clinically healthy men in Italy. *Voeding* **16**:492.

Keys, A., H. L. Taylor, H. W. Blackburn, J. Brozek, J. T. Anderson, and E. Simonson. 1963. Coronary heart disease among Minnesota business and professional men followed fifteen years. *Circulation* **28**:381.

Keys, A., C. Aravanis, H. Blackburn, F. S. P. Van Buchem, R. Buzina, B. S. Djordjevic, A. S. Dontas, F. Fidanza, M. J. Karvonen, N. Kimura, D. Lekos,

M. Monti, V. Puddu, and H. L. Taylor. 1967. Epidemiological studies related to coronary heart disease: characteristics of men aged 40–59 in Seven Countries. *Acta Med. Scand.* **460**(suppl. 180):1.

Keys, A., C. Aravanis, H. Blackburn, R. Buzina, B. S. Djordjevic, A. S. Dontas, F. Fidanza, M. J. Karvonen, N. Kimura, A. Menotti, I. Mohacek, S. Nedeljkovic, V. Puddu, S. Punsar, H. L. Taylor, and F. S. P. Van Buchem. 1980. Seven Countries. *A multivariate analysis of death and coronary heart disease.* Cambridge, Mass.: Harvard University Press.

Keys, A., C. Aravanis, F. S. P. Van Buchem, H. Blackburn, R. Buzina, B. S. Djordjevic, F. Fidanza, M. J. Karvonen, N. Kimura, A. Menotti, S. Nedeljkovic, V. Puddu, and H. L. Taylor. 1981. The diet and all-causes death rate in the Seven Countries Study. *Lancet* **2**:58.

Keys, A., A. Menotti, C. Aravanis, H. Blackburn, B. S. Djordjevic, R. Buzina, A. S. Dontas, F. Fidanza, M. J. Karvonen, N. Kimura, I. Mohacek, S. Nedelikovic, V. Puddu, S. Punsar, H. L. Taylor, S. Conti, D. Kromhout, and H. Toshima. 1984. The Seven Countries Study: 2289 deaths in 25 years. *Prev. Med.* **13**:141.

Keys, A., A. Menotti, M. J. Karvonen, C. Aravanis, H. Blackburn, R. Buzina, B. S. Djordjevic, A. S. Dontas, F. Fidanza, M. H. Keys, D. Kromhout, S. Nedeljkovic, S. Punsar, F. Seccareccia, and H. Toshima. 1986. The diet and 15 year death rate in the Seven Countries Study. *Am. J. Epidem.* **124**:903.

Kromhout, D., A. Keys, C. Aravanis, R. Buzina, F. Fidanza, A. Jensen, A. Menotti, S. Nedeljkovic, M. Pekkarinen, B. S. Simic, and H. Toshima. 1989. Food consumption patterns on the nineteen sixties in Seven Countries. *Am. J. Clin. Nutr.*, in press.

Latham, J. 1959. La maladie coronarienne en Syrie. *Acta Cardio.* **14**(suppl. 8):96.

Mariani Costantini, A. 1986. *Linee guida per l'alimentazione. Basi, opportunita', ricadute.* Doc. no. 1, Gruppo di lavoro per l'elaborazione delle "Linee guida per una sana alimenatazione Italiana." Istituto Nazionale della Nutrizione, Roma.

Mariotti, S., R. Capocaccia, G. Farchi, A. Menotti, A. Verdecchia, and A. Keys. 1982. Differences in the incidence rate of coronary heart disease between north and south European cohorts of the Seven Countries Study as partially explained by risk factors. *Eur. Heart J.* **3**:481.

Masironi, R. 1970. Dietary factors and coronary heart disease. *Bull. World Health Org.* **42**:103.

Menotti, A. 1963. Relative incidence of myocardial infarction and cerebrovascular accidents among Arabs of Tripolitania. *Acta Cardiol.* **18**:248.

Menotti, A. 1976. *La prevenzione della cardiopatia coronarica.* Rome: Pensiero Scientifico Publ.

Menotti, A. 1989. Trends in coronary heart disease in Italy. *Int. J. Epidem.* **18**(suppl. 1):S–125.

Menotti, A., and F. Seccareccia. 1986. Dati del Seven Countries Study sulle malattie cardiovascolari nelle aree del Mediterraneo. *Rev. Lat. Cardiol.* **7**:329.

Menotti, A., E. Moschini-Antinori, and G. Splendiani. 1963. Heart diseases in Tripolitania. A clinical and statistical study. *Mal. Cardiovascol.* **4**:665.

Menotti, A., R. Capocaccia, G. Farchi, and M. Pasquali. 1985. Recent trends in coronary heart disease and other cardiovascular disease in Italy. *Cardiology* **72**:88.

Menotti, A., S. Conti, F. Dima, S. Giampaoli, B. Giuli, M. Matano, and F. Seccareccia. 1985. Incidence of coronary heart disease in two generations of men exposed to different levels in risk factors. *Acta Cardiol.* **40**:307.

Miettinen, M., O. Turpeinen, M. J. Karvonen, R. Elosuo, and E. Paavilainen. 1972. Effect of cholesterol lowering diet on mortality from coronary heart disease and other causes. A twelve year clinical trial in men and women. *Lancet* **2**:835.

MRFIT Research Group. 1982. Multiple risk factor intervention trial. Risk factor changes and mortality results. *JAMA* **248**:1465.

Plavsic, C., M. Ilic, and S. Nedeljkovic. 1959. Les maladies des arteres coronaires en Yugoslavie. *Acta Cardiol.* **14**(suppl. 8):79.

Puddu, V. 1989. Aspects de la maladie coronarienne en Italie. *Acta Cardiol.* **14**(suppl. 8):60.

Puska, P., A. Nissinen, K. Koskela, A. Maclister, T. E. Kottke, N. Maccoby, and J. W. Farquhar. 1985. The community based strategy to prevent coronary heart disease: conclusions from the ten years of the North Karelia Project. *Ann. Rev. Pub. Health* **6**:147.

Uemura, K., and Z. Pisa. 1988. Trends in cardiovascular disease mortality in industrialized countries since 1950. *World Health Statistic. Quart.* **41**:155.

Wilhelmsen, L., G. Berglung, D. Elmfeldt, G. Tibblin, H. Wedel, K. Pennert, A. Vedin, C. Wilhelmsson, and L. Werko. 1986. The multifactor primary preventive trial in Goteborg, Sweden. *Eur. Heart J.* **7**:279.

World Health Organization Collaborative Group. 1986. European Collaborative Trial of multifactor prevention of coronary heart disease: final report on the 6 year results. *Lancet* **1**:869.

World Health Organization. 1982. *Prevention of coronary heart disease, Tech. Rep. Ser.* no. 678. Geneva: WHO.

13

Obesity

Ottavio Bosello
Fabio Armellini
Mauro Zamboni

Obesity is one of the principal public health problems of affluent societies. Evidence shows that an increasing number of children and adolescents are overweight; the high prevalence of obesity in the adult population and the likelihood that obesity will be an even more widespread problem in the future will demand a reassessment of the health implications of this condition (National Institutes of Health Consensus-Development Conference Statement 1985). Current knowledge of human obesity has progressed beyond the simple generalizations of the past; studies of obese subjects show that they rarely eat more or less than their lean counterparts (Trowell et al. 1985).

The availability of food is undoubtedly a fundamental factor, but it is not the only cause of obesity. Obesity was and is extremely rare in African and Asian nations even where no scarcity of foodstuffs exists. Changes in such aspects of lifestyle as diet, physical activity, smoking, and socioeconomic status can have different effects on the increase in obesity incidence. It is quite likely that the interrelation between these factors is significant. In a study begun in the early 1970s of Bantu Venda people in Africa, these interrelationships were of great interest, as was the interrelationship between changes in lifestyle and changes in diet. Obesity, a rare occurrence in this population, became more frequent when nutritional habits changed. Their diet was altered, at unchanged caloric intake levels, from one rich in fibers to a diet composed of refined foods (Trowell 1975) at the same time that they migrated from rural areas to urban centers.

Epidemiological studies dating from the beginning of the 1960s noted that the prevalence of overweight and obesity in Mediterranean countries was less than that of other industrialized nations. These populations also evidenced lower blood cholesterol and arterial pressure levels and, most significantly, a reduced rate of mortality from cardiovascular diseases. These factors were assumed to be due to a "Mediterranean advantage," which was related to a diet unique to countries in the Mediterranean basin, as well as to a particular lifestyle and, not least, to a lesser degree, industrialization (Laurenzi et al. 1989).

Much has changed since 1960 regarding both lifestyles and dietary habits, both in Europe and in the countries of the Mediterranean basin and North America. The large health associations in the United States have encouraged more healthful dietary practices among the population by promoting dietary habits that resembled, for example, those of the Mediterranean area in the 1960s. Mediterranean peoples, on the other hand, have undergone an occidentalizing trend, acquiring eating habits taken straight from North American nations.

EPIDEMIOLOGY: PREVALENCE OF OBESITY

The Western World

Surveys by the U.S. Public Health Service (1966) and subsequently by Bray et al. (1972) calculated the rate of obesity in the U.S. population at between 25% and 42% of the population. A 1980 survey of the adult population of the United Kingdom shows that the problem of excess weight and obesity is extremely common and affects all age groups. About 5–20% of the 16- to 19-year-old English population is overweight; this proportion increases with age until it reaches 40% of men in the fourth and fifth decades of life (James 1985). Waaler's data in Norway (1984) and Van Sonsbeek's in the Netherlands (1985) demonstrate less obesity in the 20 to 30 year age group than in the United Kingdom but practically identical values in the older age groups.

All the studies reported a higher prevalence of obesity among subjects of lower socioeconomic status. Low socioeconomic levels also correlate with low awareness of optimal nutritional practices and, consequently, even in conditions of ample availability of food, with the risk of incorrect diet from both quantitative and qualitative standpoints and with excessive consumption of foods of animal origin. The prevalence of obesity is similar in all the developed countries (Garrow 1974), but the data from Canada and the United States show higher rates. The prevalence of obesity, to conclude, seems to be greater in North America than in European countries, with the United Kingdom in an intermediate position.

Developing Countries

There are few references to the problem of obesity in developing countries. Development means not only economic progress but also the adoption of new lifestyles, with varying degrees of improvement in dietary and health habits. Obesity, in addition to undernutrition, is present in various degrees in developing countries. Since the Midtown Manhattan Study, most authors relate the distribution of obesity to socioeconomic and educational levels (Goldblatt et al. 1965). In poor, undeveloped countries, undernutrition mainly involves the rural populations. The biggest component in the development process is internal migration, from rural to urban areas, where the migrants adopt the city culture (Lara-Pantin 1986). The new arrivals tend to reduce their physical activity and at the same time increase their intake of food; thus, urbanization increases the prevalence of obesity. Epidemiological data demonstrate that in Venezuela, 73% of the workers in the age group between 20 and 39 years have increased their weight by 897 g/year during one recent 5-year period (Lara-Pantin 1986). The Venezuelan Institute of Nutrition reports that between 1982 and 1984, obesity in children less than 15 years of age increased from 12.8% to 16.2%. Similar data are reported for Costa Rica and other countries in Latin America.

The Mediterranean Area and Italy

Very little epidemiological data exists regarding the prevalence of obesity in Italy and in the Mediterranean countries during the 1960s. The first measurements, collected by the Seven Countries Study between 1960 and 1962 from three population samples, 40 to 59 years of age, from Crevalcore, Montegiorgio, and a quarter of Rome, demonstrated a prevalence of obesity significantly lower than in the United States (Keys et al. 1966). An interesting study conducted on military conscripts from the district of Piacenza showed an increase in obesity from 14% in 1954 to 18% in 1964 (Strata 1977). More recently, another epidemiological study in Italy showed that the body mass index (BMI) increased 3.4% in men and 1.6% in women from 1972 to 1980 (Lenzi et al. 1981). Accord-

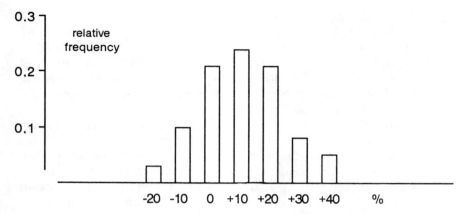

Figure 13-1.   Frequency distribution of body weight relative to standard weight in males and females of Castel D'Azzano (pers. observations).

ing to a recent study in Gubbio, half of the men between 40 and 59 years of age had a BMI equal to or greater than 26 kg/m², and that one subject in six had a BMI greater than 30 kg/m². Marked overweight is more common among women than among men: while a BMI > 26 kg/m² was found in 5.7% of the population (the same proportion in both women and men), marked obesity (BMI > 30 kg/m²) is presented among 24% of the women versus 18% of the men (Laurenzi et al. 1989). On the whole, these figures come near, if they do not equal, those found in northern European countries and in the United States. In general, the Gubbio data are similar to those recorded a few years earlier by the Italian National Research Council in nine other Italian communities (CNR 1980). A more recent epidemiological study conducted on a sample of the population of Castel d'Azzano, a town in the province of Verona, confirmed a substantial prevalence of excessive weight, noting (Fig. 13-1) that only a small percentage of subjects presented deviations below 5% from ideal weight (Bosello et al. 1989).

The prevalence of obesity in the Mediterranean basin is greater in the less socioeconomically developed regions. In fact, recent epidemiological surveys in Italy that divided the nation into four geographic zones demonstrated that the percentage of overweight subjects increases progressively from northwest and northeast toward the south (Cairella et al. 1988). In the Mediterranean basin, as in the United States, the increased prevalence of obesity is inversely correlated to socioeconomic status.

INFLUENCE OF VARIOUS NUTRIENTS
ON ENERGY BALANCE

Until recently the pathogenesis of obesity was considered the result of inappropriate dietary behavior. Actually, obesity is a complex disease with multiple causes. Environment and genetics cooperate in determining different types of obesity.

Although the etiological mechanisms that underlie obesity are not still understood, the end result is an imbalance between energy intake and energy expenditure that leads to triglyceride storage in adipocytes. Improper dietary habits and/or abnormal thermogenesis can be determinant factors in weight gain, acting as the primary causes of obesity, or they can be the consequences of obesity, promoting weight maintenance, impairing weight loss, or facilitating relapse after slimming.

There are striking individual differences in the ability to gain weight; adaptive responses to a positive caloric state also vary extensively. Apfelbaum and co-workers (Apfelbaum et al. 1971) and Sims and co-workers (Sims et al. 1973) reported that weight gain after overfeeding was lower than would have been predicted on the basis of caloric intake. Rose and William (1961) demonstrated the existence of widely varying energy requirements to maintain body weight, ranging from 1600 to 7400 kcal/day. Riumallo and co-workers (Riumallo et al. 1989) overfed (+720 kcal/day) underweight weight-stable subjects for 8 weeks; a wide range of weight gain (0.6–3.8) was observed. Poehlman and co-workers (Poehlman et al. 1988) overfed twin pairs and demonstrated significant in-pair resemblance for changes in body composition, supporting a genetic basis for changes in body fat.

In developed countries highly palatable, calorically concentrated foods are easily available and are commonly believed to be a major cause of obesity (U.S. Department of Agriculture 1962). These foods are low in complex carbohydrates, and therefore in fiber and bulk, and rich in fat and sucrose. It has been suggested that this diet could facilitate the development of obesity even when the calories consumed are not excessive (Oscai and Miller 1986). There is also evidence that caloric intake is lower in a diet high in complex carbohydrates, both in obese and lean subjects, when compared to a diet rich in fat and refined carbohydrates (Duncan et al. 1983).

Epidemiological data by West (1978) show a strong inverse relationship (Fig. 13–2) between carbohydrate intake and relative body weight. The obvious implications are that obesity could be prevented, or treated more successfully, through use of a diet rich in grains and vegetables (Danforth 1985), such as the typical Mediterranean diet.

Energy balance in obesity has been widely studied in the past and

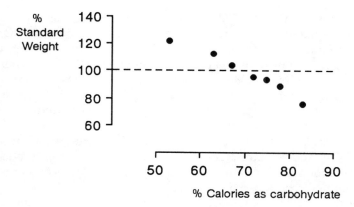

Figure 13-2.   Relationship between dietary carbohydrates and weights relative to standard weight in different populations (after West 1978).

extensive references are available (Garrow 1974: Girardier and Stock 1983; Jéquier 1984). The following sections review the interrelationships between obesity and dietary habits with respect to the Mediterranean diet, pointing out the effects of the major nutrients on energy balance.

Carbohydrates

Bandini and co-workers (Bandini et al. 1989) overfed lean and obese adolescents with carbohydrates for 2 weeks. The thermogenic response to overfeeding did not appear to be reduced in the obese subjects. The authors concluded that facultative thermogenesis does not seem to be a significant weight maintenance factor in adolescents.

Hammer and co-workers (Hammer et al. 1989) studied the long-term effects of 16-week low-fat *ad libitum* carbohydrate intake (unlimited access to complex carbohydrate food was allowed) versus low-fat restricted caloric intake (800 kcal) on body composition and resting metabolic rate (RMR) in obese women. They found that even if a greater weight loss was observed in the restricted calorie group, there was also significant weight loss in the ad libitum group. Subjects on ad libitum diets showed lower calorie intake than they did before the beginning of the study (from 1846 kcal/day to 1450 kcal/day), probably owing to the satiating effect of the large intake of complex carbohydrates. Relative RMR did not change in either group. This last finding disagrees with the majority of other authors, who encountered a reduction in RMR after calorie restriction (Apfelbaum 1976; Gillie and Raby 1984; Finer et al. 1986; Ravussin et al. 1982; Stokholm et al. 1987). This phenomenon could be explained by the use of morning measurement; in fact other authors found no reduction in RMR calculated in the morning, but reduction did become significant when evaluated as 24-hour energy expenditure (Finer et al. 1986; de Boer et al. 1987; Ravussin et al. 1985).

Elliot and co-workers (Elliot et al. 1989) have recently reported the long-term effects of massive weight loss on RMR measured before, during, and after a protein-sparing modified fast, in the last case on a maintenance diet. They found that RMR decreased during very low calorie diet (VLCD) and remained depressed for 2 months of observation after discontinuation of VLCD and despite increased caloric consumption to a level allowing body weight stabilization.

Acheson and co-workers (Acheson et al. 1984) reported that the cost of assimilation of a meal is directly proportional to the carbohydrate content of the diet. Carbohydrate content of the diet could thus be a determinant in RMR variations during caloric restriction. Its presence in calorie restricted regimens could antagonize or minimize the reduction in energy expenditure.

RMR reduction, greater than expected on the basis of fat-free mass (FFM) loss, could be at least partially due to the modified metabolic pattern (Ravussin et al. 1985) of obese women owing to VLCD-reduced peripheric monodeiodination of T4 in its more active T3 form (Barrows and Snook 1987; Bosello et al. 1981; Cavallo et al. 1990). This phenomenon could be at least partially the result of metabolic modifications induced by a specific nutrient restriction. T3 reduction, in fact, is observed when carbohydrate intake is restricted (Burger 1981); this effect would be reversed when carbohydrates are added to the diet in a sufficient amount (Hendler et al. 1983). Matzen and Kvetny (1989) studied thyroid hormones in two groups of obese women during 7 days of caloric deprivation (1100 kcal/day); one group received a high protein diet (80% protein) and the other a carbohydrate diet (100% dextrin-maltose). No thyroid hormone variations were observed in the carbohydrate group, while the first group evidenced a significant drop in T3 and free T3 with an increase in free T4.

Schutz and co-workers (Schutz et al. 1985) demonstrated that short-term overfeeding with carbohydrates induces marked and continuously increasing stimulation of energy expenditure.

A sucrose-rich diet has been thought to be more likely to induce weight gain than a diet rich in complex carbohydrates (Yudkin 1972). Sharief and Macdonald (1982) demonstrated that dietary induced thermogenesis (DIT) was greater after sucrose than after glucose but the difference was much less marked in obese subjects. Schwartz and co-workers (Schwartz et al. 1989) found that DIT and rate of carbohydrate oxidation were significantly greater with fructose than with glucose when given in a mixed meal with the same amounts of protein (20%) and lipids (33%). These results refuted the hypothesis that sucrose causes more weight gain than glucose or glucose polymers.

Protein

High-protein, low-carbohydrate diets have been used for many years and continue to be used in weight reducing regimens. The "reasoning" behind this choice was an old theory according to which proteins are characterized by high "specific dynamic action." This action would be responsible for nonspecific energy wasting. This action has been clearly demonstrated not to exist (Sims 1977). Reliable experimental studies on humans are not available, but studies in animals are very convincing.

Miller and Payne (1962) fed pigs with a low-protein diet. They observed the reduced energy efficiency of low-protein diet, which was subsequently shown to be linked to increased norepinephrine-induced thermogenetic activity (Rothwell et al. 1982). Thermogenetic studies on rats (Young et al. 1983) demonstrate that protein restriction can increase sympathetic nervous system activity.

The explanation of this phenomenon may be in the hypothesis that proteins are necessary for nitrogen balance and that they must be used only in order to do so. If a diet is poor in proteins and rich in other nutrients, principally carbohydrates, we observe an increase in wasted energy. If a diet is rich in proteins, surpassing requirements, it is obviously lacking in other nutrients and consequently less active at the thermogenetic level. The opposite effects that carbohydrates and proteins have on sympathetic nervous system activity, carbohydrates stimulating and proteins inhibiting, seem to confirm this hypothesis (Landsberg and Young 1984).

Lipids

Because of general agreement with the hypothesis that the amount of EE (basal or DIT) is positively related to the carbohydrate content of the diet, it is possible to conclude that dietary fats can reduce energy dissipating capacity.

Flatt and co-workers (Flatt et al. 1985) studied the effects of three breakfasts of different fat content on postprandial substrate oxidation in young healthy male students: (1) low-fat breakfast: 482 kcal, 27% protein, 62% carbohydrate, 11% fat; (2) high long-chain triglyceride fat breakfast: 858 kcal, 15% protein, 35% carbohydrate, 50% fat (50 g of long-chain triglyceride containing margarine); (3) high medium-chain triglyceride fat breakfast: 856 kcal, 15% protein, 35% carbohydrate, 50% fat (9 g of long-chain triglyceride and 41 g of medium-chain triglyceride margarine). The carbohydrate and protein amounts in the three meals were always the same: 75 g and 32 g respectively. During this 9-hour study the addition of fat to a fixed carbohydrate and protein content meal failed to bring about any increase in fat oxidation.

Hill and co-workers (Hill et al. 1989) tested the effects of overfeeding with medium-chain (MCT) versus long-chain triglycerides (LCT). Ten volunteers were overfed (150% of the estimated requirement) with a liquid formula diet containing 40% fat as either MCT or LCT. No differences were observed in RMR, but DIT was significantly greater in the MCT group (8% vs. 5.8%). The authors concluded that excess energy derived from MCT is stored with less efficiency than is excess energy derived from dietary LCT. Actually this research is quite different from the previous research, first because this is an overfeeding study while the other is an under-nutrition study and second because DIT was registered up until the sixth hour, while in the previously reported work up until the ninth hour. The Flatt and co-workers study with a MCT meal showed lower energy expenditure up until the fifth hour and subsequently higher than LCT. As a consequence the total thermogenic effects of MCT and LCT were similar.

Yost and Eckel (1989) studied the effects of an 800-kcal diet containing 24% calories as MCT and 6% as LCT versus an isocaloric diet containing 30% of calories as LCT. After a 12 week follow-up the amount of weight loss was similar.

Sepple and Read (1989) studied whether prefeeding lipids reduces food intake in normal weight subjects. They gave 300 ml of beef consommé with or without 60 mg of margarine followed, 20 minutes later, by either a low fat solid meal or a preselected appetizing meal. No effect on meal consumption nor on the sensation of hunger or satiation was observed. They also evaluated the effect of a high-fat (65 g), high-calorie (927 kcal) breakfast versus a low-fat (8.1 g), low-calorie (418 kcal) breakfast on a preselected appetizing lunch. Subjects who had high-fat breakfasts ate less at lunch than low-fat breakfast subjects (790 vs 1047 kcal), but total energy consumption was clearly higher in the first group.

Zed and James (1986) studied thermogenic response to fat overfeeding after low energy diet in obese and lean subjects. Fat overfeeding does lead to thermogenesis in excess of the minimum cost of fat storage; individuals with childhood-onset obesity also display metabolic differences when compared with lean subjects of comparable height and age. Subnormal thermogenic response to dietary fat supports the hypothesis that thermogenic response to high-fat diet is small in individuals with familial obesity.

Dietary Fiber

In the dietary fiber hypothesis lack of fiber is considered to be a possible factor in the genesis of obesity (Burkitt and Trowell 1975; Heaton 1973; Spiller 1986; Spiller and Amen 1976; Vahouny and Krichevsky 1986). Fiber is naturally contained in food and thus it is quite difficult to distinguish the effects of fiber from those of other fiber-containing foods. It is necessary to use a fiber-poor diet, subsequently adding fiber or a placebo. Despite these difficulties, a number of double-blind studies have been performed.

Walsh and co-workers, (Walsh et al. 1983) conducted an 8-week double-blind trial to test purified glucomannan as a food supplement (1 g 1 hour prior to three main meals) in obese subjects instructed not to deviate from their previously established eating patterns. Results showed a significant mean weight loss only in the fiber treated group.

Ryttig and co-workers completed a number of double-blind, placebo-controlled trials supporting the usefulness of fiber in weight reduction programs (Ryttig 1989). In Ryttig et al. 1989 they followed 97 mildly obese females for 52 weeks in a randomized, double-blind, placebo-controlled trial: dietary fiber (6–7 g/day: in tablets containing predominantly insoluble fiber) versus placebo. For 11 weeks both groups received a 1200 kcal diet, for 16 weeks a 1600 kcal diet, after this the placebo was withdrawn. Both groups received 6 g/day of fiber and an ad libitum diet was allowed. The fiber group lost more weight than the placebo group during the 1200 and 1600 kcal diet periods. Adherence to the treatment regime was significantly higher in the fiber group.

It is important to emphasize, in addition to the results discussed above, that fiber influences energy intake in other ways. By its very presence it can affect the physical qualities of a food and as a consequence the ease with which the food can be eaten (Heaton 1980). Differences in satiation may be due to different palatability rather than fiber content (Spitzer and Rodin 1981).

Mixed Meals

Lean and James (1988) studied the behavior of DIT in three groups of women: lean, obese, and postobese. Two isoenergetic diets were used: One was a high-fat (40%), low carbohydrate (45%) diet, the other a low-fat (3%), high-carbohydrate (82%) diet. The thermogenic effect of the high-carbohydrate diet was significantly greater than that of the high-fat diet (5.8% vs. 3.5% of the energy expenditure increase). Postobese subjects tended to have lower energy expenditure than controls when fasting and when high-fat fed, but this pattern was not shown by the obese. Sleeping energy expenditure was particularly depressed in postobese subjects when the high-fat diet was fed.

Lean and co-workers (Lean et al. 1989) studied the effects of overfeeding on the normal weight and moderately overweight postobese. Subjects were fed two baseline diets: low-fat (3% fat, 82% carbohydrate) and high-fat (40% fat, 45% carbohydrate), and then with the high-fat diet plus an extra calorie charge (50% over the amount required for energy balance) as carbohydrates. A significant increase in energy expenditure was observed only by adding extra carbohydrates to the baseline high-fat diet and only in postobese women. Carbohydrate overfeeding seems thus to increase energy expenditure only when given in a high-fat diet; furthermore, postobese subjects on high-fat diets appear more sensitive to carbohydrate supplementation than do controls as far as increased energy expenditure.

An extrapolation of these results (Lean and James 1988; Lean et al. 1989) is given in Figure 13-3. Meal carbohydrate content increases DIT over 24 hours especially in postobese subjects. Meal fat content negatively conditions sleeping metabolic rate only in postobese subjects.

Segal and co-workers (Segal et al. 1989) studied RMR and DIT after a 720-kcal mixed meal in four groups of subjects, two (obese vs. lean) matched for total body fat and two (heavier vs. lighter) matched for percent of body fat. After adjustment for differences in FFM among the four groups, no significant differences in RMR were observed. Furthermore no difference in DIT was observed between the heavier group and the lighter group when matched for body fat percentage, supporting the hypothesis that putative impaired thermogenesis in obesity is a function of relative fatness rather than body fat mass and confirming the hypothesis that RMR is determined by FFM and is not independently related to obesity.

De Palo and co-workers (De Palo et al. 1989) measured RMR and DIT in lean and obese subjects. They found similar values for RMR. However they encountered an increment in mixed-meal induced thermogenesis that was significantly greater in normal weight subjects (22% vs. 12%). Thermogenesis, after ingestion of a carbohydrate mixture, appeared slightly higher (not significant) in normal weight than in obese subjects.

Swaminathan and co-workers (Swaminathan et al. 1985) evaluated DIT induced by isocaloric (400 kcal) carbohydrate, fat, protein, and

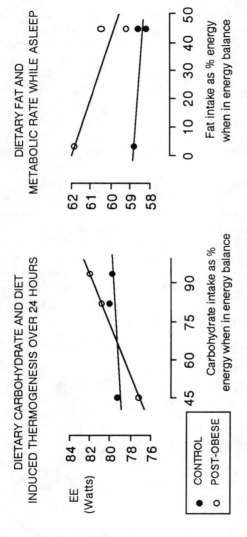

Figure 13-3. Relationships between dietary carbohydrate and diet-induced thermogenesis over 24 hours and between dietary fat and metabolic rate while asleep. Each point represents mean results of five subjects, calculated from the absolute increment in energy expenditure above fasting in relation to absolute carbohydrate or fat intake of individuals but converted to percent energy-balance for graphic presentation. Post-obese subjects showed a different relationship to controls ($p < 0.02$), with a significant increase in 24-hour energy expenditure in response to carbohydrate ($p < 0.01$). Dietary fat did not influence 24-hour EE in either group. Sleeping metabolic rate was not influenced by carbohydrate but showed an inverse relationship with dietary fat in the post-obese group ($p < 0.05$) (after Lean et al. 1989).

mixed meals in lean and obese subjects (Fig. 13–4). The thermogenetic response to the mixed meal was significantly lower in obese subjects when expressed as percentage increase (13% vs. 25%); moreover fat in-duced thermogenesis in obese subjects was dramatically reduced: no increment was observed in obese subjects (−1%) as compared to lean controls (14%). The authors observed a correlation between thermic re-sponse to fat and thermic response to mixed meal and as a consequence backed the Zed and James (1982) suggestion that the lower thermic re-sponse of obese subjects to a mixed meal is due to its fat content.

Jéquier (1989) emphasized that DIT was not found to be reduced in all obese individuals and that the thermic effect of glucose or meal inges-tion was mainly blunted in obese subjects with insulin resistance.

Increasing evidence indicates that low-fat, low-protein, high-carbo-hydrate diet could decrease the risk of onset of obesity owing to its ef-fects on energy dissipation capacity. Vegetarian communities are a good model to verify this hypothesis; in fact this kind of population permits us to verify the prevalence of obesity in subjects with different dietary habits but living in the same environment. Ophir and co-workers (Ophir et al. 1983) compared 98 randomly selected subjects of the Israeli Vege-tarian Association against 98 omnivorous controls living in the Tel Aviv urban area (Fig. 13–5). Results showed that overweight was more prev-alent in the control group. Armstrong and co-workers obtained similar results studying vegetarians (mainly Seventh-Day Adventists) in West-ern Australia (Armstrong et al. 1979). Thus there is evidence that vege-tarians are leaner than nonvegetarians and this phenomenon is espe-

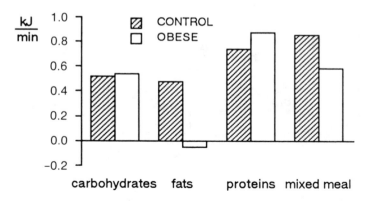

Figure 13–4.   Thermogenetic response to isocaloric (400 kcal) carbohydrate, fat, protein, and mixed meal in obese and nor-mal-weight subjects (after Swaminathan et al. 1985).

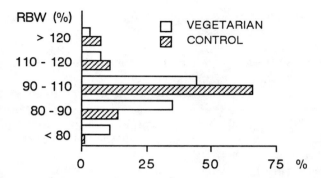

Figure 13-5.   Prevalence of vegetarian and omnivorous subjects for body weight relative to standard
weight classes (after Ophir et al. 1982).

cially evident among the strictest vegetarians, the vegans, who do not
consume animal foods at all, not even milk and eggs (Dwyer 1988).

Enhanced DIT in vegetarians could account for the reduced prevalence of obesity. Poehlman and co-workers (Poehlman et al. 1988) did
not confirm this hypothesis; they found a slightly lower DIT in vegetarians (percentage increase relative to the caloric load: 9%) in comparison
to nonvegetarians (11%). Actually, the difference was small; daily energy intake in vegetarians varied widely and only one subject among
vegetarians was vegan (consumer of no animal product). The rest consumed milk, or milk and eggs, or milk, eggs, and fish. On the other
hand vegetarians had lower body mass indexes and the same percent-
ages of body fat as omnivores. This work in any case failed to demonstrate that an elevated DIT is a contributing factor to the lower body
weight in vegetarians when compared with omnivores.

Conclusion

Total 24-hour energy expenditure, after weight reduction in obese subjects due to a hypocaloric diet, decreases by 20 to 25 kcal/day for each
kilogram of weight loss (Jéquier 1989). Failure to adapt everyday energy
intake to reduced energy needs will result in body weight gain and relapse of obesity.

Reduced DIT does not seem to be a constant feature of obesity:
Jéquier (1984) reported Dumset's observations that a defective thermogenic response to a meal was detectable in only 12 of 35 unselected

obese women. These were probably the subjects with the greatest hereditary trend toward obesity.

If obesity can, at least partially, be due to an inborn error, for example a *thrifty trait* (Neel 1962), epidemiological, clinical, and experimental results seem to indicate that a metabolic defect is linked to energy expenditure capacity in conditions where available energy exceeds energy requirements.

It may be then that certain foods can be "wrong" for obesity-prone subjects with specific metabolic defects. Blame falls increasingly on dietary fat (Lean et al. 1989).

In obesity, very little carbohydrate substance is converted into body fat and the composition of the fat in the adipose depot is similar to the fat of the diet. When entering the body fat stores, carbohydrate requires almost 25% of the starting calories; fat enters the fat stores at the cost of only 3% of the starting fat calories, indicating that fat is more *fattening* than carbohydrates (Danforth, 1989).

The use of a high-carbohydrate, low-fat diet is helpful in preventing obesity and for maintaining weight after weight loss. A high-fat diet could be a specific factor in manifesting a genetic predisposition to obesity. The Mediterranean diet by its very nature has the nutritional characteristics of a high-carbohydrate, low-fat diet and thus can be a good model for a general educational program aimed at the prevention of obesity.

COMPARISON OF DIETARY HABITS
IN DIFFERENT COUNTRIES

The Mediterranean Diet

Epidemiological studies of the 1980s have demonstrated the close links between eating habits and the incidence of degenerative and chronic pathology. These studies have shown that the populations around the Mediterranean basin have a lower incidence of cardiovascular pathologies compared to North American populations and that this advantage was even more accentuated in the southern regions of the Mediterranean. Life-style, especially the special alimentary habits of these areas, could explain this diversity. Identification of dietary practices based predominantly on bread, pasta, and unrefined foodstuffs, with little consumption of meats, characteristic of these regions, has led to recognition of the Mediterranean diet as being synonymous with healthful alimentary habits, ideal and extremely effective in preventing degenerative chronic pathologies.

Dietary Habits in Italy in the Early Twentieth Century

In 1929 the Italian National Research Center (CNR) conducted a study analyzing the dietary habits in Italy at the beginning of the century. This study was performed on a sample of families in six cities in different regions of Italy (Galeotti 1937). In 1960 EURATOM conducted another important study on a sampling of Italian and European families (Cresta et al. 1969). A comparison of results of the two studies shows that from the start of the century, but especially after the end of World War II, there has been a substantial change in dietary habits in Mediterranean countries. There has been (Fig. 13–6), in particular, an increase in con-

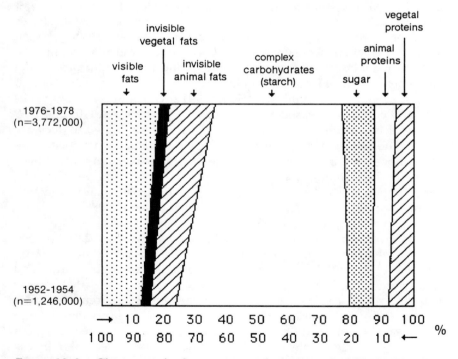

Figure 13–6. Changes in food consumption from the end of World War II in Mediterranean countries (after Cialta 1981).

sumption of meat, which quadrupled, and in refined sugar and *seasoning* fats, which have more than doubled, whereas consumption of grains remained unchanged or actually declined (Mariani Costantini 1977).

Modification of Dietary Habits in the United States During the Twentieth Century

On average, inhabitants of the United States have reduced their daily calorie intake from the beginning of the twentieth century to the present (Slattery and Randall 1988). This observation seems to be in disagreement with the observed significant increase in obesity. It is evident that the amount of daily caloric intake is not, by itself, the most important pathogenic element in the genesis of the overweight condition. After 1909 the United States saw a decrease in the relative contribution of calories from cereals and grain, which coincided with an increase in the use of sugar and syrups and fruits and vegetables. The percentage of total calories from fats also increased. The contribution of total calories from meat, fish, and poultry increased until the late 1960s when it started to level off. Consumption of dairy products increased until the 1950s when it began to decrease. Legumes and dry beans contributed a larger percentage of fat to the diet in 1980 than they did in 1909 although their contribution in terms of fat is small. Fat consumption from meat, fish, and poultry decreased in comparative terms between 1909 and 1959 after which it increased until the mid 1970s when it started to decrease again. The percentage of calories from fats remained unchanged: the consumption of butter and lard decreased and the consumption of margarine and shortening increased. Trends in animal and vegetable fat consumption showed a constant increase in vegetable fat and a constant decrease in animal fat after 1961 (Slattery and Randall 1988).

In men and women 19 to 50 years old, beef intake decreased by 35% and 45% respectively while poultry intake decreased by 22% and 8% respectively; whole milk consumption decreased by 25% and 35% respectively (Strata 1977). Conversely, intake of fish, vegetables, fruit, and low-fat milk has increased. In the final analysis it seems that dietary habits in the United States demonstrate a progressive trend toward a type of diet near that indicated by the *Dietary Goals of Americans* (Uemura and Pisa 1985). The improvement in dietary habits enacted in recent years in the United States corresponds to a significant reduction in risk factors, and above all in blood cholesterol levels, which marked a decrease in the incidence of cardiovascular pathologies. This phenomenon seems a long way from taking place in the Mediterranean regions.

Changes in the Diet in the Mediterranean Area

Dietary habits in the Mediterranean basin countries have undergone continuing and radical change in the 1980s. The "poor" diet of the first decades of the century, and especially immediately after the Second World War, has gradually changed to align with the diets of North America and northern Europe (see also chapter 1). The Seven Country Study, begun at the end of the 1950s, permits us to follow and evaluate the changes in the dietary habits of the seven countries examined and at the same time examine correlations between eating habits and cardio-vascular pathologies (Kromhout et al. 1989).

Greece, Italy, and Yugoslavia represent the Mediterranean basin countries in this study, and although they differ markedly economically, politically, and culturally, they constitute excellent elements for comparing dietary habit changes in the years following World War II. Since the mid-1960s dietary habits have changed greatly in all the countries examined. In Holland (city of Zutphen) the consumption of meat, fruit, and pastries has increased whereas that of bread, potatoes, milk products, and edible fats has decreased. Conversely in the Italian cohorts (Crevalcore and Montegiorgio) the consumption of fruit has increased and that of cereals and legumes has declined. In Montegiorgio an increase of the intake of milk, cheese, and meat was observed. In the two cohorts of Greece olive oil intake decreased and the intake of alcohol increased. In Yugoslavia the consumption of vegetables, fruit, meat, eggs, edible fats, and sugar has increased. In conclusion the differences in food consumption patterns among the countries examined have lessened during the past 25 years.

It is believed that the present-day average caloric intake by the Italian population exceeds the recommended level by about 1000 kcal/day. The current dietary pattern in Italy is characterized by a rapid evolution from what used to be a low-fat, low-animal protein, low-cholesterol, high-fiber diet toward a diet with a high contribution of fat to total energy, high saturation of dietary fats, high cholesterol and animal protein, and low dietary fiber. Mediterranean countries have moved from a diet based on cereal, vegetables, and olive oil toward a diet rich in meat and cheese: from the Mediterranean diet toward the Western diet (North European and North American).

These changes in alimentary habits are certainly caused by more than one factor. Contributing factors include a more affluent lifestyle, seen both in economic terms and in terms of increased demand for well-being, the increased availability of fast foods, and a greater variety of foods on the market.

Another important factor is an increasingly fast lifestyle, deriving undoubtedly from North American models, that has inevitably made it necessary to reduce the amount of time available for the traditional midday meal. The new work, cultural, and managerial inputs coming from North America have not been counterbalanced by the capacity to preserve a proper approach to nutrition. Mediterranean populations have quite simply adopted both positive and negative aspects of the American culture.

INTERVENTION

The most obvious nutritional anomaly of so-called Western culture is the high caloric content of the diet. Furthermore, in comparison to the accepted nutritional recommendations for healthier diets, there are striking differences in fat and carbohydrate consumption.

Consumption of fat, particularly fat derived from animal food, is almost twice as great as the recommended amount: this dietary error is the most significant of the western diet. Such a "rich" diet results in an increased incidence of obesity, diabetes, and vascular arteriosclerotic diseases (Guthrie 1987; Shiels and Young 1988).

The increased risk for some neoplastic diseases is also correlated to nutritional mistakes. Thus, correction of these errors by suitable dietetic measures is mandatory if progress is to be made in preventing nutrition-related diseases.

It is obvious that on these foundations and on what has been written in the other chapters in this book, the best diet to prevent and to correct obesity is a diet that is low in protein and fat, with high carbohydrate and fiber content. Intervention on diet composition must aim at modifying the typical Western diet, rich in animal food, to that typical of Mediterranean dietary habits based on consumption of food of plant origin.

SUMMARY

Current knowledge of human obesity has progressed beyond the simple generalizations of the past: Studies of obese subjects rarely show that they eat more than their lean counterparts.

The availability of food is undoubtedly a fundamental factor, but obesity was and is extremely rare in nations even where there is no scarcity of foodstuffs. Changes in lifestyle such as diet, physical activity, smoking, and socioeconomic status can have varying effects on the increase of the incidence of obesity. Epidemiological studies dating from the early 1960s noted that the incidence of overweight and obesity in countries of the Mediterranean area was less than that of other industrialized nations. This factor was related to a Mediterranean advantage, which was primarily linked to a special type of diet as well as to a particular life-style. Ironically, Mediterranean countries have undergone a Western-izing trend, acquiring eating habits taken directly from North American nations. The "poor" diet of the first decades of the century, and especially immediately after World War II, has gradually changed. Mediterranean countries have moved from a diet based on cereals, vegetables, and olive oil toward a diet rich in meat and cheese, from the Mediterranean diet toward the Western-style diet. Consequently, the incidence of obesity in Mediterranean countries is increasing.

If obesity can be, at least partially, due to heredity, for example a "thrifty" trait, epidemiological, clinical, and experimental results seem to indicate that a metabolic defect is linked to energy expenditure capacity in conditions where available energy exceeds energy requirements. It may be that certain foods can be wrong for obesity-prone subjects with specific metabolic defects. Dietary fat is increasingly incriminated: Fat is more fattening than carbohydrates.

Contributing factors include a rise in standard of living, seen both in economic terms and in increased expectation for physical well-being, the increased availability of fast foods, and a greater variety offered by food markets. Another important factor is an increasingly fast life-style, deriving undoubtedly from North American models. This has inevitably made it necessary to reduce the amount of time available for the traditional midday meal.

The most obvious nutritional anomaly of the Western world is the high consumption of foods from animal sources. In comparison to the nutritional guidelines there are striking differences in fat and carbohydrate contents. Consumption of fat is too high and that of vegetable foods is too low. This is the most important and significant dietary error of the Western diet.

Intervention in diet composition must aim at modifying the usual Western high animal-fat diet to approach the Mediterranean high vegetable-carbohydrate diet. An important role in modifying population dietary trends can be played by an educated mass media. They could help publicize the results of nutritional studies and encourage promotion by food manufacturers of the desirable foods of the Mediterranean diet.

REFERENCES

Acheson, K. J., Y. Schultz, T. Bessard, E. Ravussin, E. Jéquier, and J. P. Flatt. 1984. Nutritional influences on lipogenesis and thermogenesis after a carbohydrate meal. *Am. J. Physiol.* **246**:E62–70.

Apfelbaum, M. 1976. The effects of very restrictive high protein diets. *Clin. Endocrinol. Metabol.* **5**:417–430.

Apfelbaum, M., J. Bostsarran, and D. Lacatis. 1971. Effect of caloric restriction and excessive caloric intake on energy expenditure. *Am. J. Clin. Nutr.* **24**:1405–1409.

Armstrong, B., H. Clarke, C. Martin, W. Ward, N. Norman, and J. Masarei. 1979. Urinary sodium and blood pressure in vegetarians. *Am. J. Clin. Nutr.* **32**:2472–2476.

Bandini, L. G., D. A. Schoeller, J. Edwards, V. R. Young, S. H. Oh, and W. H. Dietz. 1989. Energy expenditure during carbohydrate overfeeding in obese and nonobese adolescents. *Am. J. Physiol. Endocrinol. Metabol.* **256**:E357–367.

Barrows, K., and J. T. Snook. 1987. Effect of a high-protein, very-low-calorie diet on resting metabolism, thyroid hormones, and energy expenditure of obese middle-aged women. *Am. J. Clin. Nutr.* **45**:391–398.

Bosello, O., F. Ferrari, M. Tonon, M. Cigolini, R. Micciolo, and M. Renoffio. 1981. Serum thyroid hormone concentration during semistarvation and physical exercise. *Hormone Metabol. Res.* **13**:651–652.

Bosello, O., F. Armellini, E. Arosio, L. Cominacini, T. Todesco, M. Zamboni, and I. Zocca. 1989. Contributi allo studio dei fattori di rischio nutrizionale. *Atti dell 89° Congresso della Societa Italiana di Medicina Interna*, pp. 443–465. Rome: Pozzi.

Bray, G. A., M. B. Davison, and E. Drenik. 1972. Obesity a serious symptom. *Ann. Int. Med.* **77**:792.

Burger, A. G. 1981. General comments on tissue sensitivity to thyroid hormones in starvation. *Int. J. Obesity* **5**(Suppl. 1):69–71.

Burkitt, D. P., and H. C. Trowell. 1975. *Refined Carbohydrate Food and Disease. Some Implications of Dietary Fiber.* London: Academic Press.

Cairella, M., L. Godi, and M. Pelegrino. 1988. Osservazioni sulla prevalenza regionale dell obesita in Italia. *Clin. Diet.* **15**:243–249.

Cavallo, E., F. Armellini, M. Zamboni, R. Vicentini, M. P. Milani, and O. Bosello. 1990. Resting metabolic rate, body composition and thyroid hormones; short term effects of very low calorie diet. *Hormone Metabol. Res.* **22**:632–635.

Cialta, E., and A. Mariani Costantini. 1981. Situazione ed evoluzione del consumi alimentari in Italia. In *Nutrizione Umana*, F. Fidanza and G. Liguori, eds., 390–407. Naples: Idelson.

CNR (Gruppo di Ricerca CNR-ATS-RF2) 1980. I fattori di Rischio dell aterosclerosi in Italia: La fase A del Progetto CNR-RF2. *G. It. Cardiol.* (suppl. 3):10.

Cresta, M., S. Ledermann, A. Garnier, E. Lombardo, and G. Lacourly. 1969. *Etude des consommations alimentaires des populations de onze régions de la communanté européenne en vue de la détermination des niveaux de contamination radioactive.* Rapport établi au Centre d'Etude Nucléaire de Fontenay-Aux-Roses, France: EURATOM, Commissariat à l'énergie atomique (CEA).

Danforth, E., Jr. 1985. Diet and obesity. *Am. J. Clin. Nutr.* **41**:1132–1149.

Danforth, E., Jr. 1989. Obesity and Thermogenesis. In *Diabetes 1988*, R. Larkins, P. Zimmet, and D. Chisholm, eds., pp. 308–305. New York: Elsevier.

De Boer, J. O., A. J. H. van Es. J. M. A. van Raaji, and J. G. Hautvast. 1987. Energy requirements and energy expenditure of lean and overweight women, measured by indirect calorimetry. *Am. J. Clin. Nutr.* **46**:13–21.

De Palo, C., C. Macor, N. Sicolo, R. Vettor, C. Scandelarri, and G. Federspil. 1989. Dietary-induced thermogenesis in obesity. Response to mixed and carbohydrate meals. *Acta Diabetol. Lat.* **26**:155–162.

Duncan, K. H., J. A. Bacon, and R. L. Weinsier. 1983. The effects of high and low energy density diets on satiety, energy intake and eating time of obese and nonobese subjects. *Am. J. Clin. Nutr.* **37**:763–767.

Dwyer, J. 1988. Health aspects of vegetarian diets. *Am. J. Clin. Nutr.* **48**:712–738.

Elliot, D. L., L. Goldberg, K. S. Kuehel, and W. M. Bennett. 1989. Sustained depression of the resting metabolic rate after massive weight loss. *Am. J. Clin. Nutr.* **49**:93–96.

Finer, N., P. C. Swan, and F. T. Mitchell. 1986. Metabolic rate after massive weight loss in human obesity. *Clin. Science* **70**:395–398.

Flatt, J. P., E. Ravussin, K. J. Acheson, and E. Jéquier. 1985. Effects of dietary fat on postprandial substrate oxidation and on carbohydrate and fat balances. *J. Clin. Invest.* **76**:1019–1024.

Galeotti, G. 1937. Primi risultati dell'inchiesta alimentare condotta in varie province d'Italia. *Quaderni della Nutrizione* **1**:1.

Garrow, J. S. 1974. *Energy Balance and Obesity in Man.* Amsterdam: Elsevier/North Holland.

Gillie, O., and S. Raby. 1984. *The Sunday Times ABC Diet and Bodyplan.* London: Hutchinson.

Girardier, L., and M. J. Stock. 1983. *Mammalian Thermogenesis.* London: Chapman & Hall.

Goldblatt, P., M. Moore, and A. J. Stunkard. 1965. Social factors in obesity. *JAMA* **192**:97–102.

Guthrie, H. A. 1987. *Introduction Nutrition.* St. Louis: Times Mirror/Mosby College.

Hammer, R. L., C. A. Barrier, E. S. Roundy, J. M. Bradford, and A. G. Fisher. 1989. Calorie-restricted low-fat diet and exercise in obese women. *Am. J. Clin. Nutr.* **49**:77–85.

Heaton, K. W. 1973. Food fiber as an obstacle to energy intake. *Lancet* **ii**:1418–1421.

Heaton, K. W. 1980. Food intake regulation and fiber. In *Medical Aspects of Dietary Fiber,* G. A. Spiller and R. M. Kay, eds., pp. 223–238. New York: Plenum.

Hendler, R. G., M. Walesky, and R. S. Sherwin. 1983. Isocaloric sucrose replacement reverses the fall in basal metabolic rate induced by hypocaloric feeding. *Clin. Res.* **31**:465 (abstr).

Hill, J. O., J. C. Peters, D. Yang, T. Sharp, M. Kaler, N. N. Abumrad, and H. L. Greene. 1989. Thermogenesis in humans during overfeeding with medium-chain triglycerides. *Metabol. Clin. Exp.* **38**:641–648.

James, P. 1985. Obesity: the interaction of environment and genetic predisposition. In *Dietary Fibre, Fibre Depleted Foods and Disease,* H. Trowell, D. Burkitt, and K. Heaton, eds., pp. 249–262. London: Academic Press.

Jéquier, E. 1984. Energy expenditure in obesity. *Clin. Endocrinol. Metabol.* **13**:563–580.

Jéquier, E. 1989. Energy metabolism in human obesity. *Soz. Praventivmed.* **34**:58–62.

Keys, A., C. Aravonis, H. W. Blackburn, F. S. Van Buchem, R. Buzina, B. Djordjevic, A. S. Dontas, F. Fidanza, N. Kimura, D. Lekos, M. Monci, V. Puddu, and H. Taylor. 1966. Epidemiological studies related to coronary heart disease: characteristics of men aged 40–59 in seven countries. *Acta Med. Scand.* **460**(suppl.):1–392.

Kromhout, D., A. Keys, C. Buzina, F. Findanza, S. Giampaoli, A. Jansen, A. Menotti, S. Nedeljkovic, M. Pekkarinen, B. Simic, and H. Toshima. 1989.

Food consumption patterns in the 1960s in seven countries. *Am. J. Clin. Nutr.* **49**:889–894.

Landsberg, L. L., and J. B. Young. 1984. The role of the sympathoadrenal system in modulating energy expenditure. *Clin. Endocrinol. Metab.* **13**:475–499.

Lara-Pantin, E. 1986. Obesity in developing countries. In *Recent Advances in Obesity Research: V,* E. M. Berry, S. H. Blondheim, H. E. Eliahou, and E. Shafrir, eds., pp. 5–8. London: John Libbey.

Laurenzi, M., R. Stamler, M. Trevisan, A. Dyer, and J. Stamler. 1989. Is Italy losing the Mediterranean advantage? Report on the Gubbio population study; cardiovascular risk factors at baseline. *Prev. Med.* **18**:35–44.

Lean, M. E. J., and W. P. James. 1988. Metabolic effects of isoenergetic nutrient exchange over 24 hours in relation to obesity in women. *Int. J. Obesity* **12**:15–27.

Lean, M. E. J., W. P. T. James, and P. H. Garthwaite. 1989. Obesity without overeating? Reduced diet-induced thermogenesis in postobese women, dependent on carbohydrate and not fat intake. In *Obesity in Europe 88,* P. Björntorp and S. Rössner, eds., pp. 281–286. London: John Libbey.

Lenzi, S., G. Descovic, and G. Mannino. 1981. The Brisighella Study. In *Atherosclerosis: Clinical Evaluation and Therapy,* S. Lenzi and G. Descovich, eds., pp. 357–366. Lancaster: MIT Press Limited.

Mariani Costantini, A. 1977. Profilo e motivazioni dell attuale comportamento alimentare degli Italiani. In *Atti della Conferenza Nazionale per l'Educazione Alimentare,* p. 35. Rome: Istituto Nazionale per la Nutrizione-Ministero dell Agricoltura e delle Foreste.

Matzen, L. E., and J. Kvetny. 1989. The influence of caloric deprivation and food composition on TSH, thyroid hormones and nuclear binding of T3 in mononuclear blood cells in obese women. *Metabolism* **38**:555–561.

Miller, D. S., and P. R. Payne. 1962. Weight-maintenance and food intake. *J. Nutr.* **78**:255–262.

National Institutes of Health Consensus-Development Conference Statement. 1985. Health Implication of Obesity. *Ann. Int. Med.* **103**:147–151.

Neel, J. V. 1962. Diabetes mellitus: a "thrifty" genotype rendered detrimental by "progress"? *Am. J. Human Gen.* **14**:353–362.

Ophir, O., G. Peer, J. Gilad, M. Blum, and A. Aviram. 1983. Low blood pressure in vegetarians: the possible role of potassium. *Am. J. Clin. Nutr.* **37**:755–762.

Oscai, L. B., and W. C. Miller. 1986. Dietary-induced severe obesity: exercise implications. *Med. Sci. Sports Exerc.* **18**:6–9.

Poehlman, E. T., P. J. Arciero, C. L. Melby, and S. F. Badylak. 1988. Resting metabolic rate and postprandial thermogenesis in vegetarians and nonvegetarians. *Am. J. Clin. Nutr.* **48**:209–213.

Ravussin, E., B. Burnand, Y. Schultz, and E. Jéquier. 1982. Twenty-four-hour energy expenditure and resting metabolic rate in obese, moderately obese and control subjects. *Am. J. Clin. Nutr.* **35**:566–573.

Ravussin, E., B. Burnand, Y. Schultz, and E. Jéquier. 1985. Energy expenditure before and during energy restriction in obese patients. *Am. J. Clin. Nutr.* **41**:753–759.

Riumallo, J. A., D. Scholler, G. Barrera, V. Gattas, and R. Uauy. 1989. Energy expenditure in underweight free-living adults: impact of energy supplementation as determined by doubly labeled water and direct calorimetry. *Am. J. Clin. Nutr.* **49**:239–246.

Rose, G. A., and R. T. William. 1961. Metabolic studies on large and small eaters. *Br. J. Nutr.* **15**:1-5.

Rothwell, N. J., M. J. Stock, and R. S. Tyzbir. 1982. Energy balance and mitochondrial function in liver and brown fat of rats fed "cafeteria" diets of varying protein content. *J. Nutr.* **112**:1663-1672.

Ryttig, K. R. 1989. Treatment of the mild and moderate overweight with dietary fiber. In *Obesity in Europe 88*, P. Björntorp and S. Rössner, eds., pp. 339-342. London: John Libbey.

Ryttig, K. R., G. Telines, L. Haegh, E. Boe, and H. Fagerthun. 1989. A dietary fiber supplement and weight maintenance after weight reduction: a randomized, double-blind, placebo-controlled long-term trial. *Int. J. Obesity* **13**:165-171.

Schutz, Y., J. Acheson, and E. Jéquier. 1985. Twenty-four-hour energy expenditure and thermogenesis: response to progressive carbohydrate overfeeding in man. *Int. J. Obesity* **9**(Suppl. 2):111-114.

Schwarz, J. M., Y. Schutz, F. Froidevaux, K. J. Acheson, N. Jeanpretre, H. Schneider, J. P. Felber, and E. Jéquier. 1989. Thermogenesis in men and women induced by fructose vs. glucose added to a meal. *Am. J. Clin. Nutr.* **49**:667-674.

Segal, K. R., I. Lacayanga, A. Dunaif, B. Gutin, and F. X. Pi Sunyer. 1989. Impact of body fat mass and percent fat on metabolic rate and thermogenesis in men. *Am. J. Physiol. Endocrinol. Metabol.* **256**:E573-579.

Sepple, C. P., and N. W. Read. 1989. The effect of pre-feeding lipid on food intake and satiety in humans. In *Obesity in Europe 88*, P. Björntorp and S. Rössner, eds., pp. 153-156. London: John Libbey.

Sharief, N. N., and I. Macdonald. 1982. Differences in dietary induced thermogenesis with various carbohydrates in normal and overweight men. *Am. J. Clin. Nutr.* **35**:267-272.

Sims, E. A. H. 1977. Obesità sperimentale, termogenesi dietetica e loro implicazioni cliniche. In *Obesità*, M. J. Albrink, ed., pp. 100-126. Rome: Pensiero Scientifico.

Sims, E. A. H., E. Danforth, Jr., E. S. Horton, G. A. Bray, J. A. Glennon, and L. B. Salans. 1973. Endocrine and metabolic effects of experimental obesity in man. *Rec. Prog. Hor. Res.* **29**:457-496.

Slattery, M., and E. Randall. 1988. Trend in coronary heart mortality and food consumption in the United States between 1909 and 1980. *Am. J. Clin. Nutr.* **47**:1060-1067.

Spiller, G. A. 1986. *Handbook of Dietary Fiber in Human Nutrition*. Boca Raton: CRC Press.

Spiller, G. A., and R. J. Amen. 1976. *Fiber in Human Nutrition*. New York: Plenum Press.

Spitzer, L., and J. Rodin. 1981. Human eating behaviour: a critical review of studies in normal weight and overweight individuals. *Appetite* **2**:293-329.

Stokholm, K. M., T. Andersen, and P. Lindgreen. 1987. Low serum free T3 concentrations in postobese patients previously treated with very-low-calorie diet. *Int. J. Obesity* **11**:85-92.

Strata, A. 1977. Epidemiologia dell'obesità. In *L'Obesità*, L. A. Scuro, A. Strata, P. Björntorp, O. Bosello, R. Vecchioni, and W. Montorsi, eds., pp. 9-25. Rome: Pozzi.

Swaminathan, R., R. F. G. J. King, J. Holmfield, R. A. Siwek, M. Baker, and J.

K. Wales. 1985. Thermic effect of feeding carbohydrate, fat, protein and mixed meal in lean and obese subjects. *Am. J. Clin. Nutr.* **42**:177–181.

Trowell, H. 1975. Diabetes mellitus and obesity. In *Refined Carbohydrate Foods and Disease*, H. Trowell and D. Burkitt, eds., pp. 227–289. London: Academic Press.

Trowell, H., D. Burkitt, and K. Heaton. 1985. *Dietary Fibre, Fibre Depleted Foods and Disease.* London: Academic Press.

Uemura, K., and Z. Pisa. 1985. Recent trends in cardiovascular disease mortality in 27 industrialized countries. *World Health Stat. Quart.* **38**:142–162.

U.S. Department of Agriculture. 1962. *Consumption of food in the U.S. 1909–1952*, (Agricultural handbook 62 supplement). Washington D.C.: U.S. Government Printing Office.

U.S. Public Health Service, Division of Chronic Disease. 1966. *Obesity and Health, A Source of Current Information for Professional Health Personnel.* Public Health Service Publication no. 1485. Washington, D.C.: U.S. Government Printing Office.

Vahouny, G.V., and D. Krichevsky. 1986. *Dietary Fiber. Basic and Clinical Aspects.* New York: Plenum Press.

Van Sonsbeek, J. L. A. 1985. The Dutch by height and weight, differences in height and under- and overweight in adults. *Maandbericht Gezandheidsstatist* **6**:5–18.

Waaler, H. Th. 1984. Height, weight and mortality: the Norwegian experience. *Acta Med. Scand.* **679**(suppl.):56.

Walsh, D. E., V. Vaghoubian, and A. Behforooz. 1983. Effect of glucomannan on obese patients: a clinical study. *Int. J. Obesity* **8**:289–293.

West, K. M. 1978. *Epidemiology of Diabetes and Its Vascular Lesions.* New York: Elsevier.

Yost, T. J., and R. H. Eckel. 1989. Hypocaloric feeding in obese women: metabolic effects of medium-chain triglycerides substitution. *Am. J. Clin. Nutr.* **49**:326–330.

Young, J. B., M. E. Saville, and L. Landsberg. 1983. Increased sympathetic (SNS) activity (norepinephrine turnover) in rats fed a low protein diet: evidence against a role for dietary tyrosine. *Clin. Res.* **31**:466A.

Yudkin, J. 1972. *Pure white and deadly. The Problem of Sugar.* London: Davis-Poynter.

Zed, C. A., and W. P. T. James. 1982. Thermic response to fat feeding in lean and obese subjects. *Proc. Nutr. Soc.* **41**:32A.

Zed, C. A., and W. P. T. James. Dietary thermogenesis in obesity: fat feeding at different energy intakes. *Int. J. Obesity* **10**:375–390.

14

Diabetes

Gabriele Riccardi
Angela Rivellese

The prevalence of non-insulin-dependent diabetes mellitus is very different throughout the world: It is particularly high in Western industrialized countries—the so-called affluent societies—whereas it is low in less industrialized and less wealthy countries, such as India, South America, and rural Africa. Furthermore, the incidence of diabetes sharply increased in some populations, such as the Indian tribes living in North America or the aborigines of Oceania, who were forced to a rather abrupt change in life-style as a consequence of the so-called civilization process (West 1978; WHO 1985). These populations had to adapt themselves to a new social and economic situation and, among other things, to a radical change in dietary habits. The consumption of natural unrefined foods (particularly rich in dietary fiber) declined and these people were rapidly exposed to the so-called Western diet, poor in complex carbohydrate and dietary fiber, and rich in fat, especially saturated fat. Such examples indicate that there is a close relationship between life-style, including dietary habits, and the risk of diabetes.

The Mediterranean diet is usually considered as a typical example of a healthy diet. People living in the Mediterranean region are reported to be at a particularly low risk to develop the most common degenerative diseases of the industrialized populations (coronary heart disease, cancer, etc.). Therefore, it would be of interest to gain information on the prevalence of diabetes in the Mediterranean countries in order to verify whether the Mediterranean diet is also protective with respect to the development of diabetes. Unfortunately, this task is not easy: Information on the prevalence of diabetes in the Mediterranean region is mostly anecdotal since we still lack properly designed studies. In fact, although the Seven Countries Study was able to demonstrate that the consumption of a typical Mediterranean diet, low plasma cholesterol levels and low incidence of cardiovascular disease are associated, it did not consider evaluating the incidence of diabetes.

However, even if no direct evidence proves that the Mediterranean diet protects against the development of diabetes, there are clear indications (from cross-cultural comparisons and from studies on vegetarians) that some of the most important characteristics of the Mediterranean diet—namely, the high intake of complex carbohydrate and dietary fiber and the low intake of saturated fat—may be beneficial in reducing the risk of diabetes.

The Mediterranean diet is rapidly changing. Under the effect of industrialization and/or the economic development of most Mediterranean countries, people have slowly abandoned their traditional eating habits for a diet more similar to that of other industrialized countries. This change is particularly true in large cities since the rural areas are more resistant to the effects of modernization.

Therefore, the Mediterranean diet we refer to is the type of diet consumed in the rural areas of most Mediterranean countries up to 20–30 years ago and which still has a strong influence on the present eating habits of the populations living in this region.

EPIDEMIOLOGY

Is There a Link Between Dietary Habits and Prevalence of Diabetes?

The hypothesis that differences in the prevalence of diabetes among various populations can be partly explained by dietary habits has been strongly supported by West (1974). He evaluated the prevalence of diabetes in eight selected populations (Bangor, Pennsylvania; Uruguay; Venezuela; Nicaragua; Guatemala; El Salvador; Malaya; and East Pakistan), and the results indicated a strong inverse correlation between the prevalence of diabetes and the percentage of calories deriving from carbohydrate. The highest prevalence of diabetes was found in Pennsylvania, where there was a low consumption of carbohydrate (40% of total calories), and the lowest was in East Pakistan, where the typical diet is characterized by a very high intake of carbohydrate (more than 80% of total calories). In this survey the fiber consumption of the different populations was not analyzed. However, a further examination of the diet of these populations has shown that in Pennsylvania nearly 30% of dietary energy derives from low-fiber white flour, and this leads us to speculate that almost the total amount of carbohydrates consumed in Pennsylvania (40% of energy) is represented by foods depleted of fiber. On the other hand, in East Pakistan nearly 70% of the calories is obtained by whole wheat, leguminous seeds, and vegetables. Therefore, in this study the inverse relationship between prevalence of diabetes and the percentage of calories derived from dietary carbohydrate is largely accounted for by the consumption of foods with a high carbohydrate and fiber content.

Historical data supporting the role of high-carbohydrate, high-fiber diets as a protective factor for the development of diabetes are very informative.

- Diabetes emerged as a common disease in India about 2000 years ago, along with the beginning of the production of white rice, which is low in dietary fiber (Trowell, 1981).
- Trowell (1981) reported no case of diabetes in Kenya during his stay there between 1929 and 1935; today diabetes is becoming common throughout all of East Africa at the same rate of the acquisition of lifestyles typical of the Western world.
- Trowell (1981) observed that the inhabitants of some African regions had low levels of fasting blood glucose and insulin and also a low incidence of diabetes; this was in relation with the consumption of a diet rich in lightly processed maize or in millet meal, both of which are very high in dietary fiber.
- In England in 1941–1942 mortality rates for diabetes in both sexes began to fall and continued to fall regularly until 1954–1955. The drop was about 55% for both men and women. These years (from 1942 to 1955) coincided with the so-called National Flour period, when it was mandatory to use only the national high-fiber flour instead of the white low-fiber flour generally imported from other countries. After 1954–1955 and the reintroduction of white flour, mortality rates for diabetes started to rise again.

The possibility that another feature of the Mediterranean diet, the low intake of fat (particularly saturated fat), might protect against the development of non-insulin-dependent diabetes has been suggested in some studies, but it deserves further evaluation. Most traditional diets associated with a low prevalence of diabetes are not only rich in fiber and carbohydrates but are also low in total and saturated fat. High fat intake might be associated with an increased risk of developing diabetes, since fat consumption can favor the development of obesity (which predisposes to diabetes) and can induce insulin resistance.

Studies of Vegetarians

The number of vegetarians is increasing all over the world. Their diet is based on the more or less complete avoidance of proteins derived from animal sources and by a very strong preference for cereals, legumes, and vegetables.

In the last few years some studies on the incidence of diabetes and other typical Western diseases in vegetarians have been completed. Studies on Seventh-Day Adventists have provided some very interesting data. The members of this religious group are encouraged by their church to avoid the consumption of meat, fish, eggs, alcohol, coffee, and tobacco; therefore, the majority of them can be considered real vegetarians. The rate of diabetes as an underlying cause of death in this group is half that of other white Americans. Within the male Adventist population, typical vegetarians present a significantly lower risk of developing diabetes with respect to those eating meat products only occasionally (Snowdon and Phillips 1985). Therefore, also within this selected population, eating behavior, characterized by a high intake of food rich in carbohydrates and fiber and by a low consumption of fat and protein, seems to be associated with a lower risk of developing diabetes.

Diet and Diabetes Complications

The major cause of death in diabetic patients is represented by cardiovascular disease. These patients are at increased risk to develop atherosclerotic complications in the heart, brain, and lower limbs compared to nondiabetic individuals.

A recent study has addressed the question of whether cardiovascular diseases in diabetic patients are influenced by life-style. Representative groups of diabetic patients were recruited in different countries worldwide, and a standardized assessment of cardiovascular disease was performed (Diabetes Drafting Group, 1985). The results of this study show that the prevalence of cardiovascular disease is not at all uniform in the different diabetic groups. Indeed, it can be up to 10 times higher in patients from northern Europe or from the Unites States as compared with those living in Asia or in Mediterranean Europe. The diet certainly does play a major role in explaining these differences since the prevalence of cardiovascular diseases is almost uniformly high in the diabetic groups living in countries where the consumption of saturated fat is high and the intake of carbohydrate and fiber-rich foods is low. This concept is further underlined by studies on immigrants, which show that in Japanese diabetic patients living in the United States the prevalence of cardiovascular diseases is much higher than in diabetics living in Japan (Kawate et al. 1979).

INTERVENTION

Diabetes mellitus represents a major health problem. In many Western populations the prevalence of this disease is above 5%. In some ethnic groups who have changed their traditional life-style into a typical Western one, it can be as high as 25% (WHO 1985).

In Western countries cardiovascular disease represents the leading cause of death for diabetic patients. Its importance has increased steadily in recent years and will increase even more in the future correspondingly with our ability to prevent or treat gangrene, metabolic complications, and renal failure in diabetic patients.

The objectives in the management of diabetes are not only to preserve the lives of patients and to relieve symptoms but also to try to avoid or retard the occurrence of diabetic complications by keeping the patients in good metabolic control and by correcting carviovascular risk factors, all possibly achieved without interfering with a normal social life.

Diet is still the cornerstone for treating diabetes. It represents the main treatment for non-insulin-dependent diabetes (the only treatment for many patients), and it plays a crucial role in the management of insulin dependent diabetes.

The principles on which diets for diabetics should be based recently have been illustrated in documents issued by authoritative bodies interested in this disease (Table 14–1) (American Diabetes Association 1987; National Institutes of Health 1987; DNSG 1988). Although controversies on some aspects of the nutritional management of diabetes still exist, a substantial agreement has been reached on most of the basic principles. Contrary to previous beliefs the composition of the diet for insulin dependent and non-insulin-dependent patients is, in general, the same. Moreover, the diet for diabetes closely resembles the type of diet usually advised to populations at high risk for cardiovascular disease. This simplifies dietary prescription and is, therefore, likely to improve compliance.

Considering the distribution of nutrients indicated by these recommendations, it is clear that the basic measure is represented by a reduced intake of total fat and, in particular, of saturated fat ($< 10\%$ of total energy intake). This recommendation is considered of paramount importance by all the experts since diabetic patients are exceedingly prone to atherosclerosis. Therefore, dietary measures must be primarily

TABLE 14-1. Dietary Recommendations for the Treatment of Diabetes

	ADA (1987)	NIH (1987)	DNSG (1988)
Energy	↓	↓	↓
Protein	10–15%	15–50%	↓
Fat	<30%	—	<30%
saturated	<10%	—	<10%
monounsaturated	7%	—	10%
polyunsaturated	13%	—	10%
Cholesterol	<300 mg/day	—	<300 mg/day
Complex CHO	60%	—	50–60%
Sucrose	moderate	<10 g/day	<30 g/day
Fiber	25 g/kcal	—	20 g/kcal
Alcohol	<10 g/day	—	<15 g/day

ADA = American Diabetes Association; NIH = National Institutes of Health; DNSG = Diabetes and Nutrition Study Group of the European Association for the Study of Diabetes.

aimed at cardiovascular disease prevention. A decrease in fat consumption (total fat <30% and saturated fat <10%) has to be necessarily coupled with an increase in the intake of complex carbohydrates (50–60% of total energy intake); this should be obtained by preferring foods rich in both carbohydrates and fiber, in order to reach the goal of a fiber consumption of at least 20 g/1000 kcal. According to the majority of experts, these dietary recommendations for diabetes resemble the so-called Mediterranean diet, which is low in saturated fat and rich in unsaturated fat (olive oil), complex carbohydrates, and, possibly, dietary fiber (Garg et al. 1988).

High-Carbohydrate High-Fiber Diets
For the Treatment of Diabetes

The beneficial effects of high-carbohydrate, high-fiber, low-fat diets for the treatment of diabetic patients have been generally recognized. Many controlled studies of different length performed with diets naturally enriched in fiber, or with fiber added to foods, have uniformly shown a clinically significant reduction of blood glucose values both in insulin dependent and non-insulin-dependent diabetic patients, especially during the postprandial period. Furthermore, this kind of dietary approach is proved to be effective in reducing blood cholesterol and, in some

TABLE 14-2. Metabolic Effects of High Fiber Diets (HF) or High Fiber-High Carbohydrate Diets (HCF) in Diabetic Patients

Authors	No. of Subjects	Type of Diet	Duration (days)	Blood Glucose	Cholesterol	Triglycerides
Anderson	14	HCF	1940	↓	↓	↓
Barnard	69	HCF	913	↓	↓	↓
Hjollund	9	HCF	21	↓	↓	→
Karlstrom	14	HF	21	↓	→	→
Kay	5	HF	14	↓	↓	↓
Kinmonth	10	HF	42	↓	↓	↓
Kiehm	13	HCF	21	↓	↓	↓
Lindsay	12	HCF	14	→	↓	↓
Ney	20	HCF	119	↓	↓	↓
Pedersen	40	HCF	28	↓	↓	→
Riccardi	14	HCF	10	↓	↓	↓
Rivellese	8	HCF	10	↓	↓	↓
Rosman	10	HF	91	↓	↓	↓
Simpson	27	HCF	42	↓	↓	↓
Taskinen	21	HCF	42	↓	↓	→

Source: Anderson (1988).

cases, triglyceride levels (Table 14-2), thus improving the overall lipoprotein profile in most diabetic patients (Anderson et al. 1988).

In particular we have compared the metabolic efficacy of a diet rich in complex carbohydrates and fiber and low in saturated fat (thus resembling for many aspects the traditional Mediterranean diet), with that of a low-carbohydrate, low-fiber diet often advised by many diabetologists to their patients. The Mediterranean type of diet proved to be more effective than the low-carbohydrate, high-fat diet for both insulin dependent and non-insulin-dependent patients. In particular, in the former group it was able to reduce not only glycemia but also the daily fluctuations of blood glucose levels that represent a hallmark of the metabolic instability of these patients. The Mediterranean type of diet was also more efficacious than the low-carbohydrate diet in non-insulin-dependent patients. This greater efficacy was demonstrated not only by a reduction of blood glucose levels but also by lower plasma lipids and insulin concentrations, thus ameliorating the overall profile of cardiovascular risk (Rivellese, 1980; Riccardi et al. 1984).

Even if the metabolic efficacy of these diets is almost unanimously accepted, their safety—especially in the long run—and their feasibility are still being questioned. Regarding their safety, it is now clear that the adoption of a diet containing only natural fiber-rich foods does not create special problems in relation to the absorption of vitamins, iron, and other minerals. In fact, a vitamin or mineral deficiency has never been reported in people on high-fiber diets composed of natural foodstuff, which are generally rich not only in fiber but also in vitamins and microelements.

The feasibility of adopting high-carbohydrate, high-fiber diets is supported by the observation that in many countries in East Asia and in the Mediterranean region a high-carbohydrate, high-fiber consumption does not necessarily imply a punishment for the taste. Indeed, in many industrialized countries the gastronomic interest for this type of cuisine is increasing steadily, and many traditional dishes of the Chinese and Mediterranean tradition are becoming part of everyday meals all over the world. A diet low in saturated fats and rich in vegetables has been adopted for centuries by Mediterranean populations and has never been associated with major health problems. On the contrary, it has been shown to protect against cardiovascular diseases.

CONCLUSION

Strong evidence accumulated in recent years shows that many epidemic diseases of the modern world are strongly associated with life-style and, in particular, with eating habits. There is general agreement among epidemiologists, nutritionists, and clinicians that dietary modifications might play a major role in the prevention and treatment of many common diseases of the modern world, such as diabetes, hyperlipidemia, and atherosclerosis. Unfortunately, it is not very easy to influence the eating habits of single individuals and populations. So far any attempt in this direction has been very unsuccessful. This phenomenon can be explained by considering the very strong emotional, cultural, and gastronomic facets of a diet. It is unlikely that a diet that does not consider all these aspects will be accepted and followed in the long run. Therefore, in order to be successful in our preventive and therapeutic approaches, rather than diets conceived in a metabolic ward kitchen, what we need are "eating patterns" strongly based on the population's cultural and gastronomic background.

This is why the Mediterranean diet has become so popular in recent years. In fact, the eating patterns that are common in this region are associated with a good health profile and, nevertheless, are very easily accepted by most people because they are based on a cuisine that has a strong tradition of delicacy, taste, flavor, and that is able to offer hundreds of interesting recipes. Unfortunately, eating habits are also changing in the Mediterranean region, and in order to find the characteristics of the Mediterranean diet we must go back to the eating habits that were common in the rural areas of this region up to some decades ago.

Strong evidence suggests that the Mediterranean diet protects against the development of cardiovascular disease, therefore it can be proposed as a nutritional model for the prevention of this condition.

This chapter has reviewed the evidence of the relationship between the Mediterranean diet and diabetes. Unfortunately, there is no clear proof that diabetes can be prevented by implementing a Mediterranean type of nutrition. However indications are that a diet low in fat (especially in saturated fat) and high in complex carbohydrates and fiber (as the Mediterranean diet is and was, especially in the past), is probably useful in the prevention of diabetes and, moreover, is certainly the best available diet to treat diabetic patients.

REFERENCE

American Diabetes Association. 1987. Nutritional recommendations and principles for individuals with diabetes mellitus. *Diabetes Care* **10**:126–132.

Anderson, J. W. 1988. Nutritional management of diabetes mellitus. In *Modern Nutrition in Health and Disease*, M. E. Smils and V. R. Young, eds., pp. 1201–1229. Lea and Febiger.

Diabetes Drafting Group. 1985. Prevalence of small vessel and large vessel disease in diabetic patients from 14 centres: the World Health Organization multinational Study of Vascular Disease in Diabetics. *Diabetologia* **28** (Suppl.1): 615–640.

Garg, A., A. Bonamane, S. M. Grundy, et al. 1988. Comparison of a high carbohydrate diet with a high monounsaturated fat diet in patients with non-insulin dependent diabetes mellitus. *New Engl. J. Med.* **34**:819–829.

National Institutes of Health. Consensus development conference on diet and exercise in non-insulin dependent diabetes mellitus. 1987. *Diabetes Care* **10**:639–644.

Kawate, R., M. Yamakido, and Y. Nishimoto. 1979. Diabetes Mellitus and its vascular complication in Japanese migrants on the island of Hawaii. *Diabetes Care* **2**:161–170.

DNSG (Diabetes and Nutrition Study Group of the European Association for the Study of Diabetes). 1988. Nutritional recommendations for individuals with diabetes mellitus. *Diabetes Nutr. Metab.* **1**:145–149.

Riccardi, G., A. Rivellese, D. Pacioni, et al. 1984. Separate influence of dietary carbohydrate and fibre on the metabolic control in diabetes. *Diabetologia* **26**:116–121.

Rivellese, A., G. Riccardi, A. Giacco, et al. 1980. Effect of dietary fibre on glucose control and serum lipoproteins in diabetic patients. *Lancet* II:447–450.

Snowdon, D. A., and R. L. Phillips. 1985. Does a vegetarian diet reduce the occurrence of diabetes? *Am. J. Public Health* **75**:507–512.

Trowell, H. 1981. Emergence of Western disease in sub-Saharal Africans: Hypertension, obesity, diabetes mellitus and coronary heart disease. In *Western Diseases: Their Emergence and Prevention,* H. C. Trowell and D. P. Burkitt, eds., pp. 3–32. London: Edward Arnold.

West, K. 1974. Epidemiologic observation on 13 populations of Asia and Western hemisphere. In *Is the Risk of Becoming Diabetic Affected by Sugar Consumption?* S. S. Hillebrand, ed., pp. 33–43. Proc. 8th Symp. of Int. Sugar Research Foundation, Bethesda, Md.: International Sugar Research Foundation.

West, K. 1978. Prevalence and incidence. In *Epidemiology of Diabetes and Its Vascular Lesions,* pp. 127–157. New York: Elsevier.

WHO. 1985. *Diabetes Mellitus.* Technical report series 727. Geneva: WHO.

15

Diet and Cancer

Adriano Decarli
Carlo La Vecchia

Diet plays an important role in cancer etiology, although quantification of the importance of various components of diet is still largely uncertain. The figures in Table 15-1 reflect both the relevance attributed to diet in the etiology of cancer and the difficulties connected with its quantification. The wide range of the estimate—10% to 70%—of the proportion of cancer deaths attributed to dietary factors has different explanations, including the inferential nature of the available information and the wide variation in dietary habits in different countries. In fact, although strong correlations have been found between cancer and dietary habits throughout the world, it is well known that correlation does not necessarily mean causation.

Besides ecological studies, information on the diet-cancer relationship in humans derives from case-control and cohort studies, while very little is known at present about the impact of diet supplements or modifications on subsequent cancer rates. Unfortunately, the evidence from various types of data is largely inconsistent. For example, Table 15-2 compares the results of different analytical studies on diet and breast cancer (Berrino et al. 1989). Similar tables exist for many other cancers. This lack of consistency can be partly ascribed to the heterogeneity of diet within and between populations, to the varying precision achieved by different studies, and to the diverse methods of dietary data collection.

SUMMARY OF KNOWLEDGE

In an effort to summarize the results from different studies on various cancers, it is possible to formulate some basic working hypotheses. The following were derived from those expressed by the National Research Council (1982) and are similar to those given by other institutions (Palmer 1986):

TABLE 15-1. Various Factors in Cancer Deaths

	Best Estimate (%)	Range (%)
Tobacco	30	25–40
Diet	35	10–70
Alcoholic Beverages	3	2–4
Reproductive–Sexual Habits	7	1–13
Occupation	4	2–8
Radiation	3	2–4
Viruses	10?	1–?
Pollution	2	1–5
All Others	6	—

Source: Doll and Peto (1981).

Total Caloric Intake.   Studies conducted on animals show that a reduction in the total food intake decreases the incidence of cancer. The specific effect of such reduction on the risk is not evident from the results of epidemiological studies except for selected cancer sites, that is, gallbladder, endometrium and postmenopausal breast, which are related to overweight.

Fats and Lipids.   Epidemiological and experimental evidence suggests a relationship between high fat intake and increased occurrence of selected cancers, for example, colorectum. The role of cholesterol in carcinogenesis is not clearly understood.

Protein.   High protein consumption may be related to an increased risk of cancer. However, because of the strong correlation between fat and protein, no firm conclusion can be drawn about an independent effect of protein.

Carbohydrates.   The role of carbohydrates in cancer etiology is questionable since the information is limited and inconclusive.

Dietary Fibers.   Although descriptive epidemiology has suggested a potential protection by fiber, mainly on colorectal cancer, no firm evidence is available from analytical studies.

Alcoholic Beverages.   Excessive alcohol consumption and cigarette smoking appear to act synergistically in increasing the risk for some cancers, for example, mouth, esophagus, and upper respiratory tract, but the independent effect of alcohol is proven only for a few cancer sites, for example, esophagus or liver.

Fruits and Vegetables.   Different epidemiological studies suggest that high consumption of vegetables, such as cabbage, broccoli, and cauliflower, and fruits is associated with a lower cancer risk.

TABLE 15-2. Analytical Studies on Diet and Breast Cancer

	First Author	Design	No. Cases	Total or Saturated Fats	Meat	Milk and Dairy	Vegetable Fats	Fruit or Vegetables
1987	Willett	P	601	na			na	
1989	Toniolo	N	250	+	sp	+	na	na
1978/85	Miller/Howe	N	400	+*			-*	
1985	Hirohata	N,H	212	sp			sn	
1987	Hirohata	N,H	344	sp			na	
1986	Hislop	N	861		+*	+*		-*
1982	Kinlen	P	62		sp			
1988	Mills	P	186		na	na		
1986	Lubin, F.	N,H	818	+*				sn*
1986/88	Katsouyanni	H	120		na	na		-
1982	Graham	H	2024	na	na			-*
1984	Talamini	H	368		na	+		
1986	Lé	H	1010			+	sn	
1987	Jones	P	99	-				
1978	Hirayama	P	139		+			
1978	Nomura	P	86		+	+		
1981	Lubin, J.	N	577		+	+		
1975	Phillips	N,H	77		na	sp		
1985	Zemla	N	328		sp*			-*
1985	Sarin	H	68	+				

Source: Berrino et al. (1989).

H = Hospital-based case-control study; P = Cohort study; + = Significant (p<.05) positive association; − = Significant (p<.05) negative association; na = No association; N = Case-control study with population or neighboring controls; sp = Suggestive of positive association; sn = Suggestive of negative association; * = Association limited to subgroups.

289

Vitamins.   Vitamin A and retinoids have an antioxidant effect in laboratory experimentations. The epidemiological evidence suggests that foods rich in carotene and vitamin A can be associated with a reduction in risk for some cancers, although it is not known whether this apparent protection simply reflects the role of other components of a vegetable-rich diet. There is some evidence that vitamin C can inhibit the action of some carcinogens. In the epidemiological field, consumption of foods rich in vitamin C is associated with a lower risk of some cancers such as stomach and esophagus. Not enough information exists about the effect of vitamins E and B on cancer in humans to formulate any conclusions.

Minerals.   There is only scattered evidence about a protective effect of selenium. Epidemiological data on the effect of iron, zinc, and copper are insufficient.

The information collected until the present on the relation of diet to cancer has allowed only general guidelines of disease prevention to be defined. For example, the American Cancer Society makes the following recommendations for controlling and possibly reducing the risk of cancer (Holleb 1984):

Avoid obesity.
Cut down on total fat intake.
Eat more high-fiber foods (cereals, vegetables, etc.).
Include foods rich in vitamins A and C in daily diet.
Include cruciferous vegetables in the diet.
Be moderate in consumption of alcoholic beverages.
Be moderate in consumption of salted, smoked, and nitrite-cured foods.

These are similar to general recommendations made by other institutions and agree with indications from other fields of public health (see, for example, dietary habits suggested to reduce risk of cardiovascular diseases). These general guidelines are based on a number of studies conducted principally in the United States and in other English-speaking populations. Mediterranean countries have become involved in this research area only in the past few years.

CHARACTERISTICS OF MEDITERRANEAN DIET

The diet in Mediterranean countries is characterized by a high availability of potentially "protective" food items, such as those rich in vitamin

C, fruits, fresh vegetables, vegetable fats, and items of "suspected" risk, such as cheese and salami (with a different method of preservation) (Mariani Costantini 1987). Still, the average diet in Mediterranean countries appears not very different from the recommendations of the American Cancer Society, except for the elevated alcoholic beverage consumption. For these reasons, the Mediterranean region can provide an interesting setting for analyzing the role of different foods and/or macro- and micro-nutrients in carcinogenesis.

Several features from descriptive epidemiology indicate that Italy is probably now an excellent environment for etiological analyses of lifestyle features and cancer risk. First, there are marked and systematic north/south gradients in cancer incidence and mortality rates for most common sites, rates being almost invariably considerably higher in the northern part of the country. This gradient applies to cancer of the lung and other tobacco-related sites, for which the differences may to a large extent be associated with different smoking habits in the past. This north/south gradient also is associated with several nontobacco-related sites, such as stomach, colorectum, breast, and prostate, for which a "natural" interpretation is probably to be sought in the variations in dietary habits in various Italian regions (Cislaghi et al. 1986; La Vecchia and Decarli 1986; Mezzanotte et al. 1986).

On a national scale in Italy, recent changes have occurred in mortality for several cancer sites with potentially important dietary correlates. Stomach cancer declined as in other developed countries, but there were considerable upward trends, at least between the 1950s and 1970s, for cancers of the intestines and breast, which are largely at variance with data from other countries and again suggest a potential role for recent changes in the composition of the Italian diet (Decarli and La Vecchia 1985; La Vecchia and Decarli 1985; La Vecchia and Decarli 1986).

Some typical results were obtained for the Mediterranean area by studies of the relationship between dietary factors and cancer; we have summarized and discussed some of the major findings from a large multicentric gastric cancer study conducted in seven areas of Italy, with markedly different mortality rates for the disease (Buiatti et al. 1989a; Buiatti et al. 1989b) and from a case-control surveillance of several neoplasms conducted in northern Italy.

GASTRIC CANCER AND DIET IN ITALY

Gastric cancer is estimated to be the most common cancer worldwide and the second leading cause of cancer death (Parkin et al. 1988). Among western European countries, Italy has one of the highest rates of gastric cancer mortality (Decarli et al. 1986). Within Italy, a peculiar geographic pattern of gastric cancer mortality is observed, with lower rates being registered in the south, which is the poorest part of the country (Cislaghi et al. 1986). A few well-defined provinces in northern and central Italy, however, show gastric cancer rates in both sexes around and over twofold higher than the national average.

To investigate the reasons for these regional differences, a large, multicenter case-control study was conducted in high- and low-risk areas. Personal interviews were conducted on 1,016 histologically confirmed gastric cancer cases and 1,159 population controls of similar age and sex. Cases were most often of low social class, resided in rural areas, and frequently reported a family history of gastric cancer. After adjusting for these effects, case-control differences were found for several dietary variables, assessed by asking about the usual frequency of consumption of 146 food items and beverages. A significant trend of rising gastric cancer risk was found with increasing consumption of traditional soups, meat, salted and/or dried fish, and a combination of cold cuts and seasoned cheeses. The practice of adding salt and the preference for salty foods were associated with elevated gastric cancer risk, while frequently

TABLE 15-3. Relative Risks (RR) of Gastric Cancer According to Refrigeration and Salt-Use Practices

Variable	Strata	Cases	Controls	RR	CI
Ever had freezer	No	504	511	1.0	—
	Yes	512	648	0.8	0.7–0.9
Age obtained refrigerator	<32	308	385	1.0	—
	32–42	304	389	1.0	0.8–1.3
	43+/never	404	385	1.4	1.0–1.9
Storing in refrigerator	Often/always	598	742	1.0	—
	Never/seldom	418	417	1.3	1.0–1.5
Use of frozen foods	1 (low)	442	374	1.0	—
	2 (medium)	419	490	0.7	0.4–0.9
	3 (high)	155	295	0.5	0.4–0.6
Add salt	Never/seldom	629	820	1.0	—
	Often always	387	339	1.5	1.3–1.9
Taste for foods	Low salt	220	175	1.0	—
	Normal	549	676	1.4	1.1–1.7
	Salty	292	263	1.4	1.1–1.9

Source: Buiatti et al. (1989).
Note: CI = 95% confidence interval.

the storing of foods in a refrigerator, the availability of a freezer, and the use of frozen foods lowered the risk (Table 15–3).

Reduced gastric cancer risk was associated with increasing intake of raw vegetables and fresh fruit, including citrus. Lowered risk was also associated with consumption of spices, olive oil, and garlic. The high-risk areas tended to show higher consumption of food related to elevated risk and lower consumption of foods associated with reduced risk. Independent effects of the various food groups are illustrated in Table 15–4. Part A shows that the risks of gastric cancer declined with increasing fruit intake (citrus and other fresh fruit) and with increasing intake in each category of raw vegetables; conversely, risks rose with decreased intake. Those with high intake of both had only 30% of the risk of those with low intake of both. Similarly, a nearly fourfold difference in gastric cancer risk was found between those with high versus those with low intake of traditional soup, meat, fish, cold cuts, and seasoned cheeses (part B). A more than fivefold difference was found between those reporting a high consumption of traditional soup, meat, fish, cold cuts and seasoned cheeses, and high fruit and raw vegetable intake (part C).

TABLE 15-4. Relative Risks of Gastric Cancer Associated with Tertile Level of Intake of Selected Pairs of Groups of Food

| A | | Raw vegetables | | |
		1 (low)	2	3
Fruit	1 (low)	1.0	0.8	0.5
	2	0.7	0.5	0.4
	3	0.5	0.5	0.3

| B | | Meat, fish, cold cuts, seasoned cheeses | | |
		1 (low)	2	3
Traditional soups	1 (low)	1.0	1.1	1.6
	2	1.6	2.1	2.4
	3	1.9	3.0	3.9

| C | | Traditional soups, meat, fish, cold cuts, seasoned cheeses | | |
		1 (low)	2	3
Fruit and raw vegetables	1 (low)	1.0	2.0	2.4
	2	0.7	1.1	1.9
	3	0.4	1.0	1,2

Source: Buiatti et al. (1989a).

A CASE-CONTROL SURVEILLANCE STUDY
IN NORTHERN ITALY

Major urban concentrations in northern Italy provide a particularly favorable situation for epidemiological studies of diet and cancer risk since there has been considerable immigration from several other regions throughout this current century and chiefly after World War II. Therefore, widespread heterogeneity exists in the dietary habits of the population and other potential life-style correlates of cancer risk (Vigotti et al. 1989).

In the framework of the northern Italy surveillance study, information was obtained using structured questionnaires, which included the frequency of consumption per week of selected food items. The 14 items considered for neoplasms other than those of the digestive tract included the major sources of vitamin A, fat, and fibers in the Italian diet; the 37-item list used for digestive tract neoplasms included, in addition, major sources of starches, protein, and nitrates/nitrites. Information was also collected on consumption of the same foods over about 10 years before diagnosis (La Vecchia et al. 1987a; La Vecchia et al. 1988).

The cases considered were patients below the age of 75 with histologically confirmed cancers of the mouth or pharynx, esophagus, stomach, colon, rectum, liver, pancreas, breast, female genital tract, prostate, or bladder, who had been admitted to a network of university and general hospitals in the greater Milan area. The comparison groups comprised patients below age 75 admitted for a wide spectrum of acute conditions to the same network of hospitals where patients with various cancers had been diagnosed. The numbers of cases and controls considered are listed in Table 15-5.

Although it is difficult in such a widely heterogeneous group of neoplasms to identify a single common denominator in terms of risk factors, it is still of interest to note the generalized protection conveyed by frequent green-vegetable consumption against the risk of most cancer sites. The relative risk estimates in the upper tertile ranged between 0.21 for cervix or 0.33 for stomach and 0.89 for pancreas, and the trends in risk were statistically significant for all sites considered except mouth or pharynx, bladder (possibly on account of limited absolute numbers), and pancreas (Table 15-6).

In contrast to the strong and consistent connection of green vegetables with most cancers studied, the association with other foods or nutrients frequently considered in the etiology of various cancer sites was much less clear (Weisburger and Horn 1985). For instance, frequent consumption of fresh fruit, particularly citrus fruits, appeared to provide some protection against oral, esophageal, laryngeal, and gastric cancers,

TABLE 15-5. Number of Cases and Controls Available for Analysis for Each Specific Cancer Site, Milan, Italy, 1983 to 1987

Type of Cancer	Cases	Controls
Mouth or Pharynx	50	1051
Esophagus	105	348
Stomach	206	474
Colon	339	778
Rectum	236	778
Liver	151	1051
Pancreas	215	1051
Breast	1108	1281
Cervix, uteri	392	392
Endometrium	434	1385
Ovary	455	1385
Prostate	44	129
Bladder	163	181

TABLE 15-6. Relation Between Green-Vegetable Intake and Various Neoplasms, Milan, Italy, 1983 to 1987

| Type of Cancer | Multivariate Relative Risk Estimates for Approximate Intake Tertiles | | |
	1 (low)	2 (Intermediate)	3 (High)
Mouth or Pharynx	1	0.93	0.73
Esophagus	1	1.07	0.62
Stomach	1	0.58	0.33
Colon	1	0.75	0.50
Rectum	1	0.86	0.51
Liver	1	0.83	0.58
Pancreas	1	0.82	0.89
Breast	1	0.76	0.42
Cervix, uteri	1	0.67	0.21
Endometrium	1	1.07	0.38
Ovary	1	1.10	0.61
Prostate	1	0.77	0.50
Bladder	1	0.76	0.49

Note: Reference category = 1.

but little consistent association was observed with many other neoplasms considered. Likewise, subjective measures of fats in seasonings showed only a slight positive association with breast cancer, or borderline statistical significance, and no material relation with colon cancer (Table 15-7). Similar results were borne out by detailed analyses performed on each single type of fat: butter, olive, and other oils. Frequency of meat consumption was positively related to the risk of colon and rectal cancers but not with breast cancer (Table 15-7), nor to most of the other sites considered with the possible exception of endometrium and ovary.

Pasta and rice, which represent important sources of starches in the Italian diet, were positively linked with cancers of the stomach (relative risk (RR) for the upper versus lower tertile = 1.65), colon (RR = 3.01), and rectum (RR = 1.80). If the association with gastric cancer could, at least in part, be explained in terms of lower socioeconomic status of the cases (and hence generally poorer quality diet), it is difficult to identify plausible confounding factors for the increased risk of intestinal cancer with starchy foods. The association observed, therefore, may well be real, and tentatively explainable in terms of modifications of the digestive tract flora by starches. One specific starchy food, polenta, a porridge made of maize commonly eaten in northern and chiefly northeastern Italy, showed a strong positive association with gastric cancer risk (RR = 2.3–2.5 for the upper tertile) (Table 15-8).

Whole grain foods are not widely eaten in Italy, and it is therefore not surprising that little association emerged with any neoplasm considered

TABLE 15-7. Relation Between Measures of Seasoning Fats and Meat Consumption and Cancers of the Colon, Rectum, and Breast, Milan, Italy, 1983 to 1987

| Nutrient | Type of Cancer | Multivariate Relative Risk Estimates for Approximate Intake Tertiles | | |
		1 (Low)	2 (Intermediate)	3 (High)
Fat in seasoning, total	Breast	1	1.27	1.27
	Colon	1	0.94	1.25
	Rectum	1	0.85	0.94
Meat	Breast	1	1.05	1.39
	Colon	1	1.35	2.13
	Rectum	1	1.23	2.26

Note: Reference category = 1.

TABLE 15-8.   Relation Between Frequency of Consumption of Polenta and Gastric Cancer Risk, Milan, Italy, 1983 to 1987

	Relative Risk Estimates for Approximate Intake Tertiles		
	1	2	3
M-H[a]	1	1.61	2.45
M-H[b]	1	1.54	2.26
M-H[c]	1	1.45	2.32

Note: Reference category = 1.

[a] Mantel-Haenszel estimates adjusted for age and sex.

[b] Estimates from multiple logistic regression; allowance was made for age, sex, education, and area of residence.

[c] Estimates from multiple logistic regression, with simultaneous allowance for all other significant food items besides the above listed nondietary variables.

except as a protection against that in the stomach but, again, this result might be due to some uncontrolled confounding by socioeconomic status, since whole grain foods are consumed more frequently by higher social classes in Italy.

This case-control survey provided the opportunity to reassess the role of various other components of the diet in cancer risk. Alcohol and coffee, for instance, show a pattern of use in Italy different from that in northern Europe or North America (La Vecchia et al. 1987b; Pagano et al. 1988). Alcohol, besides the expected associations with cancers of the mouth or pharynx, esophagus, and liver, was strongly related to breast cancer too, and this study offered a particularly interesting opportunity for analyzing this association, since wine is commonly drunk by Italian women at meals (La Vecchia et al. 1987b).

The evidence on coffee, whose utilization, again, is peculiar in terms of frequency and type of preparation, is summarized in Table 15-9. There was no association with cancers of the stomach, pancreas, and breast, and only a slight and inconsistent relation with ovarian cancer. Colorectal neoplasms, in contrast, were inversely related with measures of coffee consumption, confirming the results of some but not all previous studies and, hence, supporting the hypothesis that the reduced bile acid and neutral sterol secretion induced by coffee can modify the risk of intestinal cancer (Jacobsen and Thelle 1987). Likewise, the direct association

**TABLE 15-9.   Relation Between Measures of Coffee
Consumption and Risk of Selected Neoplasms, Milan,
Italy, 1983 to 1987**

	Multivariate Relative Risk Estimates for Approximate Intake Tertiles		
Type of Cancer	1 (Low)	2 (Intermediate)	3 (High)
Stomach	1	0.83	1.00
Colon	1	0.80	0.56
Rectum	1	0.89	0.65
Pancreas	1	1.24	1.17
Breast	1	0.98	0.84
Ovary	1	1.04	1.12
Bladder	1	2.39	2.21

Note: Reference category = 1.

with bladder cancer, despite the lack of any dose-risk trend, is consistent with most previous evidence (Matanoski and Elliott 1981).

Table 15–10 is a sort of numerical exercise to show the extent of variation in risk for gastric and colorectal cancers that can be observed using scores obtained simply through algebraic combinations of four risk factors. Since these scores are derived *a posteriori* from the data, the results should be interpreted with the utmost caution and viewed simply as a confirmation that a four- to seven-fold difference in risk for some common cancers can be correlated to the pattern of use of an extremely limited number of foods. The obvious implication of this finding is in interpretation of the geographical differences in cancer incidence and mortality in Italy, which are approximately of this magnitude for most common cancer sites (Cislaghi et al. 1986; Mezzanotte et al. 1986).

**TABLE 15-10.   Relation Between a Combined Risk
Score[a] and the Risk of Cancers of the Stomach, Colon,
and Rectum, Milan, Italy, 1983 to 1987**

	Score Quintiles				
Type of Cancer	1	2	3	4	5
Stomach	1	2.66	3.03	3.10	6.92
Colon	1	1.22	2.02	4.18	5.05
Rectum	1	1.13	1.71	2.96	3.84

[a] Based on the simple algebraic sum of the four strongly related food items for each cancer site.
Note: Reference category = 1.

In contrast, for some neoplasms the variation in risk in regard to any of the specific food items considered was limited. This was the case with liver cancer, whose risk estimates tended to be inversely associated with most of the nutrients in a fairly specific pattern, indirectly suggesting that a diet deficient in several aspects is probably related to hepatocellular carcinoma. In relation to pancreatic cancer, no obvious association emerged on preliminary analysis, thus further confirming the difficulties in obtaining clues for the etiology of this neoplasm. These data give a summary overview of some of the most interesting findings obtainable using very simple instruments for dietary data collection in a study from a heavy populated area in northern Italy, where food habits are largely an intermixture of typical Mediterranean and other, more Western, components.

The most striking finding was the substantial protection given by frequent green-vegetable consumption against the risk of neoplasms at most sites considered. However, the results on fats, meats, alcohol, and coffee are also interesting, particularly because they are often at least quantitatively different from those obtained by studies in North American populations. A major problem with the American studies, in fact, is the limited variety in diet, so that the studies do not provide information on the effect of modifying the intake of common nutrients outside a very narrow range. For instance, in a large prospective study of fat and breast cancer, the cut-off point for extreme quintiles of total fat was 32% and 44% of total calorie intake, which is conceivably too narrow an interval to observe any biological effect (Willett et al. 1987).

Some of the apparent discrepancies between these results and evidence from North America may be due to real differences in dietary habits and pattern of risk in various populations. In fact, when attention is restricted to Mediterranean countries, there are reassuring similarities between the results of this survey and those from case-control studies of esophageal (Tuyns et al. 1987), gastric (Trichopoulos et al. 1985; Buiatti et al. 1989a), colorectal (Macquart-Moulin et al. 1986; Manousos et al. 1983), and breast cancer (Katsouyanni et al. 1986, 1988) conducted in Italy, France, and Greece.

In this overview, we were inclined to interpret the results in terms of food items or food nutrients, although we could derive measurements of retinoid, carotenoid, and ascorbic acid intake from the data collected. These vitamins, in fact, appeared to convey some protection at various cancer sites: esophagus (Decarli et al. 1987), stomach (La Vecchia et al. 1987c), and cervix uteri (La Vecchia et al. 1984), but not others; such as breast (La Vecchia et al. 1987a), colon (La Vecchia et al. 1988), or prostate, but we believe that any inference on micronutrients requires the utmost caution. In fact, the associations were often weaker than for their single components, and there are obvious problems of collinearity for the interpretation of any model including, simultaneously, these overall weighted indices and their components.

Even if attention is restricted to frequency of use of selected foods as indicators of dietary patterns, and hence a more reductive and simplistic interpretation of these findings is accepted, this circumstance does not obscure, in our view, the interest and importance of some of these results and of studying the relation between diet and cancer in Mediterranean countries or, more in general, in areas where appreciable heterogeneity and change in dietary patterns and cancer rates have taken place over recent decades.

CONCLUSIONS

Within the context of this series of studies, it is of particular interest that not only the most frequent cancers but also a number of less common neoplasms may have important dietary correlates. This observation, besides helping to understand the epidemiology of the neoplasms, justifies further efforts in the area. Both the cultural and scientific skills and the population characteristics and dietary patterns in southern Europe, however, justify such an effort. This may not be true in a few years' time if the process towards homogenizing dietary patterns (Mariani Costantini 1983) across European populations continues. We should, therefore, not miss such a unique opportunity.

Acknowledgments

We wish to thank the Group for Research on Diet and Gastric Cancer, coordinated by Dr. E. Buiatti, for allowing us to use the data discussed on pages 292–293. The contributions of the Italian Association for Cancer Research and the Italian League Against Tumors are gratefully acknowledged. We also wish to thank Mrs. Angela Simm for editorial assistance.

REFERENCES

Berrino, F., S. Panico, and P. Muti. 1989. Dietary Fat, Nutritional Status and Endocrine Associated Cancers. In *Diet and Cancer Etiology*, A. B. Miller, ed., ESO Monography, pp. 1–10. New York, Heidelberg: Springer Verlag.

Buiatti, E., D. Palli, A. Decarli, et al. 1989a. A case-control study of gastric cancer and diet in Italy. *Int. J. Cancer* **44**:611–616.

Buiatti, E., D. Palli, D. Amadori, et al. 1989b. Methodological issues in a multicentric study of gastric cancer and diet in Italy: Study design, data sources and quality controls. *Tumori* **75**:410–419.

Cislaghi, A. Decarli, C. La Vecchia, N. Laverda, G. Mezzanotte, and M. Smans. 1986. *Statistics and Maps on Cancer Mortality. Italy 1975–1977.* Bologna: Pitagora Ed.

Decarli, A., and C. La Vecchia. 1985. Cancer mortality in Italy, 1979. *Tumori* **71**:519–526.

Decarli, A., C. La Vecchia, C. Cislaghi, G. Mezzanotte, and E. Marubini. 1986. Descriptive epidemiology of gastric cancer in Italy. *Cancer* **58**:2560–2569.

Decarli, A., P. Liati, E. Negri, S. Franceschi, and C. La Vecchia. 1987. Vitamin A and other dietary factors in the etiology of esophageal cancer. *Nutr. Cancer* **10**:29–37.

Doll, R., and R. Peto. 1981. The causes of cancer: Quantitative estimates of avoidable risks of cancer in United States today. *J. Natl. Cancer Inst.* **66**:1191–1308.

Graham, S., J. Marshall, C. Mettlin, et al. 1982. Diet in the epidemiology of breast cancer. *Am. J. Epidermiol.* **116**:68–75.

Hirayama, T. 1978. Epidemiology of breast cancer with special reference to the role of diet. *Prev. Med.* **7**:173–195.

Hirohata, T., T. Shigematsu, A. Nomura, et al. 1985. Occurrence of breast cancer in relation to diet and reproductive history: A case-control study in Fukuoka, Japan. *Natl. Cancer. Inst. Monogr.* **69**:187–190.

Hirohata, T., A. M. Y. Namura, J. H. Haukin, L. N. Kolonel, and J. Lee. 1987. An epidemiologic study on the association between diet and breast cancer. *JNCI* **78**:595–600.

Hislop, T. G., A. J. Coldman, J. M. Elwood, G. Braner, and L. Kan. 1986. Childhood and recent eating patterns and risk of breast cancer. *Cancer Detect. Prev.* **9**:47–58.

Holleb, A. I., ed. 1984. Nutrition and Cancer. Cause and Prevention. An American Cancer Society Special Report. Reprinted in *Ca-A Cancer J. for Clinicians,* 1984, **34**:121–126.

Jacobsen, B. K., and D. S. Thelle. 1987. Coffee, cholesterol and colon cancer: Is there a link? *Br. Med. J.* (Clin Res) **294**:4–5.

Jones, Y. D., A. Schatakin, S. B. Green, et al. 1987. Dietary fat and breast cancer in the National Health and Nutrition Examination Survey. I. Epidemiologic follow-up study. *JNCI* **79**:465–471.

Katsouyanni, K., D. Trichopoulous, P. Boyle, et al. 1986. Diet and breast cancer: A case-control study in Greece. *Int. J. Cancer* **38**:815–820.

Katsouyanni, K., W. Willett, D. Trichopoulos, P. Boyle, A. Trichopoulos, S. Vasilaros, J. Papadiamantis, and B. MacMahon. 1988. Risk of breast cancer among Greek women in relation to nutrient intake. *Cancer* **61**:181–185.

Kinlen, L. 1982. Meat and fat consumption and cancer mortality: A study of strict religious order in Britain. *Lancet* **1**:946–949.

La Vecchia, C., and A. Decarli. 1985. Trends in cancer mortality in Italy, 1955–78. *Tumori* **71**:201–218.

La Vecchia, C., and A. Decarli. 1986. Cancer mortality in Italy: Temporal trends and geographical distribution. *Eur. J. Cancer Oncol.* **22**:1425–1429.

La Vecchia, C., S. Franceschi, A. Decarli, A. Gentile, M. Fasoli, S. Pampallona, and G. Tognoni. 1984. Dietary vitamin A and the risk of invasive cervical cancer. *Int. J. Cancer* **34**:319–322.

La Vecchia, C., A. Decarli, S. Franceschi, A. Gentile, E. Negri, and F. Parazzini. 1987a. Dietary factors and the risk of breast cancer. *Nutri. Cancer* **10**:205–214.

La Vecchia, C., R. Pagano, E. Negri, and A. Decarli. 1987b. Determinants of alcohol consumption in Italy. *Int. J. Epidemiol.* **16**:295–296.

La Vecchia, C., E. Negri, A. Decarli, B. D'Avanzo, and S. Franceschi. 1987c. A case-control study of diet and gastric cancer in Northern Italy. *Int. J. Cancer* **40**:484–489.

La Vecchia, C., E. Negri, A. Decarli, B. D'Avanzo, L. Gallotti, A. Gentile, and S. Franceschi. 1988. A case-control study of diet and colorectal cancer in Northern Italy. *Int. J. Cancer* **41**:492–498.

Lé, M. G., L. H. Moulton, C. Hill, and A. Kramar. 1986. Consumption of dairy produce and alcohol in a case-control study of breast cancer. *JNCI* **77**:633–636.

Lubin, F., Y. Wax, and B. Modan. 1986. Role of fat, animal protein and dietary fiber in breast cancer etiology: A case-control study. *JNCI* **77**:605–612.

Lubin, J. H., P. E. Burns, W. J. Blot, R. G. Ziegler, A. W. Lees, and J. F. Fraumeni Jr. 1981. Dietary factors and breast cancer risk. *Int. J. Cancer* **28**:685–689.

Macquart-Moulin, G., E. Riboli, J. Corne, B. Charnay, P. Berthezene, and N. Day. 1986. Case-control study on colorectal cancer and diet in Marseilles. *Int. J. Cancer* **38**:183–191.

Manousos, O., N. Day, D. Trichopoulos, F. Gervassilis, A. Tzonou, and A. Polychronopoulou. 1983. Diet and colorectal cancer: a case-control study in Greece. *Int. J. Cancer* **32**:1–5.

Mariani Costantini, A. 1983. Dietary trends in Western Europe. *Prev. Med.* **12**:218–221.

Mariani Costantini, A. 1987. Energia. In *Atti del Convegno Nazionale Alimentazione Mediterranea e Salute, May 1986 at Tabiano Terme*, pp. 17–25. Parma: Barilla.

Matanoski, G. M., and E. A. Elliott. 1981. Bladder cancer epidemiology. *Epidemiol. Rev.* **3**:203–229.

Mezzanotte, G., C. Cislaghi, A. Decarli, C. La Vecchia. 1986. Cancer mortality in broad Italian geographical areas 1975–1977. *Tumori* **72**:145–152.

Miller, A. B., A. Kelly, N. W. Choi, et al. 1978. A study of diet and breast cancer. *Am. J. Epidemiol.* **107**:499–509.

Mills, P. K., and P. C. MacDonald. 1988. Animal product consumption and subsequent fatal breast cancer risk among Seventh-Day Adventists. *Am. J. Epidemiol.* **127**:440–453.

National Research Council. 1982. *Diet, Nutrition, and Cancer.* Washington, D.C.: Commission on Life Sciences, National Academy of Sciences.

Nomura, A., B. E. Henderson, and J. Lee. 1978. Breast cancer and diet among the Japanese in Hawaii. *Am. J. Clin. Nutr.* **31**:2020–2025.

Pagano, R., E. Negri, A. Decarli, and C. La Vecchia. 1988. Coffee drinking and prevalence of bronchial asthma. *Chest* **94**:386–389.

Palmer, S. 1986. Dietary considerations for risk reduction. *Cancer* **58**:1949–1953.

Parkin, D. M., E. Laara, and C. S. Muri. 1988. Estimates of the worldwide frequency of sixteen major cancers in 1980. *Int. J. Cancer* **41**:184–197.

Phillips, R. L. 1975. Role of lifestyle and dietary habits in risk of cancer among Seventh-Day Adventists. *Cancer Res.* **35**:3513–3522.

Sarin, R., R. K. Tandon, S. Paul et al. 1985. Diet, body fat and plasma lipids in breast cancer. *Indian J. Med. Res.* **81**:493–498.

Talamini, R., C. La Vecchia, A. Decarli et al. 1984. Social factors, diet and breast cancer in a northern Italian population. *Br. J. Cancer* **49:**723–729.

Toniolo, P., E. Riboli, F. Protta, M. Charrel, and A. P. Cappa. 1989. Calorie-providing nutrients and risk of breast cancer. *J. Natl. Cancer Inst.* **81:**278–286.

Trichopoulos, D., G. Ouranos, N. E. Day, A. Tzonou, O. Manousos, Ch. Papadimitriou, and A. Trichopoulos. 1985. Diet and cancer of the stomach: a case-control study in Greece. *Int. J. Cancer* **36:**291–297.

Tuyns, A. J., E. Riboli, G. Doornbos, and G. Pequignot. 1987. Diet and esophageal cancer in Calvados (France). *Nutr. Cancer* **9:**81–92.

Vigotti, M. A., C. Cislaghi, D. Balzi, D. Giorgi, C. La Vecchia, A. Decarli, and R. Zanetti. 1989. Cancer mortality in migrant populations within Italy. *Tumori* **74:**107–128.

Weisburger, J. H., and C. L. Horn. 1985. Modern preventive medicine: Update on elements of value in clinical practice, with emphasis on tobacco use and nutrition as causative factors for cancer and cardiovascular disease. *IM—Int. Med. for Specialists* **12:**6–13.

Willett, W. C., M. J. Stampfer, G. A. Colditz, et al. 1987. Dietary fat and the risk of breast cancer. *New Engl. J. Med.* **316:**22–28.

Zemla, B. 1985. The role of selected dietary elements in breast cancer risk among native and migrant populations in Poland. *Nutr. Cancer* **6:**187–190.

INDEX

Acetaldehyde, in fermented milks, 141
Acetic acid, in fermented milks, 141
Acid-alcoholic mesophilic products, 142
Acid mesophilic products, 142
African regions, low fasting blood glucose and insulin, 279
Alcohol, 269
Aleura, wheaten flour, 22
Algeria, total fat intake, 8
Alica, 27
Alkali cooking, corn, 92
Alkaline drying, neutralizing, and washing of oils, 133
Alkaline treatment of foods and side chains of amino acid, 92
Alkaloids, 106
Almonds, 54, 183
  and cholesterol, 188
  and lipoproteins, 188
Alphita, barley-meal, 22
Amino acid(s)
  balance in oats, 97
  in breads, 81
  composition of cereals, 62
  diffusion of, 161
  in wheat endosperm, 69
Ammonia nitrogen, fixation, 166
Amphoras, for wine, 50
Amylopectin, in barley, 94
Amylopectin starch, 162
Amylose, in barley, 94
Amylose starch, 162, 172
Anatolia, 17
Ancient Greece, bread shops, 32
Ancient Rome, bread-making, 31
Animal fats, 126
Animal foodstuffs, annual consumption, 117

Animal proteins, in Mediterranean diets, 267
Antigone, 10
Apo A-I, 206
Apo A-II, 206
Apoprotein A, 204
Apoprotein A-I, 205
Apoprotein A-II, 205
Apoproteins and monounsaturated fats, 186
Apples, 43, 111
  of China, 40
  native European fruit, 43
  sweet, 45
Apricots, 44
Arabinoxylans, in barley, 94
Aromatic herbs, 119
Ascorbic acid, 299
Atherosclerosis, risk factors, 220, 221
Atherosclerotic heart disease, 234
Autopyros, 34
Avena, 37
Avocados, 183

Bakers, professional, 31
Barley, 11, 59, 168, 170
  amino acid composition, 62
  beer, 24
  cakes, 20
  composition, 61, 94–95
  crop failure, 18
  crushed, 20
  endosperm proteins, 69
  flaked, 95
  gruel, 13, 23–24
  husked, 30
  milled, 95–96
  chemical composition, 95
  minerals, 65, 95
  naked, 17

Barley (*cont.*)
 pearl, pearled, 93, 95–96
 pot, 93
 roasted, roasting, 19
 as staple diet, 16
 vitamin content, 64
 water, 13
 and wheat, 16
Barley-bread, Roman, 24
Barley-cakes, 19
Barley-grain, in water, 19
Barley-meal, 16, 22, 24
 alphita, 22
Beans
 chemical composition, 103–106
 dried, 162
 fara, 172
 kidney, 102, 172
 white, 172
Beer manufacture, 32
Beta-glucan
 in cereals, 73
 oats, 97
Blackberries, 54
Black currants, 54
Black mulberries, 54
Bladder cancer, 297
Bleaching, of oils, 133
Blood glucose response, 162
Blood lipids, lower, 164
Blood pressure, 220, 222
 diastolic and systolic, 224
 and fiber, 227
 and lipids, 222
 and Mediterranean diet, 225
 and potassium, 225, 226
 and Western diet, 225
Botanical families of vegetables and
  fruits, 115
Book of Ruth, 17, 18
Bread, 12, 20, 36, 200
 with cheese and olives, 36
 composition, 27, 79
 European-type, 80
 Jewish, 37
 with milk, 151
 with onions, 36
 protein content, 81
 Syrian, 36
 unleavened, 18
 varieties in ancient times, 33
 and wine, 33

Bread-making
 Ancient Rome, 31
 shaping dough in ancient times, 33
Bread shops, in Ancient Greece, 32
Bread-wheat, 28
Breast cancer and diet, 289
Britain, 160
Briza, 37
Broad bean, 102
Broccoli, 288
Bronze Age, 15
Brown rice, 86
Bulgur, 168
 physiological effects, 170
Butter, 4, 142
 and olive oil, 48
Butter fat, 126
Butyrate, 166

Cabbage, 288
Cakes
 in ancient times, 36
 in the shape of animals, 37
Calories, from fat, 199
Cancer, 288–289. *See also specific types*
 alcoholic beverages, 288, 297
 of breast
  and meat consumption, 296
  and seasoning fats, 296
 and carotene, 289
 coffee, 298
 of colon, 288
  and combined risk score, 298
  and meat consumption, 296
  and seasoning fats, 296
 deaths, 288
 etiology, 287
 of pancreas, 299
 of rectum
  and combined risk score, 298
  and meat consumption, 296
  and seasoning fats, 296
 of stomach, and combined risk
   score, 298
 and vitamin A, 289
Canola oil, 188
Carbohydrates. *See also* Complex carbohydrates; Dietary carbohydrates
 absorption, 160, 165
 complex, 201
 contents, of cereal grains, 63
 conversion to fat, 266

and death rates, 239
   fermentation, 166
   lente, 160–175
   low, and weight reduction, 261
   metabolism, 161–162
   and mortality, 237
Cardiovascular disease, 232–248, 282
β-Carotene, 122
Carotenoids, 299
Casein, 206
Cassia, 15
Cattle, domestication of, 11
Cauliflower, 288
Cellulose, in cereals, 73
Cereals
   amino acid composition, 62
   carbohydrate fraction, 60
   composition of, 61
   consumption of, 5
   dietary fiber, 72, 79
   extrusion of, 81
   fatty acids, 60
   foods, 59
   lignin in, 73
   linoleic acid in, 60
   Mediterranean, 59
   mineral content, 70–71
   noncellulosic polysaccharides in, 73
   NPU, 62
   PER, 62
   physiological effect, 167–168
   phytic acid, 73, 74, 75
   porridges, physiological effects, 171
   as a staple food, 59
   total protein, 62
CHD. See Coronary heart disease
Cheese, 142, 144–146, 156
   with bread, 155
   histamine in, 148
   low-cholesterol or low-fat, 151
   marinated in oil or vinegar, 136
   in Middle Ages, 136
   tyramine in, 148
Cheesecake, 136
Cherries, 42
Chestnuts, 54
Chick-peas, 24, 102, 160, 172
Cholesterol
   content of dairy products, 151
   and diets, 185
   socioeconomic development and, 8
Cholestyramine, 196
Chondrites, 34

Cilento study, 4
   and hypertension, 223
Cinnamon, 15
Citrus Aurantium amarum, 40
Citrus Aurantium dulce, 40
Citrus fruit, 111, 112
CNR study, 198
Colonic fermentation, increased, 165
Colorectal neoplasms, 297
Complex carbohydrates. See also Car-
      bohydrates; Dietary carbohy-
      drates
   in Mediterranean diets, 267
   and obesity, 257
Consumption
   annual, animal and vegetable food-
      stuffs, 117
   of dairy products, 138
   of dietary fat, 203
   of fruits and vegetables, 110–113
Copper, in cereals, 70
Corn, 89–93
   alkali cooking, 92
   amino acid composition, 62
   calcium content, 93
   composition, 61, 88–90
   deficiencies, 92
   dietary fiber, 93
   dry milling, 89, 90–92
   endosperm proteins, 69
   lime-treated, 92
   milled, chemical composition, 90
   minerals, 65, 89, 91
   nutritional value, 92–93
   ornithine residues in, 92
   protein content, 91
   resistant starch in, 93
   starch, 89
   trace elements, 91
   vitamin content, 64
   wet processing, 89
   zein in, 91
Corn meal
   coarse, 168
   fine, 90
Corn oil and lipoproteins, 187
Coronary heart disease
   and death rates, 238–239, 243, 246
   morbidity, 245
   mortality data, 234
   prevention of, 6, 197
Coronary Primary Prevention Trial,
      195

Cottonseed oil, 126
Couscous, physiological effects, 171
Cowpea, 102
Cracked grain, physiological effects, 170
Cracked wheat, parboiled, 170
Cream, cream derivates, 142
Creta praeparata, 27
Cribrum pollinarium, 31
Cuckoo-apple, 46
Cyanogenetic glucosides, 106

Dairy products
  combinations with nondairy foods, 156
  composition, 149
  consumption of, 5, 135, 154
  in Mediterranean diets, 219
Dairying, in Ancient Rome, 135
Damson plum, 46
Death rates, from coronary heart disease, 238, 243, 246
Degermed grits, composition, 91
Degumming, of oils, 133
Dextrins, in cereals, 60
Diabetes mellitus, 277, 279, 282
  complications and diet, 281
  and high-carbohydrate, high-fiber diets, 283
  non-insulin-dependent, 277
  treatment of, 162
  and vegetarians, 281
Dietary carbohydrates. *See also* Carbohydrates; Complex carbohydrates
  and induced thermogenesis, 263
  and weights, 257
Dietary fats
  and metabolic rate, 263
  and plasma lipids, 203
Dietary fatty acids, and HDL, 204
Dietary fibers, 208
  in cereals, 72
  from fruits and vegetables, 121
  in grains, 65
  intake, daily, 121
  in legumes, 104
Dietary habits
  and incidence of diabetes, 278
  lipid-lowering effects of, mechanisms, 208
  in Mediterranean area, 115

Dietary induced thermogenesis. *See* DIT
Dietary proteins, and plasma lipids, 206
Dietary variations, geographical, 196–197
Diet–cancer relationship, 187
Diets. *See also* Mediterranean diet
  and breast cancer, 289
  and complications from diabetes, 281
  in East Asia, 284
  high in animal fats, 270
  high carbohydrate, 185
    and HDL, 202
  high fat, and weight reduction, 261
  high monounsaturated fat, 185
  high potassium, 221
  high protein, and weight reduction, 259
  high vegetable-carbohydrate, 270
  Holland, 269
  Italy, 269
  low fat, 202
  Western, 277
    and blood pressure, 225
DIT (dietary induced thermogenesis), 258, 262, 265
Donkey-millstone, 31
Dough, shaping in ancient times, 33
Dried beans, 162
Dried legumes, 172
  amylase starch in, 162
Dry milling, corn, 90
Durum wheat semolina, 82
Dyacetil, in fermented milks, 141

East Asia, diets in, 284
Eggs, consumption of, 5
Egypt, 160
  total fat intake, 8
Egyptian sycamore, 54
Einkorn, 25
Eleusinian Mysteries, 24
Embryo, 65
Emmer, 25, 26, 28, 59
Emmer cake, symbol of wedding vows, 60
Emmer farinata, 59
Emmer-groats, porridge, 27
Endosperm, 65
Enzyme inhibitors, 160
Ethanol, in fermented milks, 141

Etrog groves, 42
EURATOM (European Atomic En-
    ergy Community), 204, 207
European Atomic Energy Commu-
    nity Study, 4, 198–199
Exclusion colitis, 167
Extraction rate, 74
Extrusion cooking, 83

Farina, 27, 59
Farrago, 59
Fats. *See also* Dietary fats; Mono-
    unsaturated fats
  corn, 89
  edible, 125–134
  invisible, in diets, 267
  in Mediterranean countries, 128,
    267
  polyunsaturated, and mortality,
    237, 239
  safe level, 189
  vegetable and animal ratios, 198
Fatty acid composition, of grains, 63
Fatty acid patterns, 184
Fatty acids, dietary, and HDL, 204
Fava beans, 172
Favism, 172
FFM (fat-free mass), 262
Fiber. *See also* Dietary fibers
  corn, 89
  hypothesis, 207
  intake of, 8
  insoluble, in flours, 73
  soluble, 160
    in flours, 73
  water-insoluble, 207
  water-soluble, 208
Figs, 16, 21, 23, 43, 47, 51
  as ancient laxatives, 51
  dried, 51
  first fruit ever cultivated, 52
Finland, 3
  levels of serum cholesterol, 197
Finnish trials, and hypertension, 223
Flatulence, and legumes, 103
Floors, malting, 26
Flour, 27, 75, 76, 78
Fluid milks, 137–140
Food, of animal origin, 219
Food consumption
  in five Mediterranean cohorts, 241
  in three northern European co-
    horts, 241

Food shortages, ancient times, 14
Foxtail millet, 38
Framingham Heart Study, 195
Free-threshing, wheat, 29
Fructosans, in barley, 94
Fruits, 110–123, 160–175, 288
  classification of, 113, 116
  consumption of, 110–113
  indigenous Mediterranean, 43, 47
  in the Italian diet, 118
  native European, 43
  nonindigenous, 40
  nutritional content, 120
  sources of vitamins, 121
  sources of fiber, 120
  fruits and vegetables, physiological
    effects, 173

Garlic, 23
Gastric cancer, 290–293, 297
Geographical dietary variations,
    196–197
Germ, 65, 89
Gioddu, 142
Globulin, in oats, 97
Glucose, diffusion of, 161
Glucose response, 201
Glucoxidase inhibitors, 160
Glucuronoarabinoxylans, in cereals,
    73
Gluten, 68
  intolerance, 83
Glycemic index, 165
  definition, 162
  and legumes, 173
  pasta, 201
Glycolipids, in cereals, 60
Goat milk, 20, 148
Goats, domestication of, 11
Goitrogenic factors, 106–107
Gooseberries, 54
Gorging, 160
Grain merchants, 40
Grains, 160–175
  grinding, 31
  and obesity, 256
  structure of, 65
Grain shortages, in ancient times, 39
Grapes, 16, 47, 48
  native European fruit, 43
Greece
  diets, 269
  total fat intake, 8

Greek comedy, 12
Greek moussaka, 157
Greek pastitsio, 157
Green-vegetable consumption
  protection by, 299
  and various neoplasms, 295
Grits, degermed, composition of, 91
Groundnut, 102
Gruel, medicinal, 38
Gubbio, study, 255
G-6-P dehydrogenase deficiency, 172

Hazelnuts, 183
HDL. See High-density lipoprotein
Hemagglutinins, 107
Hepatic lipogenesis, 164
Hepatocellular cardinoma, 299
High-density lipoproteins, 182, 185,
    195, 202
  cholesterol, 206
    and olive oil, 205
  subfractions, 206
High-density lipoprotein^2, 206
High-density lipoprotein^3, 206
Hippocratic corpus, 13
Histamine, in cheeses, 148
HMG CoA reductase, 164
Holland, diets, 269
Honey, 53
Hopper-rubber, 30
Hops, 24
Horse gram, 102
Hot stones, baking on, 33
Hummus, 24, 172
Hyperlipoproteinemia, type IV, 204
Hypertension, 219, 220
Hypertriglyceridemia, 201

IgA, of milk, 152
Immune suppression, 183
Immunoglobulins, of milk, 152
Inhibitor, 106
Insulin, 163, 164, 201
INTERSALT study, 222
Ipnites, 34
Iron, in cereals, 70
Israel, total fat intake, 8
Italian cannelloni, 157
Italian sartu, 157
Italy
  caloric intake, 269
  dietary habits in early twentieth
    century, 265
  diets, 269
  total fat intake, 8
Italy, southern, 15

Jam, quince, and honey, 53
Japan, levels of serum cholesterol,
    197
Japanese populations in California,
    Hawaii, and Japan, 197
Jesus, on leavening, 32
Jewish bread, 37

Kammata, 21
Karelia, 223
Keys, Ancel, 232
Kidney beans, 102, 172
Kidney disease, 173
Kingdom of Naples, 219

Lactase deficiency, secondary, 150
Lactic acid, in fermented milks, 141
Lactobacillus acidophilus, 139
Lactose, 149
Lard, 4
Lathyrus pea, 102
Laxatives, 51
LCT (long-chain triglycerides), 260
LDL. See Low-density lipoprotein
Leaven, as symbolic force, 32
Leben, 142
Lectins, 162, 172
Legumes, 160–175
  chemical composition, 103, 106
  consumption of, 5
    and colonic cancer, 173
  in the diet, 107–108
  dietary fiber, 104
  disease prevention and treatment,
    173
  dried, 172
    consumption of, 103, 105
    essential amino acid content, 108
    production of, 104
  and flatulence, 103
  and glycemic index, 173
  in the Mediterranean diet, 102
  nutritive value, 103
  physiological effects, 182
  proteins, 108
  in southern Italy, 173
  world production, 102
  toxic substances in, 106
Lehem, 17

Lemons, 41, 42
Lente carbohydrate, 160–175
Lentils, 102, 172
Lentil soup, 160
Leuconostoc cremoris, 143
Levant, 15
Librum, 136
Libya, 233
  total fat intake, 8
Life style and disease, 284
Lignin, in cereals, 73
Lima beans, 102
Linoleic acid, 182, 204
  in cereals, 60
  and HDL, 182
  in olive oil, 127
  physiological effect, 182
  and tumors, 183
Lipase system, in oats, 96
Lipid hypothesis, 195–196
Lipid Research Clinics Program, 195
Lipoprotein-lipase-induced catabo-
      lism, 202
Liver disease, 173
Long-chain triglycerides (LCT), 260
Low glycemic indexes, 160, 162, 170
Low-density lipoprotein (LDL), 195
  cholesterol, 197, 206
  and diets, 186
Low-fat diet, 202
Lysine, in barley, 94

Macaroni, 168
Maize, 39
Malta, total fat intake, 8
Maltase activity, 161
Malthouth, 168
Malting floors, 26
Malus, 43
Manganese, in cereals, 70
Margarine, 4
  consumption of, 127
Masa, 92
Mascarpone, 142
Maza, 21, 22
MCT (medium-chain triglycerides),
      and weight reduction, 260
Meals
  frequency, 160
  midday, 270
  number of, per day, 163
Meat
  boiled, 12

consumption of, 5
  northern Europe, 16
Mediterranean advantage, 270
Mediterranean areas
  changes in the diet, 269
  dietary habits, 4, 115
  and fat consumption, 239
Mediterranean countries
  consumption of olive oil, 6
  France, 7
  milk consumption, 137
  prevalence of diabetes in, 277
  saturated fatty acids, 7
Mediterranean diet, 5, 198, 199, 206,
      219, 266
  animal proteins in, 267
  and blood pressure, 225
  carbohydrate fraction, 8
  changes in, 278
  characteristics of, 198, 289
  and dairy products, fish, and meat,
      219
  and diabetes, 283
  as a healthful diet, 3
  historical description, 219
  legumes, 102
  nutritional characteristics, 4
  and olive oil, 219, 221
  and saturated fatty acids, 203
  and vegetables, 221
  and wine, 219
Mediterranean food, 10
Mediterranean population, nine-
      teenth century, 219
Mediterranean regions, epidemiol-
      ogy, 189
Melon, 43
Mesopotamia, 16
Metabolic effects
  of high-fiber diets, 283
  of high-fiber–high-carbohydrate
      diets, 283
Middlings, 69
Milk, 138–142
  additives, 147
  concentrated and dried, 140
  consumption of, 5
    in Mediterranean countries, 137
    of different species, 149
  fat and cholesterol, 150
  fermented, 140–141
    lactic acid in, 141
  fluid, 137–140

Milk (*cont.*)
  goat, 20, 148
  health hazards, 147
  immunoglobulins of, 152
  lactose-reduced, 139
  lipids, intolerance to, 150
  microflora, 145–146
  minerals in, 152
  partial hydrolysis, 150
  proteins, 151
  raw, 137
Milk-boiling pots in Etruscan civilization, 135
Milled fractions, amino acid content, 78
Millet, 59 ,
  in the ancient Mediterranean, 38
  foxtail, 38
Millet-eaters, 38
Milling, 30, 85
  of corn, 91
  effect on rice composition, 85
  of wheat, 74
Mills, 30
Millstones, 30
  donkey, 31
Mineral contents of grains, 65, 71, 75
Minerals
  bioavailability, 70
  and growing conditions, 70
Monounsaturated fats
  consumption, 239
  foods, 184
  and mortality, 237, 239
  and saturated fatty acids, ratio, 199
Monounsaturated fatty acids, 199
Monounsaturated oils, physiological effects, 182
Morocco
  hospital statistics, 233
  total fat intake, 8
Mortality data, 234
Mortality rates, 235
Mortars, 30
Mount of Olives, 47
MRFIT. *See* Multiple Risk Factor Intervention Trial
Mulberry, black, 54
Multiple Risk Factor Intervention Trial, 195
Mushrooms, 21
Myceneans, 15
Myocardial infarction, 232

M/S (monounsaturated/saturated) ratio, and death rates, 239

Na-K pump and cell membrane, 228
Narang, 40
Neoplasms, and coffee consumption, 298
Neoplastic diseases and diet, 270
Neutral lipids, in cereals, 60
Niacin, bound in corn, 92
Nibbling, 160
Nitrogen metabolism, 164
Noncellulosic polysaccharides, in cereals, 73
Nonvegetarians and body weight, 265
Northern Europe and fat consumption, 239
Northern Italy surveillance study, 294
NPU, of cereals, 62
Nutrients
  and all causes of mortality, 241
  and death rates, 238
  levels of, and incidence of disease, 236
Nuts, 53

Oatmeal, 96
Oats, 37, 59, 168
  amino acid composition, 62
  antioxidant activity, 97
  beta-glucan, 97
  composition of, 61, 96–97
  endosperm proteins, 69
  groats, 96
  globulin in, 97
  lipase system in, 96
  lipids, 97
    in endosperm, 97
  as medicinal gruel, 38
  mineral content, 65
  mineral distribution, 98
  nutritive value, 97–98
  phytate in, 98
  prolamins, 97
  protein, 97
  tocopherols in, 97
  vitamin content, 64
Obesity, 252–271
  and carbohydrates, 256, 257
  in African nations, 252
  in Asian nations, 252
  in developed countries, 256

in developing countries, 254
and dietary fiber, 261
influence on energy balance, 256
influence of various nutrients, 256
and lipids, 259
in the Mediterranean area, 254–255
prevalence of, 253
and protein, 259
and relative body weight, 256
and RMR, 258
and sucrose-rich diet, 258
and the western world, 253–254
Oil of roses, 54
Oils
bleaching of, 133
consumed in the Mediterranean
countries, 128–129
degumming of, 133
edible, 125–134
monounsaturated, physiological effects, 182
physical deodorizing/neutralizing, 133
preservation, 133
vegetable, refining of, 133
winterizing, 133
Olefinic compounds, 92
Oleic acid
and olive oil, 228
of the plasma membrane, 228
Olive oil, 47, 52, 125, 182, 205, 269
and butter, 48
consumption of, 5–6
extraction, 129
fatty acid composition, 128
and HDL-C or LDL-C, 184
and lipoproteins, 184, 187
and membrane lipid composition, 228
and perfumes, 48
production, 125
refined, 126
studies, 184
types of, 132
and unguents, 48
virgin, 126
extraction of, 131
"Olive oil strip," 125
Olives, 16, 47, 59, 183
native European fruit, 43
Omega-3 fatty acids, 204
Onions, 36
Oranges, in the Mediterranean, 41

Ornithine residues, in corn, 92
Oslo Study, 196
Ovens, portable, 34

Palestine, 16
Pancreatic amylase activity, 161
Panis hordaceus, 24
Pasta, 29, 81, 168, 200
ancient practice, 82
from durum wheat, 82
and gastric cancer, 296
high protein, 82
limiting amino acid, 82
physiological effects, 168–170
protease inhibitors in, 83
starch gelatinization, 82
Peaches, 42
Peanut oil, 187
Pears, 44, 45, 111
native European fruit, 43
Pecorino, 155
Pellagra and corn, 92
Pentosans
in cereals, 60
in rice, 84
PER, of cereals, 62
Perfumes, and olive oil, 48
Phoenician, 15
Phospholipids, in cereals, 60
Phytate, in oats, 98
Phytates, 162, 172
Phytic acid
in cereals, 73
destruction, in breads, 80
Pigs, domestication of, 11
Pizza, 156
Placenta, 27
Plants, 21
Plasma cholesterol, 3
Plums, 44
damson, 46
native European fruit, 43
Polenta, 25, 168
and gastric cancer, 296
physiological effects, 171
roasted, 25
Pollen, 31
Polyphenols, 107
Polyunsaturated fats, and mortality, 237, 239
Pomegranates, 16, 47
native European fruit, 43

Porridge, 59
  emmer-groats, 27
  Greek, 19
Porridge-making, toasting, 26
Portugal, total fat intake, 8
Post-systemic encephalopathy, 173
Potassium, 222
  high, 225
  lower blood pressure, 222
Potatoes, consumption of, 112
Prolamin, 69
  in oats, 97
Propionate, 167
Protease inhibitors, in pasta, 83
Proteins
  corn, 89
  dietary, and plasma lipids, 206
  digestibility
    in breads, 81
    in pasta, 83
  milk, 151
  sources and insulin responses, 163
Puls, 26, 59
Pulse, 102
Pushing-mill, 30
Pyros, 28
P/S (polyunsaturated/saturated) ra-
    tio, 222
  and death rates, 239

Quince, 53

Raffinose, in beans, 103
Rapeseed, 126
Raspberries, 54
Recommended dietary intakes (RDI),
    153
Reference food, 163
Refined husk olive oil, 126
Refined sugars and plasma lipids, 200
Resistant starch, in corn, 93
Resting metabolic rate (RM), 262
  and obesity, 258
  and T3, 258
  and T4, 258
Retinoids, 299
Rheumatic fever, and heart disease,
    233
Riboflavin and European-type
    breads, 80
Rice
  in ancient times, 38
  bran, 84

brown, 84, 87–88
  amino acid composition, 62
characteristics, 84
composition of, 61, 84
dehulling, 85
endosperm proteins, 69
essential amino acids, 86
and gastric cancer, 296
lipids, 87
long-grain, amylose starch in, 162
milling and shelling, 85
mineral content, 65
nutritional value, 87–88
paddy rice, 84, 85
parboiling, 86–87
pentosans in, 84
physiological effects, 171
polished, 84
protein, 87
rough rice, 84, 85
starch, 84, 87
vitamin content, 64
Ricotta cheese, 151
RMR. See Resting metabolic rate
Roman grainary buildings, 39
Romano beans, 172
Rome, 160
Roses, oil of, 54
Rotary mill, 30
Rough rice, 86
Rye, 37, 59
  amino acid composition, 62
  composition of, 61
  endosperm proteins, 69
  mineral content, 65
  vitamin content, 64

Sacramental drink, 24
Saddle-querns, 30
Sadziki, 155
Safflower oil, and lipoproteins, 187
Salt intake, 223
Saponins, 106
Saturated fats
  CHD-mortality, 237
  and death rates, 239
  in Mediterranean diet, 279
Savillum, 136
SCFA (short-chain fatty acids), 166
Scutellum, 65
Secale, 37

Seed oils, 125
  extraction, 132–133
  in Italy, 129
Selenium, in cereals, 70
Semidalites, 34
Semolina, 29, 82
Serum cholesterol, 242
Seven Countries Study, 3, 183, 197,
    198, 205, 233, 235–244, 277
  calories from saturated fats, 240
  changes in dietary habits, 244
Seventh-Day Adventists and body
    weight, 264
Seville orange, 40
Sheep, domestication of, 11
Short-chain fatty acids (SCFA), 166
Slow absorption, 160
Slow release starch, 161
Soap, ancient, 47
Soda bread, 32
Soft wheat, 69
  gliadins, 83
Sophocles, 10
Sorghum, mineral content, 65
Sow-thistle, 21
Soybean, 102
Soy protein, 206
Spaghetti, 168
Spain, total fat intake, 8
Spanakopita, 155
Spelt, 37, 102
Spit-baked bread, 33
Stachyose, in beans, 103
Staple diet, barley, 16
Starch, 200
  in cereals, 60
  consumption of, 5
  corn, 89
  gelatinized, 83
  linear structure, 162
  loss, 165
  and plasma lipids, 200
  in rice, 84
Starchy foods, 163
Strawberries, Alpine, 54
Streptococcus lactis, 141
  var. diacetylactis, 141
Subaleurone layer, corn, 89
Sucrase activity, 161
Sucrose-rich diet, and obesity, 258
Sugar
  in cereals, 60
  in Mediterranean diets, 267

Sunflower, 126
Symposia, as wine parties, 49
Synkomistos, 34
Syria, 233
Syrian bread, 36

Tannins, 172
Tetraploid emmer, 25
Thermogenetic response to diet, 264
Thermogenic response to overfeed-
    ing, 257
Thiamine and European-type breads,
    80
Toasting, as part of porridge-making,
    26
Tocopherols, in oats, 97
Tomatoes, consumption of, 112
Tomato sauce, 117
Tortillas, 92
  processing, 92
Total fat, and mortality rate, 237, 239
Total fat intake, 8
Total protein, of cereals, 62
Toxic substances, in legumes, 106
Trahanas, 142
Tripolitania, 233
Triticum spp., 28, 59, 61
  monococcum, 25
  spelta, 37, 102
  turgidum, 25
Trypsin, 106
Tsampa, 22
Tunisia, total fat intake, 8
Turkey, total fat intake, 8
Turning-mill, 30
Tyramine, in cheeses, 148

Unguents, and olive oil, 48
United States
  consumption of olive oil, 6
  dietary habits, 268
  and fat consumption, 239
  total fat intake, 8
Unleavened bread, 18

Vegetable foodstuffs, annual con-
    sumption, 117
Vegetables, 110–123, 160–175
  classification of, 113, 116
  consumption of, 110–113, 117
  and fruits, combined with other
    foods, 118
  garden, consumption of, 112

Vegetables (*cont.*)
 green, 295, 299
 nutritional content, 120
 and obesity, 256
 proteins, 173
  in Mediterranean diets, 117, 267
 sources of vitamins, 121
Vegetarians, 219
 and body weight, 264
 and diabetes, 280
 and hypertension, 220
Verbascose, in beans, 103
Very low-density lipoprotein (VLDL)
  apo B, 207
Vetch, 24
Vitamin A, 122
Vitamin C, sources, 122
Vitamin contents of grains, 64
Vitamin E, 123
Vitamins. *See also specific vitamins*
 in cereals, 60, 71
 distribution in wheat kernel, 71
 fruits, 121
 of milk, 154
 vegetables, 121
VLDL. *See* Very low-density lipoprotein

Walnuts, 54
Western diet, 277
 and blood pressure, 225
Westernizing of Mediterranean countries, 271
Wheat, 11
 aleurone layer, 67
 ash content, 75
 and barley, 16
 bran, 69
 composition of, 61
 cracked, parboiled, 170
 diploid einkorn, 25
 distribution of nutrients, 66
 durum, amino acid composition, 62

endosperm, amino acid, 69
 failure, 18
 flour, 74, 76, 77
 free-threshing, 29
 and gluten intolerance, 83
 grain, longintudinal section, 66
 hard, 29, 62, 69
 hexaploid, 83
 hulled, 25
 kernel, nutrient distribution, 67
 milling and nutritive value, 73
 millings of, 76
 mineral content, 65, 70, 71, 75
 as preferred for human food, 16
 processing and nutritive value, 73
 production, 61
 products, mineral content, 71
 proteins, 68, 75
 soft, 69, 83
 tetraploid, 83
 vitamin content, 64, 78
 whole, amino acid content, 78
Wheaten flour, 16
 aleura, 22
Whey proteins
 lactoalbumin, 151
 lactoglobulin, 151
White beans, 172
Whole grain, physiological effects,
  170, 171
Whole wheat, amino acid content, 78
Wine, 12, 21, 49, 50
 and bread, 33
 as daily staple, 49
 sweetened, 23

Yogurt, 140–141
Yugoslavia
 diets, 269
 total fat intake, 8

Zein, in corn, 91
Zinc, in cereals, 70